# Encyclopedia of Hemodialysis: Diagnosis, Management and Methods

## Volume II

# Encyclopedia of Hemodialysis: Diagnosis, Management and Methods
# Volume II

Edited by **Frank Kesley**

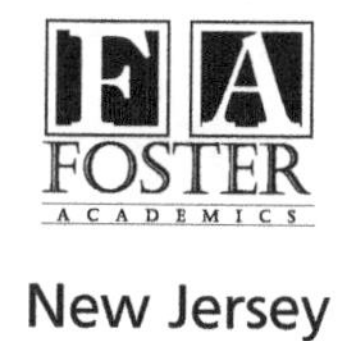


New Jersey

Published by Foster Academics,
61 Van Reypen Street,
Jersey City, NJ 07306, USA
www.fosteracademics.com

**Encyclopedia of Hemodialysis: Diagnosis, Management and Methods**
**Volume II**
Edited by Frank Kesley



International Standard Book Number: 978-1-63242-154-8 (Hardback)



Printed in the United States of America.

# Contents

# Preface

I am honored to present to you this unique book which encompasses the most up-to-date data in the field. I was extremely pleased to get this opportunity of editing the work of experts from across the globe. I have also written papers in this field and researched the various aspects revolving around the progress of the discipline. I have tried to unify my knowledge along with that of stalwarts from every corner of the world, to produce a text which not only benefits the readers but also facilitates the growth of the field.

This book elucidates several aspects of hemodialysis therapy; particularly, its diagnosis, management and techniques for treatment. From these reviews, the readers will gain precious information and suggestions in daily practice. In this book several experts have discussed hemodialysis, producing vital and fruitful suggestions. The information provided in this book will be of help for those who are interested in the field of hemodialysis therapy.

Finally, I would like to thank all the contributing authors for their valuable time and contributions. This book would not have been possible without their efforts. I would also like to thank my friends and family for their constant support.

**Editor**

Section 1

# Pathogenesis and Management of Anemia

Chapter 1

# Current Anemia Treatment in Hemodialysis Patients: The Challenge for Secure Use of Erythropoietin-Stimulating Agents

Paulo Roberto Santos

Additional information is available at the end of the chapter

## 1. Introduction

Anemia is the poor capacity of blood to carry oxygen. Anemia is diagnosed by measuring hemoglobin (HB) level (g/dL) and hematocrit (HT) (percentage of erythrocytes in the blood). Normal limits vary in the general population [1]. According to the World Health Organization, normal HB is defined as 13 g/dL in men and 12 g/dL in women [2]. In clinical practice, HB lower than 11 g/dL is widely accepted as abnormal. For didactic purposes, the several causes of anemia can be placed into three groups: blood loss, increased destruction of erythrocytes or decreased production of erythrocytes.

The main regulatory mechanism for erythrocyte production is the action of the hormone erythropoietin (EPO) in the bone marrow. EPO acts in bone marrow to promote the development of red blood cells and also stimulates the synthesis of HB. In adults, EPO is mainly produced by interstitial fibroblasts in the kidneys and is secreted when specialized cells sense low oxygen level. Independently of etiology, chronic kidney disease (CKD) provokes anemia by decreasing EPO production. In clinical practice, it is useful to classify CKD in five stages according to glomerular filtration rate (GFR) [3]. Based on a normal GFR of 90 ml/min,

- stage 1 refers to CKD with normal GFR, which means GFR of 90 ml/min or higher;
- stage 2 corresponds to GFR between 60 and 90 ml/min;
- stage 3 to GFR between 30 and 60 ml/min;
- stage 4 to GFR between 15 and 30 ml/min; and
- stage 5, the most advanced, to GFR lower than 15 ml/min.

Usually anemia appears in stage 3, worsens with the further decrease of GFR and is universally present and usually symptomatic in stage 5.

In stage 5, CKD patients need some kind of renal replacement like peritoneal dialysis, hemodialysis (HD) or kidney transplantation. Each of these treatment modalities imposes particular factors contributing to anemia in addition to the main cause, decreased renal production of EPO. The focus of this chapter is anemia treatment of patients with CKD in stage 5 undergoing conventional HD.

Among HD patients, several factors besides decreased renal production of EPO contribute to anemia, such as: increased destruction of red blood cells due to chemical effects of uremic toxins; platelet dysfunction provoking blood loss, usually due to occult bleeding; blood loss due to clotting inside hemodialyzers and sets during HD sessions; hemolysis associated with contamination of dialysate water; and water-soluble losses of folate and $vitamin_{12}$ through hemodialyzer membranes, affecting red blood cell production [4]. In summary, anemia is multi-factorial in patients undergoing HD because besides the central role of decreased EPO production, HD therapy per se negatively affects production and survival of red blood cells. Moreover, typical comorbidities associated with stage 5 CKD also act as causal factors of anemia, mainly bone disease (secondary to hyperparathyroidism or aluminum intoxication) and high inflammatory activity.

Anemia must be highlighted among the main challenges of CKD treatment. In this context, anemia's effects on cardiovascular outcomes and quality of life deserve especial attention. Anemia decreases physical function and vitality, worsening quality of life [5]. Cardiovascular problems are the main causes of death among HD patient, and anemia imposes an overload on cardiac function, ultimately provoking left ventricular hypertrophy, a well-recognized marker of morbidity and mortality [6]. Nonetheless, there is no certainty about the optimal HB level in order to improve quality of life and decrease cardiovascular risk. Paradoxically, higher HB levels seem to cause side effects and, concerning quality of life, higher HB is only associated with a small and not clinically significant improvement [7,8]. Presently, there is substantial discussion about the ideal level of anemia control. This is a topic of this chapter.

Before the start of the clinical use of erythropoietin stimulating agents (ESAs) in the early nineties, anemia had been the main stigma of CKD and its treatment was based on repeated blood transfusions, which caused many HD patients to be infected with C virus. Now the use of ESAs is widespread. They can correct EPO deficiency and control anemia among HD patients. Basically, there are three generations of ESAs: epoetin (first generation), darbepoetin (second generation) and methoxy polyethylene glycol-epoetin (a long-acting EPO receptor activator of the third generation, recently introduced). Successive generations acquired longer half-lives (see Table 1, based on [9]). ESAs are able to increase HB to normal levels, but their clinical use during the past 20 years has brought unexpected questions: Why is complete anemia correction associated with worse clinical outcomes? Are ESAs toxic? And, how should patients be managed patients who do not respond to ESA?

| Erythropoietin-stimulating agents | Half-lives in hours | |
|---|---|---|
| | Intravenous route | Subcutaneous route |
| Epoetin | 6.8 | 19.4 |
| Darbepoetin | 25.3 | 48.8 |
| Methoxy polyethylene glycol-epoetin | 134 | 139 |

**Table 1.** Half-lives of erythropoietin-stimulating agents

The next sections summarize the literature evidence on "side effects" of complete correction of anemia, review the current recommendations on anemia treatment and discuss the main obstacles to efficient anemia control among HD patients, with focus on the condition of patients who do not respond to usual ESA doses.

## 2. Why partial and not complete anemia correction?

After 20 years of clinical use of ESAs, the question about the optimal HB target for CKD patients remains unanswered. ESAs allow complete correction of anemia, but at the end of the nineties a study indicated a higher risk of death when targeting complete anemia correction compared to partial anemia control among HD patients [7]. This study, comprising high-risk patients (either with congestive heart failure or ischemic heart disease), showed more death, more myocardial infarction and more vascular thrombosis among patients treated to reach complete anemia correction (HT of 42%) when compared to patients treated to achieve partial anemia correction (HT of 30%). In fact, bad outcomes were present even among patients assigned to the high-HT group who did not really achieve the target of 42% HT. These findings posed three questions:

Are CKD patients in general at danger when they have anemia completely corrected or only HD cardiac patients with characteristic similar to the sample studied?

Since patients in the high-HT group were submitted to high epoetin dose and were at risk even when the high-HT target was not reached, is the risk due to high HT level or high ESA dose?

Since to reach higher HT, the patients were also submitted to higher replacement of iron, is iron the villain?

At least three controlled random trials were conducted trying to answer some of these questions, using first and second ESA generations [10-12]. All three studies focused on comparing partial versus complete anemia correction among CKD patients, not only in high risk HD, like typical cardiac patients from the Besarab study [7], but also among CKD patients in stages 3 and 4 under conservative treatment (not yet undergoing HD). Two studies [10,11] were published in the same year and comprised all-cause CKD patients. One study [10] showed benefits regarding quality of life among patients under complete anemia correction when compared to partial anemia correction. However, there were more hypertensive episodes and headaches among patients under complete anemia correction. Due to the main objective of the study, if complete correction could improve cardiovascular outcomes, the result was neutral. Cardiovascular events and death rates were the same between the two groups. The conclusion was that even not showing a risk, complete anemia correction did not seem to be beneficial related to cardiovascular outcomes for CKD patients under conservative treatment. Thus, this study did not give support to the clinical practice of targeting complete anemia correction. The other study [11] showed a greater risk of death and congestive failure hospitalization among patients for whom the target was HB of 13.5 g/dL compared to patients with HB target of 11.3 g/dL. Moreover, no improvement in quality of life was found among higher-HB patients. Consequently, complete anemia correction was discouraged. The third study [12] was specifically designed to investigate the effects of different patterns of anemia correction only among diabetics. Even though high risk of death or cardiovascular events associated with complete anemia correction was found, patients treated to achieve higher HB experienced more episodes of stroke and thromboembolism. Taken together, these studies show no advantage and even potential risks of targeting higher HB/HT in CKD patients. Concerning HD patients, the safety of targeting higher HB level using higher ESA doses requires even more attention, because HD patients present more comorbidities than those under conservative treatment, with a profile closer to the high-risk patients that took part in the Besarab study [7] than the patients in the other studies [10-12]. The consequence is the current adoption in clinical practice of partial anemia correction among HD patients. These studies did not address the possible causes of adverse outcomes observed with complete anemia control, but cast doubt on the safety of high ESA doses and high iron replacement.

There are more convergent findings coming from observational studies. As known, randomized controlled trials are suitable for hypothesis-testing and observational studies work to generate hypotheses. However, in the nephrology area, observational studies are able to comprise more typical patients under regimens found in daily practice. Here I comment on three observational studies which demonstrated higher risk of all-cause mortality associated with higher ESA doses [13-15]. In North America, based on the United States Renal Data System, comprising a sample of 94,569 prevalent HD patients, the patients were stratified in four groups according to ESA dose quartiles and also according to five HT levels: < 30%, 30-<33%, 33-<36%, 36-<39 and ≥39 [13]. The finding was higher risk of all-cause death associated with the fourth quartile of ESA dose (higher ESA doses), regardless of HT level achieved. A similar result was found in another study among 139,103 patients treated in DaVita dialysis clinics in the United States [14]. In this more recent study, patients were classified in four groups according to weekly ESA dose: <10.000 IU, 10-<20.000 IU, 20-<30.000 IU, ≥30.000 IU, and also according to HB level: <10 g/dL, 10-<11g/dL, 11-<12 g/dL, 12-<13 g/dL, ≥13 g/dL. The result was higher risk of death among patients submitted to more than 30.000 units of ESA for any of the five HB levels. In both studies [13,14], the group with highest mortality was that of patients using higher ESA doses and presenting lower HT/HB levels.

It must be stressed that the association between high ESA dose and high risk of death is not only found in observational studies comprising large samples. Last year in Brazil, the research group I lead performed a study encompassing HD patients from a single unit [15]. In our study, we divided patients into two groups according to anemia control profile: excellent/good and moderate/bad control, taking into consideration of HT and HB levels during a period of one year. Also, patients were divided into two groups according to ESA dose: usual ESA dose and high ESA dose (=epoetin dose higher than 400 units per kg per month). Patients submitted to high ESA dose presented a five-fold risk of death, independent of anemia control profile. Again, as found in the other studies [13,14], most of the patients submitted to high ESA dose were those with worse anemia control. Unlike inconclusive results coming from randomized controlled trials, data from observational studies strongly indicate higher mortality among HD patients submitted to high ESA dose, especially those not reaching good anemia control.

A detailed discussion of the mechanisms involved in the genesis of bad outcomes related to complete anemia correction is beyond the scope of this chapter. Indeed, these mechanisms are not clear in the literature. Further knowledge of such mechanisms is essential to propose safer approaches to anemia in the future. The suggested mechanisms are: ESA toxicity, effects of hyperviscosity, iron toxicity or merely a selection bias of patients (patients submitted to high ESA are sicker). Probably there is not a single mechanism, but rather an interaction of factors leading to adverse clinical outcomes. The main points involved in the supposed mechanisms are summarized below and are shown in Table 2. High HT results in higher blood viscosity, which might explain the higher risk of thromboembolism [16]. Targeting high HB demands greater replacement of iron. High intravenous replacement of iron is linked to cardiovascular disease and susceptibility to bacterial infections [17,18]. ESAs have hypertensive effects but no studies have shown a link between arterial hypertension and bad outcomes. More attractive is the biological plausibility of ESA toxicity due to activation of extra-bone marrow receptors of EPO distributed in myocardium, brain and endothelial cells. These receptors are only activated by a high EPO concentration, as occurs with the clinical use of ESA. Theoretically, unphysiologic EPO spikes in plasma could activate extra-bone marrow receptors and be harmful [19,20]. Finally, patients submitted to high ESA dose may die more just because they are sicker, without any role of blood hyperviscosity and ESA or iron toxicity.

## 3. Current recommendations

The National Kidney Foundation describes the initial evaluation of anemia in HD patients, consisting of measurement of HB, HT, reticulocyte count, serum iron, total iron binding capacity, percent transferring saturation, serum ferritin and a test for occult blood in stools [21]. My opinion is that analysis of peripheral blood smears can be added to the initial evaluation. This simple analysis can give important clues on underlying factors contributing to anemia (see Table 3).

There is general consensus that the target of anemia treatment is to achieve partial anemia correction, which means HB in the range of 11 to 12 g/dL and HT between 33% and 36%

[21]. Currently this is a target for all patients, including children, CKD patients under conservative treatment, peritoneal dialysis patients and kidney transplant recipients. The data supporting partial anemia control in HD patients and CKD patients under conservative treatment were provided in the previous topic. However, less information is available on the effects of high HB level on peritoneal dialysis outcomes. A difference in the effects of a higher level in peritoneal dialysis patients could be possible due to the fact that most peritoneal dialysis patients receive lower ESA doses for the same achieved HB level when compared to HD patients. In support of this hypothesis, a recent study did not find any association between higher achieved HB and all-cause mortality among ESA-treated peritoneal dialysis patients [22]. On the other hand, it seems that among kidney transplant recipients the risks are similar to those of HD patients. There are studies suggesting that targeting HB more than 12.5 g/dL is associated with increased mortality risk in kidney transplant recipients [23,24]. In my view, it is probable that in the coming years an individualized target according to specific patient profiles will be a better way of controlling anemia. Based on this opinion, I make some suggestions of individualized approaches in the conclusion of this chapter.

| Variable | Mechanism |
|---|---|
| Hyperviscosity | More episodes of thromboembolism because of platelet activation and increased proacoagulant activity |
| High ESA dose | Activation of hematopoietic receptors, producing highly active platelets, and/or<br>Activation of extra-hematopoietic receptors, triggering adverse events |
| High iron replacement | Cardiovascular disease, and/or susceptibility to bacterial infections |

**Table 2.** Possible mechanisms involved in bad clinical outcomes related to complete anemia correction

| Finding | Factors |
|---|---|
| Microcytosis | Iron deficiency |
| Macrocytosis | Folate or Vitamin $B_{12}$ deficiency |
| Echinocytes | Hypomagnesemia or hypophosphatemia |
| Stomatocytosis | Over-hydration |
| Heinz bodies | Acute hemolysis |
| Howell-Jolly bodies | Iron deficiency |
| Basophilic stippling | Lead toxicity |

**Table 3.** Correlation of red cell morphology in peripheral blood smears with contributing factors of anemia

Iron depletion is found in nearly all patients undergoing HD. Thus, in order to achieve and maintain the HB/HT target, the recommended treatment is initial replacement of 100 mg of iron intravenously at every HD session for a total of 10 doses, and then 100 mg of iron intravenously once a week for maintenance replacement [20]. In the case of patients presenting iron overload (percent transferring saturation ≥ 50% or serum ferritin ≥ 800 ng/mL) withholding of initial iron replacement is recommended until iron comes back to normal. For those who develop iron overload during the maintenance phase, re-introduction of half the previously used maintenance dose can be tried when iron levels return to normal.

After certifying iron status, HD patients presenting HB < 11 g/dL may be submitted to ESA replacement. The most used ESAs are epoetin and darbepoetin, and for both subcutaneous administration is the most efficient route for replacement in HD patients. More recently, C.E.R.A (continuous EPO receptor activator) was introduced. The usual dose for initial replacement with epoetin should be 80 to 120 units/kg/week (typically 6,000 units/week) in two to three doses per week [21]. In a monthly control, if the increase of HB is less than 2%, the epoetin dose should be increased by 50%. On the other hand, if the increase of HB is more than 8% or exceeds the target, a 25% decrease in the epoetin dose should be tried [21]. The initial dose for darbepoetin is 0.45 μg/kg once a week and 20 to 30% of the initial dose can be used as maintenance dose [25]. C.E.R.A can be started using 0.60 μg/kg each 15 days and maintained using120 to 360 μg/kg once a month [25].

The most common causes of hyporesponsiveness to ESAs are iron deficiency, infection and inflammatory states, mainly due to access infections and surgical inflammation, but also due to some primary causes of CKD like acquired immunodeficiency syndrome and systemic lupus erythematosus. The other possible causes to be ruled out in case of hyporesponsiveness are: chronic blood loss, osteitis fibrosa, aluminum intoxication, hemoglobinopathies, folate or vitamin B12 deficiency, multiple myeloma, malnutrition, and hemolysis. For didactic purposes, these various causes are grouped according categories in Table 4.

| Categories | Variables |
|---|---|
| Related to dialysis therapy | Less biocompatible hemodialyzers |
| | Poor quality of water |
| | Contamination of dialysate |
| | Hemolysis and clotting |
| | Recurrent infection of vascular access |
| | Inadequate dialysis dose |
| Related to nutritional status | Iron, folate or vitamin $B_{12}$ deficiency |
| | Low protein intake |
| Related to kidney disease | Hyperparathyroidism |
| | Inflammation |
| | Failed renal transplant graft |
| | Drugs (see Table 5) |

**Table 4.** Causes of hyporesponsiveness to erythropoietin-stimulating agents related to dialysis therapy, nutritional status and kidney disease

Hyporesponsiveness to ESA is the main obstacle to anemia treatment among HD patients. Nonetheless, a consensus about the definition for resistance to ESA is lacking. The definition of resistance by the European Best Practice Guidelines can be mentioned, which is the failure to reach the target using more than 20.000 IU/week of epoetin or more than 100 μg/week of darbepoetin, or the need for consistently high doses to maintain the target HB [26]. For others, the erythropoietin resistance index (weight-adjusted dose of ESA divided by HB g/dL) is a better way to evaluate the resistance to ESA [27]. Indeed, it is not a lack of a widely accepted definition for resistance the main problem; it is the lack of efficient approaches to treat cases of resistance.

The initial approach to hyporesponsiveness may be to rule out some common and modifiable conditions, like iron deficiency, blood loss (reticulocyte count can help), catheter infection, inadequate dialysis (check Kt/V, discard access malfunction), and to search for occult malignancy, evaluate nutritional status and check drugs in use that can aggravate anemia (see Table 5, based on [28]). Routine laboratory follow-up can diagnose hyperparathyroidism. There is a strong association between hyporesponsiveness to ESA and high parathyroid hormone levels [29]. Sometimes a bone marrow examination is necessary to confirm osteitis fibrosa or aluminum toxicity. In case of absence of the previous conditions, micronutrients can be suspected. Response to folic acid replacement remains the gold-standard diagnosis if there is suspicion of folate deficiency. More controversial is the replacement of vitamin C. It leads to the release of iron from ferritin and enhances movement of iron to the erythrocytes [30]. Even without broad recommendation, some clinicians replace vitamin C in patients with poor response to ESA, using a scheme of intravenous replacement of vitamin C after each HD session [31]. L-carnitine deficiency has been extensively studied in nephrology area, but there are no conclusive recommendations about its replacement in HD anemic patients, basically because no large clinical trials have been conducted. Based on the Carnitine Consensus Conference [32], the recommended dose of L-carnitine in the context of anemia is 20 mg/kg administered intravenously after each HD session. The results of this treatment must be evaluated at 3-month interval and be discontinued if no results are reached after 9 months.

Unfortunately, most patients that are unresponsive to ESA do not present one of the conditions mentioned above that can be modified. CKD, especially in stage 5, is a chronic disease characterized by a very high activated inflammatory status. Thus, CKD itself is a central cause of hyporesponsiveness to ESA, and because it is irreversible, it cannot be significantly modified. In fact, inflammation occurs in many other chronic diseases and is responsible for the so-called anemia of chronic disease. The difference is the magnitude of inflammation in CKD, which is much higher than in other morbid conditions. The understanding of the pathophysiology of anemia due to inflammation is useful to suggest possible approaches to anemia in CKD. Basically, inflammation is a stimulus to hepatic production of hepcidin, a small cysteine-rich polypeptide that is a regulator of iron homeostasis. Hepcidin acts to suppress iron release into plasma by decreasing ferroportin and the resulting iron accumulation within the cell. Hepcidin also inhibits the small intestine's absorption of iron. A final consequence is reduced availability of iron for erythropoiesis [33]. This all corresponds to a very usual and well-known profile of patients found in daily activities by nephrologists: patients being supplied with iron or with iron store in the upper limits without response to ESA. It should be borne in mind that despite being a good physiological explanation, in fact hepcidin has failed to predict ESA responsiveness in HD patients [34].

| Groups | Drugs |
|---|---|
| Antibiotics | Penicilins<br>Cephalosporins<br>Bactrim<br>Furadantin<br>Ciprofloxacim<br>Vancomycin |
| Anti-hypertensive | Angiotensin-converting enzyme inhibitors |
| Antifungals | Amphotericin<br>Fluconazole<br>Ketoconazole |
| Antivirals | Vanganciclovir<br>Didanosine |
| Analgesics | Aspirin<br>Non-steroidal anti-inflammatory drugs |
| Antacids | Esomeprazole<br>Ranitidine<br>Cimetidine |
| Miscellaneous | HMG-CoA reductase inhibitors<br>Lorazepam |

**Table 5.** Drugs that can contribute to anemia

Current guidelines do not give attractive options for the treatment of patients with inadequate response to ESA. In our practice we are forced to treat hyporesponders as done in the era before ESA. Virtually all symptomatic anemic patients must be submitted to red cell transfusions, with well-known risks of blood transfusions [21]. The National Kidney Foundation guidelines [21] recommend the use of L-carnitine and androgen, but their effects are limited. In summary, there are no new or special approaches to resistance to ESA, at least in the guidelines. Practitioners will have to wait for results from studies testing novel therapeutic agents. These new potential agents are: the protein product of the growth arrest-specific gene 6, known as Gas6, only tested in an animal model [35]; a natural mixture of herbs called Juzen-taiho-to (TJ-48), which showed good results in a small HD sample [36]; and oxpentifyline, with significant results in small samples [37,38] and undergoing further testing in a multi-center randomized clinical trial [39]. In my view, among these drugs oxpentifyline is the most promising because it works to decrease inflammation, which plays a central role in the genesis of anemia and also in the resistance to ESA.

## 4. Hyporesponders: The challenge

It is necessary to distinguish two groups of hyporesponders among HD patients. The first group consists of patients with an identified cause of hyporesponsiveness, like iron deficiency, infection, neoplasia, malnutrition, hyperparathyroidism, aluminum intoxication, vitamin $B_{12}$ or folate deficiency or inadequate dialysis. For this first group, most causes of hyporesponsivennes are modifiable with well-established approaches. The second group consists of patients without a clearly defined cause for hyporesponsiveness, who are called here primary hyporesponders. This group comprises very high-risk patients. Since they do not present an identified and modifiable cause, the usual approach is to increase ESA dose, trying to reach the HB/HT target. Thus, this group of patients is usually submitted to high ESA dose whether or not they reach a minimum control of anemia. These patients were identified in the observational studies as having a high risk of death [13-15]. In the literature, it is estimated that at least 10% of HD patients are primary hyporesponders [40]. From my personal experience of nearly 20 years treating HD patients in clinical practice, I believe this figure of 10% is low.

Primary hyporesponders fit the profile of patients with normal iron reserves, but with their release for erythorpoiesis somehow being blocked, leading to failure of the actions of erythropoeisis-stimulating agents. It seems reasonable to explain primary hyporesponsiveness by the previously mentioned model where the inflammatory status interferes with iron hemostasis via hepcidin. If this is the case, the proper approach to ESA resistance would be anti-inflammatory treatment. But drugs with potent anti-inflammatory effects in the context of CKD are still lacking. Oxpentifyline (pentoxifyline), a drug used for more than 20 years in the treatment of vascular disease due to its haemorrheological properties, is a promising option for therapy. It has been proved to have potent anti-inflammatory properties mediated by inhibition of phosphodiesterase [41]. Oxpentifyline acts as anti-apoptic, anti-oxidant, anti-TNF-alpha and anti-IFN-gama [42-44] agent. In small and not randomized studies, oxpentifyline was able to significantly increase HB among HD resistant patients [34,35]. Oxpentifyline is not cited in anemia guidelines yet. It is necessary to wait for results of a multicenter double-blind randomized placebo controlled phase 3 trial in progress [36]. Meanwhile, I believe it is advisable to consider ESA resistance as a useful and powerful marker of morbidity and mortality and to avoid at all costs large increases in ESA dose for hyporesponders.

## 5. Conclusion

Many crucial questions about optimal anemia control among HD patients are not adequately answered yet. However, the central role of anemia in the context of morbidity of CKD and dialytic therapy requires continuing to work with the available data. Guidelines are very general and there is an urgent need to attend to the particularities of patients. In medicine, successful treatments are usually individualized therapy. I believe it is possible to consider a few individualized approaches based on the present data. For experienced clinicians it is clear that the general target of HB between 11 and 12 g/dL is not suitable for all patients. Patients with type-2 diabetes or advanced cardiovascular or cerebrovascular disease can be treated for HB level near the lower limit or even with limits of 10-11 g/dL when concerning risks. On the other hand, for young and highly active patients, aiming better quality of life, vitality and physical functioning, the possibility should be considered of pursuing a higher hemoglobin target, but at the moment nothing allows a target exceeding 13 g/dL. When thinking about individualized HB-targets with concern for quality of life, it is advisable to perform follow-up of quality of life level using one of the several validated instruments to evaluate life quality in HD samples. Care must be taken for all patients not to exceed the upper limits of ESAs and stay below 20.000 IU/week of epoetin or 100 μg/week of darbepoetin. ESA resistance should be routinely used in dialysis units as a powerful marker of morbidity and mortality. Finally, the complexity of the management of anemia among HD patients cannot blind us to simple tasks, like routine screening for infection, evaluation of malnutrition and avoidance of sub-dialysis. Due to the characteristics of intense inflammation inherent to CKD, it will be hard to find new drugs that can reduce inflammation enough to make anemia treatment easy. Thus, anemia will continue a challenge all professionals involved in the care of CKD patients on dialysis.

## Author details

Paulo Roberto Santos

Federal University of Ceará, Brazil

## References

[1] Zakai, N. A., Katz, R., Hirsch, C., Shlipak, M. G., Chaves, P. H. M., Newman, A. B., & Cushman, M. (2005). A prospective study of anemia status, hemoglobin concentration, and mortality in an elderly cohort: the Cardiovascular Health Study. *Archives of Internal Medicine*, 165(19), 214-220.

[2] World Health Organization. (1968). Nutritional anaemias. *Report of a WHO scientific group. World Health Organization Technical Report Series*, 405, 5-37.

[3] National Kidney Foundation. (2012). Definition and stages of chronic kidney disease. http://www.kidney.org/professionals/KDOQI/guidelines_ckd/4 class_g1.htm, accessed 23 July.

[4] Bowry, S. K., & Gatti, E. (2011). Impact of hemodialysis therapy on anemia of chronic kidney disease: the potential mechanisms. *Blood Purification*, 32(3), 210-219.

[5] Lasch, K. F., Evans, C. J., & Schatell, D. (2009). A qualitative analysis of patient-reported symptoms of anemia. Nephrology Nursing Journal , 36(6), 621-622.

[6] Foley, R. N., Parfrey, P. S., Harnett, J. D., Kent, G. M., Murray, D. C., & Barre, P. E. (1996). The impact of anemia on cardiomyopathy, morbidity, and mortality in end-stage renal disease. *American Journal of Kidney Diseases*, 28(1), 53-61.

[7] Besarab, A., Bolton, W. K., Browne, J. K., Egrie, J. C., Nissenson, A. R., Okamoto, D. M., Schwab, S. J., & Goodkin, D. A. (1998). The effects of normal as compared with low hematocrit values in patients with cardiac disease who are receiving hemodialysis and epoetin. *New England Journal of Medicine*, 339(9), 584-590.

[8] Clement, F. M., Klarenbach, S., Tonelli, M., Johnson, J. A., & Manns, D. J. (2009). The impact of selecting a high hemoglobin target level on health-related quality of life for patients with chronic kidney disease. *Archives of Internal Medicina*, 169(12), 1105-1112.

[9] Ohashi, N., Sakao, Y., Yasuda, H., & Kato, A. Fujigaki. (2012). Methoxy polyethylene glycol-epoetin beta for anemia with chronic kidney disease. *International Journal of Nephrology and Renovascular Disease*, 5, 53-60.

[10] Drueke, T. B., Locatelli, F., & Clyne, N. (2006). Normalization of hemoglobin level in patients with chronic kidney disease and anemia. *New England Journal of Medicine*, 355(20), 2071-2084.

[11] Singh, A. K., Szczech, L., Tang, K. L., Barnhart, H., Sapp, S., Wolfson, M., & Reddan, D. (2006). Correction of anemia with epoetin alfa in chronic kidney disease. *New England Journal of Medicine*, 355(20), 2085-2098.

[12] Pfeffer, M. A., Burdmann, E. A., Chen, C. Y., Coper, M. E., Zeeun, D., Eckardt, K., Feyzi, J. M., Ivanovich, P., Kewalamani, R., Levey, A. S., Lewis, E. F., Mc Gill, J. B., Mc Murray, J. J. V., Parfrey, P., Parving, H., Remuzzi, G., Singh, A. K., Solomon, S. D., & Toto, R. (2009). A trial of darbepoetin alfa in type 2 diabetes and chronic kidney disease. *New England Journal of Medicine*, 361(21), 2019-2032.

[13] Zhang, Y., Thamer, M., Stefanik, K., Kaufman, J., & Cotter, D. J. (2004). Epoetin requirements predict mortality in hemodialysis patients. *American Journal of Kidney Disease*, 44(5), 866-876.

[14] Duong, U., Kalantar-Zadeh, K., Molnar, M. Z., Zaritsky, J. J., Teitelbaum, I., Kovesdy, CP, & Mehrotra, R. (2012). Mortality associated with dose response of erythropoiesis-stimulating agents in hemodialysis versus peritoneal dialysis patients. *American Journal of Nephrology*, 35(2), 198-208.

[15] Santos, P. R., Melo, A. D. M., Lima, M. M. B. C., Negreiros, I. M. A. H., Miranda, J. S., Pontes, L. S., Rabelo, G. M., Viana, A. C. P., Alexandrino, M. T., Barros, F. A., Neto, B. R., Brito, AA, & Silva Costa, A. (2011). Mortality risk in hemodialysis patients accord-

ing to anemia control and erythropoietin dosing. *Hemodialysis International*, 15(4), 493-500.

[16] Stohlawetz, P. J., Dzirlo, L., Hergovich, N., Lackner, E., Mensik, C., Eichler, H. G., Kabrna, E., Geissler, K., & Jilma, B. (2000). Effects of erythropoietin on platelet reactivity and thrombopoiesis in humans. *Blood*, 95(9), 2983-2989.

[17] Feldman, H. I., Santana, J., Guo, W., Furst, H., Franklin, E., Joffe, M., Marcus, S., & Faich, G. (2002). Iron administration and clinical outcomes in hemodialysis patients. *Journal of the American Society of Nephrology*, 3(3), 734-744.

[18] Hoen, B., Paul-Dauphin, A., Hestin, D., & Kessler, M. (1998). EPIBACDIAL: a multicenter prospective study of risk factors for bacteremia in chronic hemodialysis patients. *Journal of the American Society of Nephrology*, 9(5), 869-876.

[19] Arcasoy, M. O. (2008). The nonhaematopoietic biological effects of erythropoietin. *British Journal of Haematology*, 141(1), 14-31.

[20] Brines, M. (2010). The therapeutic potential of erythropoiesis-stimulating agents for tissue protection: a tale of two receptors. *Blood Purification*, 29(2), 86-92.

[21] National Kidney Foundation. (2006). Clinical practice guidelines and clinical practice recommendations for anemia in chronic kidney disease adults. *American Journal of Kidney Diseases*, 47(3), S16-S85.

[22] Molnar, M. Z., Mehrotra, R., Duong, U., Kovesdy, C. P., & Kalantar-Zadeh, K. (2011). Association of hemoglobin and survival in peritoneal dialysis patients. *Clinical Journal of the American Society of Nephrology*, 6(8), 1973-1981.

[23] Heinze, G., Kainz, A., Horl, W. H., & Oberbauer, R. (2009). Mortality in renal transplant recipients given erythropoietins to increase haemoglobin concentration: cohort study. *British Medical Journal*, 339, b4018.

[24] Molnar, M. Z., Czira, M., Ambrus, C., Szeifert, L., Szentkiralyi, A., Beko, G., Rosivall, L., Remport, A., Novak, M., & Mucsi, I. (2007). Anemia is associated with mortality in kidney-transplanted patients: a prospective cohort study. *American Journal of Transplantation*, 7(4), 818-824.

[25] Romao Jr, J. E., & Bastos, M. G. (2007). Uso de medicamentos estimuladores da eritropoiese. *Jornal Brasileiro de Nefrologia*, 29(4), S12-S16.

[26] Locatelli, F., Aljama, P., Bárány, P., Canaud, B., Carrera, F., Eckardt, K. U., Horl, W. H., Mac Dougal, I. C., Mac Leod, A., Wiecek, A., & Cameron, S. (2004). Revised European Best Practice Guidelines for the management of anemia in patients with chronic renal failure. *Nephrology Dialysis Transplantation*, (2), ii1-ii47.

[27] Chung, S., Song, H. C., Shin, S. J., Ihm, S., Park, C. S., Kim, H., Yang, C. W., Kim, Y., Choi, E. J., & Kim, Y. K. (2012). Relationship between erythropoietin resistance index and left ventricular mass and function and cardiovascular events in patients on chronic hemodialysis. *Hemodialysis International*, 16(2), 181-187.

[28] Bamgbola, O. (2011). Resistance to erythropoietin-stimulating agents: etiology, evaluation, and therapeutic considerations. *Pediatric Nephrology*, 27(2), 195-205.

[29] Al-Hilali, N., Al-Humoud, H., Ninan, V. T., Nampoory, M. R., Puliyclil, MA, & Johny, K. V. (2007). Does parathyroid hormone affect erythropoietin therapy in dialysis patients? *Medical Principles and Practice*, 16(1), 63-67.

[30] Keven, K., Kutlay, S., Nergizoglu, G., & Erturk, S. (2003). Randomized, crossover study of the effect of vitamin C on EPO response in hemodialysis patients. *American Journal of Kidney Diseases*, 41(6), 1233-1239.

[31] Canavese, C., Marangella, M., & Stratta, P. (2008). Think of oxalate when using ascorbate supplementation to optimize iron therapy in dialysis patients. *Nephrology Dialysis Transplantation*, 23(4), 1463-1464.

[32] Eknoyan, G., Latos, D. L., & Lindberg, J. (2003). Practice recommendations for the use of L-carnitine in dialysis-related carnitine disorder. *American Journal of Kidney Diseases*, 41(4), 868-876.

[33] Babitt, J. L., & Lin, H. Y. (2010). Molecular mechanisms of hepcidin regulation: implications for the anemia of chronic kidney disease. *American Journal of Kidney Disease*, 55(4), 726-741.

[34] Kato, A., Tsuji, T., Luo, J., Sakao, Y., Yasuda, H., & Hishida, A. (2008). Association of prohepcidin and hepcidin-25 with erythropoietin response and ferritin in hemodialysis patients. *American Journal of Nephrology*, 28(1), 115-121.

[35] Angelillo-Scherrer, A., Burnier, L., Lambrechts, D., Fish, R. J., Tjwa, M., Plaisance, S., Sugamele, R., De Mol, M., Martinez-Soria, E., Maxwell, P. H., Lemke, G., Goff, S. P., Matsushima, G. K., Earp, H. S., Chanson, M., Collen, D., Izui, S., Schapira, M., Conway, E. M., & Carmeliet, P. (2008). Role of Gas6 in erythropoiesis and anemia in mice. *Journal of Clinical Investigation*, 118(2), 583-596.

[36] Nakamoto, H., Mimura, T., & Honda, N. (2008). Orally administered Juzen-taiho-to/TJ-48 ameliorates erythropoietin (rHuEPO)-resistant anemia in patients on hemodialysis. *Hemodialysis International*, (2), S9-S14.

[37] Cooper, A., Mikhail, A., Lethbridge, M. W., Kemeny, D. M., & Macdougall, I. C. (2004). Pentoxifylline improves hemoglobin levels in patients with erythropoietin-resistant anemia in renal failure. *Journal of the American Society of Nephrology*, 15(7), 1877-1882.

[38] Navarro, J. F., Mora, C., Garcia, J., Rivero, A., Macia, M., Gallego, E., Mendez, M. L., & Chahin, J. (1999). Effects of pentoxifylline on the haematologic status in anaemic patients with advanced renal failure. *Scandinavian Journal of Urology and Nephrology*, 33(2), 121-125.

[39] Johnson, D. W., Hawley, C. M., Rosser, B., Beller, E., Thompson, C., Fasset, R. G., Ferrari, P., Mac Donald, S., Pedagogos, E., & Cass, A. (2008). Oxpentifylline versus pla-

cebo in the treatment of erythropoietin-resistant anaemia: a randomized controlled trial. *BMC Nephrology*, 9, 8.

[40] Macdougall, I. C., & Cooper, A. C. (2002). Erythropoietin resistance: the role of inflammation and pro-inflammatory cytokines. *Nephrology Dialysis Transplantation*, 17(11), S39-S43.

[41] Semmler, J., Gebert, U., Eisenhut, T., Moeller, J., Schonharting, Allera. A., & Endres, S. (1993). Xanthine derivatives: comparison between suppression of tumour necrosis factor-alpha production and inhibition of cAMP phosphodiesterase activity. *Immunology*, 78(4), 520-525.

[42] Bienvenu, J., Doche, C., Gutowski, M. C., Lenoble, M., Lepape, A., & Perdrix, J. P. (1995). Production of proinflammatory cytokines and cytokines involved in the TH1/TH2 balance is modulated by pentoxifylline. *Journal of Cardiovascular Pharmacology*, (2), S80-S84.

[43] Freitas, J. P., & Filipe, P. M. (1995). Pentoxifylline. A hydroxyl radical scavenger. *Biological Trace Element Research*, 47(3), 307-311.

[44] Belloc, F., Jaloustre, C., Dumain, P., Lacombe, F., Lenoble, M., & Boisseau, M. R. (1995). Effect of pentoxifylline on apoptosis of cultured cells. *Journal of Cardiovascular Pharmacology*, (2), S71-S74.

**Chapter 2**

# Management of Anemia on Hemodialysis

Konstantinos Pantelias and Eirini Grapsa

Additional information is available at the end of the chapter

## 1. Introduction

The definition of anemia is controversial. The WHO defines anemia as hemoglobin (Hb)<13 g/dL for men and <12 g/dL for women [1]. The National Kidney Foundation's Kidney Disease Outcomes Quality Initiative, which is the criteria used for Medicare reimbursement, defines anemia in adult men and postmenopausal women as Hb<12 g/dL, or <11 g/dL in a premenopausal woman [2]. Anemia represents a significant problem to deal with in patients with chronic kidney disease (CKD) on hemodialysis (HD). Renal anemia is typically an isolated normochromic, normocytic anemia with no leukopenia or thrombocytopenia [3]. This is a frequent complication and contributes considerably to reduced quality of life (QoL) [4-6] of patients with CKD. It has also been associated with a number of adverse clinical outcomes, increased morbidity and mortality [5, 7-13]. In general, there is a progressive increase in the incidence and severity of anemia with declining renal function. The reported prevalence of anemia by CKD stage varies significantly and depends, to a large extent, on the definition of anemia and whether study participants selected from the general population, are at a high risk for CKD. Data from the National Health and Nutrition Examination Survey (NHANES) showed that the distribution of Hb levels starts to fall at an estimated glomerular filtration rate (eGFR) of less than 75 ml/min per 1.73 $m^2$ in men and 45 ml/min per 1.73 $m^2$ in women [14]. Among patients under regular care and known to have CKD, the prevalence of anemia was found to be much greater, with mean Hb levels of 12.8 ± 1.5 g/dl (CKD stages 1 and 2), 12.4 ± 1.6 g/dl (CKD stage 3), 12.0 ± 1.6 g/dl (CKD stage4), and 10.9 ± 1.6 g/dl (CKD stage 5) [15]. Although renal anemia is independent of the etiology of kidney disease, there are two important exceptions. Renal anemia in diabetic patients develops more frequently, at earlier stages of CKD, and more severely at a given level of renal impairment [16-18]. In patients with polycystic kidney disease, Hb is higher than in other patients with similar degrees of renal failure, and polycythemia may occasionally develop [19]. Many patients not yet on dialysis still receive no specific treatment for their anemia. In contrast, in patients on dialysis,, average Hb values have steadily increased during the past 15 years, following the advent of erythropoietin (EPO) and the development of clinical practice guidelines for anemia management [16, 17]. Anemia contributes to significant healthcare costs associated with CKD [20]. The average Hb value, however, varies considerably between countries, reflecting variability in practice patterns [21]. Before the availability of recombinant human erythropoietin (rhuEPO, or epoetin), patients on dialysis frequently required blood transfusions, exposing them to the risks of iron overload, transmission of viral hepatitis, and sensitization, which reduced the chances of successful transplantation. Anemia in CKD patients except from the lack of EPO [22, 23], is a multifactor process. Shorter lifespan of red blood cells, iron and vitamin deficiency due to dietary restrictions, and rarely bleeding that accompanies uremia seem to be other important factors [24, 25]. Adequate dialysis can contribute to anemia correction through many mechanisms, including the removal of molecules that may inhibit erythropoiesis using high-flux dialyzers [26-30]. It also seems that residual renal function is important in dialysis patients and its decline also contributes significantly to anemia, inflammation, and malnutrition in patients on dialysis [31, 32]. It is also affected by the underlying disease, co morbid conditions, malignancy, infection, heart failure, as mentioned above, the environment and several other factors (therapeutic treatment with angiotensin-converting enzyme(ACE) inhibitors, [33-37] increased PTH, [38-43] osteodystrophy [44, 45]) that differ among patients. Thus, anemia management in these patients needs an individualized approach. Each patient should be treated according to an Hb target with the lowest effective Erythropoiesis Stimulating Agents (ESA) dose, while avoiding large fluctuations in Hb levels or prolonged periods outside the target. This strategy may necessitate changes to the ESA dose, dosing frequency and iron supplementation over the course of a patient's treatment, and proactive management of conditions that can affect ESA responsiveness. While all ESAs effectively increase Hb levels, differences with respect to route of administration, pharmacokinetics, and dosing frequency and efficiency should be considered to maximize the benefits of ESA treatment for the individual patient [46]. Substitution of the subcutaneous route of administration for the intravenous route for epoetin-alfa can reduce drug acquisition and costs, the two largest components of healthcare costs in CKD patients [20]. Hence, treating anemia in CKD patients on HD seems to be very complex and has to be managed step by step correcting all the factors that affect this process.

## 2. Diagnostic approach of anemia in hemodialysis patients

The diagnosis of anemia and the assessment of its severity are best made by measuring the Hb concentration rather than the hematocrit. Hb is a stable analyte measured directly in a standardized fashion, whereas the hematocrit is relatively unstable, indirectly derived by automatic analyzers, and lacking of standardization. Within-run and between-run coefficients of variation in automated analyzer measurements of Hb are one half and one third those for hematocrit, respectively [16]. There is considerable variability in the Hb threshold used to define anemia in CKD patients. According to the definition in the Kidney Disease Outcomes Quality Initiative (KDOQI) guidelines, anemia should be diagnosed at Hb concentrations of less than 13.5 g/dl in adult men and less than 12.0 g/dl in adult women [16].These values represent the mean Hb concentration of the lowest 5th percentile of the sex-specific general adult population. In children, age-dependent differences in the normal values have to be taken into account. Normal Hb values are increased in high-altitude residents [16]. The end of the short interdialytic period is the most appropriate timing for anemia assessment [47]. Although renal anemia is typically normochromic and normocytic, [48, 49] deficiency of vitamin B12 or folic acid may lead to macrocytosis, whereas iron deficiency or inherited disorders of Hb formation (such as thalassemia) may produce microcytosis. Macrocytosis with leucopenia or thrombocytopenia suggests a generalized disorder of hematopoiesis caused by toxins, nutritional deficit, or myelodysplasia. Hypochromia probably reflects iron-deficient erythropoiesis. An absolute reticulocyte count, which normally ranges between 40,000 and 50,000 cells/μl of blood, is a useful marker of erythropoietic activity. Iron status tests should be performed to assess the level of iron in tissue stores or the adequacy of iron supply for erythropoiesis. Although serum ferritin is so far the only available marker of storage iron, several tests reflect the adequacy of iron for erythropoiesis, including transferrin saturation, MCV, and MCHC; the percentage of hypochromic red blood cells (PHRC); and the content of Hb in reticulocytes (CHr) [50]. Storage time of the blood sample may elevate PHRC, MCV and MCHC are below the normal range only after long-standing iron deficiency. It is important to identify anemia in CKD patients because it may signify nutritional deficits, systemic illness, or other conditions that warrant attention, and even at modest degrees, anemia reflects an independent risk factor for hospitalization, cardiovascular disease, and mortality [16, 51]. Drug therapy such as ACE inhibitors may reduce Hb levels by: firstly, direct effects of angiotensin II on erythroid progenitor cells, [52] secondly, accumulation of N-acetyl-seryl-lysyl-proline (Ac-SDKP), an endogenous inhibitor of erythropoiesis, [53] and thirdly, reduction of endogenous EPO production, potentially due to the hemodynamic effects of angiotensin II inhibition [54]. Myelosuppressive effects of immunosuppressants may further contribute to anemia [55].The measurement of serum EPO concentrations is usually not helpful in the diagnosis of renal anemia because there is relative rather than absolute deficiency, with a wide range of EPO concentrations for a given Hb concentration that extends far beyond the normal range of EPO levels on healthy, non-anemic individuals. Abnormalities of other laboratory parameters should be investigated, such as a low MCV or MCHC (may indicate an underlying hemoglobinopathy), a high MCV (may indicate vitamin B12 or folic acid deficiency), or an abnormal leukocyte or platelet count (may suggest a primary bone marrow problem, such as myeloma or myelodysplastic syndrome).

## 3. Clinical manifestations

Due to the fact that anemia reduces tissue oxygenation, it is associated with widespread organ dysfunction and hence an extremely varied clinical picture. In mild anemia there may be no symptoms or simply increased fatigue and a slight pallor. As anemia becomes more marked the symptoms and signs gradually appear. Pallor is best discerned in the mucous membranes; the nailbeds and palmar creases, although often said to be useful sites for detecting anemia, are relatively insensitive for this purpose. Cardiorespiratory symptoms and signs include dyspnea, tachycardia, palpitations, angina or claudication, night cramps, increased arterial pulsation, capillary pulsation, a variety of cardiac bruits, reversible cardiac enlargement. Neuromuscular involvement is reflected by headache, vertigo, light-headedness, faintness, tinnitus, roaring in the ears, cramps, increased cold sensitivity. Acute anemia may occasionally give rise to papilledema. Gastrointestinal symptoms include loss of appetite, nausea, constipation, and diarrhea. Genitourinary involvement causes menstrual irregularities, urinary frequency, and loss of libido. There may also be a low-grade fever. In the elderly, to whom associated degenerative arterial disease is common, anemia may be manifested with the onset of cardiac failure. Alternatively, previously undiagnosed coronary narrowing may be unmasked by the onset of angina [56].

In the early clinical trials of EPO performed in the late 1980s, the mean baseline Hb concentration was about 6 to 7 g/dl, and this progressively increased to about 11 or 12g/dl after treatment. Patients subjectively felt much better, with reduced fatigue, increased energy levels, and enhanced physical capacity, and there were also objective improvements in cardiorespiratory function [57]. Thus, it is now clear that many of the symptoms previously attributed to the "uremic syndrome" are indeed due to the anemia associated with CKD. Although the avoidance of blood transfusions and improvement in quality of life are obvious early changes, there are also possible effects on the cardiovascular system. The physiologic consequences of long-standing anemia are an increase in cardiac output and a reduction in peripheral vascular resistance. Anemia is a risk factor for the development of left ventricular hypertrophy in CKD patients and exacerbate left ventricular dilation. Sustained correction of anemia in CKD patients results in a reversal of most of these cardiovascular abnormalities, with the notable exception of left ventricular dilation. Once the left ventricle is stretched beyond the limits of its elasticity, correction of anemia cannot reverse this [58]. It may, however, prevent the development of LV dilation, and this leads to improved quality of life [59]. Anemia correction may improve QoL, [60, 61] cognitive function, sleep patterns, nutrition, sexual function, menstrual regularity, immune responsiveness, and platelet function [62-66].

## 4. Therapeutic approach

As mentioned above, renal anemia is a multifactor process and its treatment has to focus on a step by step correction of all factors which are involved in this process [67]. First of all, iron deficiency has to be treated before adding more expensive therapies such as EPO therapy.

### 4.1. Iron deficiency

Iron is an essential ingredient for heme synthesis, and adequate amounts of this mineral are required for the manufacture of new red cells. Thus, under enhanced erythropoietic stimulation, greater amounts of iron are used, and many CKD patients have inadequate amounts of available iron to satisfy the increased demands of the bone marrow [68]. Patients with CKD, on HD treatments, may lose up to 3gr of iron each year because of frequent blood losses, so they are at particularly high risk of iron store depletion with subsequent iron deficiency anemia [17]. Even before the introduction of ESA therapy, many CKD patients were in negative iron balance as a result of poor dietary intake, poor appetite, and increased iron losses due to occult and overt blood losses. Losses on HD patients are up to 5 or 6 mg a day, compared with 1 mg on healthy individuals, and this may exceed the absorption capacity of the gastrointestinal tract, particularly when there is any underlying inflammation. Iron deficiency can be defined as absolute or functional [17, 68, 69]. Absolute iron deficiency develops as the body's iron stores become depleted to such a low level that not enough iron is available for the production of Hb [70, 71]. This is usually indicated by a decline in serum ferritin levels to ~<15 μg/l in patients with normal kidney function, [70, 71] or <12 ng/mL [72] according to other studies and TSAT levels below 16% [73]. Absolute iron deficiency in CKD patients has been defined as serum ferritin levels <100 ng/mL and TSAT levels <20%. The functional iron deficiency describes the state when iron cannot be mobilized from stores (despite an adequate dietary supply) to meet the demand for erythropoiesis [70]. Serum ferritin levels can appear normal (200–500 μg/l) or increased in chronic inflammatory disorders, [70] while levels of transferrin saturation (TSAT), which is serum iron divided by total iron-binding capacity, [68] will be low (typically <20%), indicating limited transport of iron to the erythron for erythropoiesis [70, 74, 75] and increased hypochromic red cells (>10%). The distinction between absolute and functional iron deficiency is crucial to understanding what constitutes adequate TSAT and serum ferritin levels on Epoetin-treated patients. The iron deficit limits the effectiveness of EPO therapy, and, to optimize the treatment, patients must receive an oral or intravenous (IV) iron supplement [76-78]. Thus, higher doses of ESAs may worsen iron depletion and lead to an increased platelet count (thrombocytosis), ESA hyporesponsiveness, and hemoglobin variability. Hence, ESA therapy requires concurrent iron supplementation [17, 79]. On the other hand, serum ferritin <200 ng/mL suggests iron deficiency in CKD patients, ferritin levels between 200 and 1,200 ng/mL may be related to inflammation, latent infections, malignancies, or liver disease. In part, this is due to the fact that, in addition to reflecting body iron stores, serum ferritin is also an acute phase reactant. As such, it can increase in the setting of either acute or chronic inflammation. Available data demonstrate that the lower the TSAT and the serum ferritin, the higher the likelihood that a patient is iron deficient, and the higher the TSAT and the serum ferritin, the lower the likelihood that a patient is iron deficient [77, 80]. A serum ferritin concentration of 100-500 ng/mL is the target during oral and intravenous (i.v.) iron therapy for pre-dialysis and peritoneal dialysis patients, but use of the i.v. route of administration and a target serum ferritin concentration of 200-500 ng/mL is recommended for HD patients by NKF [81]. Due to the fact that parenteral iron administration has potential risks that are immediate (eg, toxic effects and anaphylactic reactions) and long-term (e.g., decreased polymorphonuclear leukocyte function, increased risk of infections, organ damage), it is essential to select patients who need iron supplementation. Although oral iron administration is the primary treatment for iron deficiency, it has also disadvantages, such as poor iron absorption and adverse gastrointestinal reactions, which often lead to poor compliance. Oral iron is ineffective in many CKD patients, and parenteral iron administration is required, particularly on those receiving hemodialysis [68]. Nevertheless, even with these limitations of oral iron absorption, the cheap costs of using this route, along with convenience for the patient, often persuade physicians to try oral iron supplementation first on non-dialysis patients; if, however, there is insufficient response after 2 to 3 months, intravenous iron should be administered. However, the use of IV iron reduces the risk of adverse gastrointestinal reactions and overcomes the problem of poor compliance with oral therapy [82, 83]. Another advantage of the i.v. route is that the iron will not be eliminated by first-pass effects or by high efficiency dialysis membranes and the iron can be quickly released into the reticuloendothelial system and used for erythropoiesis, thus increasing its bioavailability. Intravenous iron administration may not only decrease hemoglobin variability and ESA hyporesponsiveness, it may also reduce the greater mortality associated with the much higher ESA doses that have been used in some patients when targeting higher hemoglobin levels [84]. Other, longer term concerns about intravenous administration of iron include the potential for increased susceptibility to infections and oxidative stress. Much of the scientific evidence for this has been generated in *in vitro* experiments, the clinical significance of which is unclear. There is emerging evidence that intravenous iron may improve the anemia of CKD in up to 30% of patients not receiving ESA therapy and have a low ferritin level [85]. Abnormalities of iron metabolism and anemia in chronic renal failure seem to correlate with levels of serum Hepcidin [86]. Hepcidin is a recently discovered protein of expeditious action produced in the liver and that may play an important role in iron homeostasis [87-89]. Hepcidin limits the absorption of iron from the intestine and iron release from macrophages and hepatocytes [90]. Iron absorption capacity in patients with CKD is considerably lower than in non-uremic individuals, particularly in the presence of systemic inflammatory activity, and this is probably mediated by Hepcidin up-regulation [91, 92]. The data in CKD and particularly in ESRD is limited both in hemodialysis and in peritoneal dialysis [93]. Because of its excretion in the urine [94, 95] and regulation by the presence or absence of inflammation, it is likely that its metabolism is affected by renal function and consistently influences the absorption of iron from the intestine and the stores of iron [96-99]. Originally due to the inability to measure serum levels of Hepcidin, its role in chronic kidney disease had not been adequately studied and most studies involved hepcidin's levels in urine. It has been attempted to measure prohepcidin a precursor peptide of Hepcidin in CKD patients [100, 101]. According to our recently unpublished data Hepcidin levels were increased in hemodialysis patients in relation to normal individuals. The U.S. [16] and European [17] guidelines on renal anemia management suggest that the ferritin level be maintained in the range of 200 to500 μg/l, with an upper limit of 800 μg/l. Levels of ferritin above this threshold usually do not confer any clinical advantage and may exacerbate iron toxicity. The optimal transferring saturation is above 20% to 30% to ensure a readily available supply of iron to the bone marrow. Several studies support the maintenance of the percentage of hypochromic red cells at levels of less than 6%. Other measures of iron status, such as serum transferring receptor levels [102] and erythrocyte zinc protoporphyrin levels, are mainly research tools and have not been established in routine clinical practice. Intramuscular administration of iron is not recommended in CKD, given the enhanced bleeding tendency, the pain of the injection, and the potential for brownish discoloration of the skin. Thus, intravenous administration of iron has become the standard of care for many CKD patients, particularly those receiving hemodialysis [17, 68, 69, 103]. An important advantage of i.v. iron over oral iron is that it may bypass hepcidin actions by directly loading transferrin and making iron available to macrophages. Despite a reduction in the short-term risks, there is still concern about the potential for long-term toxicity of i.v. iron use (e. g. atherosclerosis development, infection and increased mortality) [104, 105] .The association of atherosclerosis with iron overload remains unclear. Alternatively, the relative risk for mortality or hospitalization from infection in patients undergoing HD and receiving i.v. iron was shown not to be higher than that observed in the overall HD population. Indeed, doses of i.v. iron up to 400 mg/month were associated with improved patient survival. There are several intravenous iron preparations available worldwide, including iron dextran, iron sucrose, and iron gluconate and Ferric carboxymaltose (table 1).

| AVAILABLE IRON PREPARATIONS | IVMAXIMUM DOSE | ADMINISTRATION | TEST DOSE |
|---|---|---|---|
| Dextran Iron* | 1000mg | 0.0442 (Desired Hb - Observed Hb) x LBW + (0.26 x Lean body weight in kg) (For males: LBW = 50 kg + 2.3 kg for each inch of patient's height over 5 feetFor females: LBW = 45.5 kg + 2.3 kg for each inch of patient's height over 5 feet.) | A test dose of 25 mg diluted in 50 ml normal saline and infused over 5 minutes should be given. Infusion should then be stopped for 1 hour. If there is no reaction after 1 hour continue. |
| Gluconate Iron* | 125mg | The recommended dosage of Sodium Ferric Gluconate for the repletion treatment of iron deficiency in hemodialysis patients is 10 mL of Ferrlecit (125 mg of elemental iron). Ferrlecit may be diluted in 100 mL of 0.9% sodium chloride administered by intravenous infusion over 1 hour per dialysis session | No test |
| Iron Sucrose* | 500mg | Administer Venofer 100 mg undiluted as a slow injection over 2 to 5 minutes, or as an infusion of 100 mg diluted in a maximum of 100 mL of 0.9% NaCl over a period of at least 15 minutes, per consecutive session. Venofer should be administered early during the dialysis session. | No test dose |

| AVAILABLE IRON PREPARATIONS | IVMAXIMUM DOSE | ADMINISTRATION | TEST DOSE |
|---|---|---|---|
| Ferric Carboxymaltose** | A cumulative iron dose of 500 mg should not be exceeded for patients with body weight < 35 kg. A single dose of Ferinject should not exceed 1000 mg of iron (20 ml) per day. Do not administer 1000 mg of iron (20 ml) more than once a week. | 1000 mg of iron during a minimum administration time of </=15 minutes. | No test dose |

**Table 1.** Avalaible i.v. iron preparations. *: www.globalrph.com - **: www.medicines.org.uk

All of these preparations contain elemental iron surrounded by a carbohydrate shell, which allows them to be injected intravenously. The liability of iron release from these preparations varies, with iron dextran being the most stable, followed by iron sucrose and then iron gluconate. Iron is released from these compounds to plasma transferrin and other iron-binding proteins and is eventually taken up by the reticulo-endothelial system. In hemodialysis patients, it is easy and practical to give low doses of intravenous iron (e.g., 10 to 20 mg every dialysis session) or, alternatively, 100 mg weekly. The more stable the iron preparation, the larger the dose administration rate that can be used. For example, 1gr of iron dextran may be given by intravenous infusion, whereas the maximum recommended dose of iron sucrose at any one time is 500 mg. For iron gluconate, doses in excess of 125 to 250 mg are best avoided. A 100 mg dose of iron sucrose is administered at 10 consecutive HD sessions. If after the end of the first 10-dose cycle patients remain iron deficient they complete another 10-dose cycle. If TSAT is 20-50% and SF 100-800 ng/mL, the patients start the maintenance regimen. If TSAT>50% or SF> 800 ng/mL then no further iron supplementation was deemed necessary. Iron replete patients received the iron maintenance regimen, consisting of 10 one weekly doses of up to 100 mg iron sucrose over 5 minutes. Iron repletion is defined as TSAT

20-50% and SF 100-800 ng/mL [106, 107]. Iron sucrose appears to offer the most favorable safety profile when compared to iron dextran and sodium ferric gluconate in treating hemodialysis patients. Oxidative stress and hypersensitivity reactions are common problems encountered when administering intravenous iron [108]. Therapy with dextran-free iron formulations is an essential part of anemia treatment protocols, and was not found to be associated with either short- or long-term serious side-effects [109]. Results suggest that 200 mg/FeIV/month is effective and that, of the markers tested, TSAT would be the most suitable one to the practicing nephrologist so as to optimize intravenous iron in the long run [110]. Sodium ferric gluconate is well tolerated when given by intravenous push without a test dose [111]. SFGC has a significantly lower incidence of drug intolerance and life-threatening events as compared to previous studies using iron dextran. The routine use of iron dextran in hemodialysis patients should be discontinued [112]. Nevertheless, older i.v. iron formulations have their limitations, including the potential for immunogenic reactions induced by dextran molecules (iron dextran) [113], dose limitations, a slow rate of administration (to prevent acute, labile iron-induced toxicity and vasoactive reactions) [70, 113] and the compulsory requirement for a test dose (iron dextrans in USA [114] and Europe. All-event reporting rates were 29.2, 10.5 and 4.2 reports per million 100 mg iron dose equivalents, while all-fatal-event reporting rates were 1.4, 0.6 and 0.0 reports per million 100 mg dose equivalents for iron dextran, sodium ferric gluconate and iron sucrose, respectively [115]. Recently, two new iron preparations have become available for intravenous use (ferumoxytol in the United States and ferric carboxymaltose in Europe) [116]. Both of these compounds allow higher doses of intravenous iron to be administered rapidly as a bolus injection, without the need for a test dose. Ferric carboxymaltose [FCM; FerinjectR; Vifor (International) Inc., St Gallen, Switzerland] is a next-generation parenteral, dextran-free iron formulation designed to overcome the limitations of existing i.v. iron preparations. The FCM is a macromolecular ferric hydroxide carbohydrate complex, composed of a poly-nuclear iron(III) hydroxide complexed to carboxymaltose [117]. As FCM is a strong and robust iron complex, and it can be administered in high doses, it does not release large amounts of reactive ('free') iron into the circulation and does not trigger dextran- associated immunogenic reactions [111, 117-119]. All intravenous iron preparations carry a risk for immediate reactions, which may be characterized by hypotension, dizziness, and nausea. These reactions are usually short-lived and caused by too large a dose given during too short a time. Iron dextran also carries the risk for acute anaphylactic reactions due to preformed dextran antibodies, and although this risk may be less with the lower molecular weight iron dextrans, the potential for anaphylaxis still remains. In such patients, a response to intravenous iron alone may occur within 2 to 3 weeks of iron administration. In those already receiving ESAs, there is considerable evidence that concomitant intravenous iron may enhance the response to the ESAs and result in lower dose requirements [17, 21, 68]. Ferric carboxymaltose also replenishes depleted iron stores and improves health-related quality-of-life (HR-QoL) on patients with iron-deficiency anemia. FCM is at least as effective as iron sucrose and as ferrus sulfate with regards to end point relative to serum ferritin, transferrin saturation and HR-QoL. Commonly reported drug-related adverse events include headache, dizziness, nausea, abdominal pain, constipation, diarrhea, rash and injection-site reactions. The incidence of drug-related adverse events on patients receiving intravenous FCM was generally similar to that in patients receiving oral ferrous sulfate. In general, rash and local injection-site reactions were more common with ferric carboxymaltose, whereas gastrointestinal adverse events were more frequent with ferrous sulfate [120]. Based on the No-Observed-Adverse-Effect-Levels (NOAELs) found in repeated-dose toxicity studies and on the cumulative doses administered, FCM has good safety margins. Lastly, no evidence of irritation was found in local tolerance studies with FCM [70]. Ferric carboxymaltose may represent a cost-saving option compared with the most likely alternative existing therapies used for the management of anemia [121, 122].

### 4.2. Correction of vitamin B and Acid Folic

Vitamin abnormalities in patients with CKD are frequent and appear early even with mild renal failure; fat-soluble vitamin supplements (A and E) should be avoided and their dietary intake limited [123]. Deficiency and/or altered metabolism of vitamins in ESRD is caused by uremic toxins, dietary restrictions, catabolic illness, losses during dialysis and drug interaction. In patients with polyneuropathy high doses of thiamine pyrophosphate (Cocarboxylase), given i.v., can be helpful in this respect. There are conflicting reports concerning plasma level of vitamin B2 (riboflavin) in ESRD patients. Some authors recommend its supplementation. The majority of patients with ESRD exhibit biochemical and clinical signs of vitamin B6 deficiency. A univocal opinion exists that supplementation of this vitamin effects the cellular immune system and the amino acid metabolism as well. An adequate dose of vitamin B6 is still a matter of dispute. Evidence of vitamin B12 deficiency has been reported rarely, thus, only few authors recommend the supplementation of it, mainly in CAPD patients. According to most authors the losses of folic acid and ascorbic acid during dialysis require oral supplementation. Despite the divergences in opinions concerning the deficiency of water-soluble vitamins in ESRD patients, the supplementation of these vitamins is practiced in many nephrological centers. The amount and the route of vitamins, administered to ESRD patients, should be individualized [124-126]. In ESRD patients under maintenance hemodialysis, oral L-carnitine supplementation may reduce triglyceride and cholesterol and increase HDL and hemoglobin and subsequently reduce needed erythropoietin dose without effect on QoL [127]. Adjuvant therapy includes: iron, vitamin C and D, L-carnitine, folic acid, cytokines and growth factors. Vitamin C (500 mg, after every hemodialysis) is very helpful in cases of functional iron deficiency. L-carnitine stabilizes the membrane of erythrocytes and prolongs their lives. Folic acid (10 mg/day) enhances response to EPO [128]. According to other authors supplementations of pyridoxine in the dose of 20 mg/day and of folic acid 5 mg/week in hemodialyzed patients during erythropoietin treatment are necessary [129].

### 4.3. Erythropoiesis Stimulating Agents

Erythropoiesis is a complex physiologic process through which homeostasis of oxygen levels in the body is maintained. It is primarily regulated by EPO, a 30-kD, 165–amino acid hematopoietic growth factor that is produced primarily by renal tubular and interstitial cells. Under normal conditions, endogenous EPO levels change according to O2 tension. EPO gene expression is induced by hypoxia-inducible transcription factors (HIF) [130]. In the presence of EPO, bone marrow erythroid precursor cells proliferate and differentiate into red blood cells. In its absence, these cells undergo apoptosis [131]. Endogenous EPO and rHuEPO share the same amino acid sequence, with slight but functionally important differences in the sugar profile. In clinical practice, rHuEPO is typically administered as a bolus injection, and the dosage is titrated to give the desired effect [131]. There is no significant difference between once weekly versus thrice weekly subcutaneous administration of rHu EPO. Once weekly administration of rHu EPO would require an additional 12U/kg/week for patients on hemodialysis [132].

Recombinant human erythropoietin has been used for more than 20 years for the treatment of renal anemia, revolutionizing its treatment in patients with CKD when it was approved for use in the United States in 1989, [133, 134] with epoetin-alfa and -beta representing the common traditional preparations. By the modification of the molecule's carbohydrate moiety or structure a longer duration of erythropoietin receptor stimulation was achieved. The administration of darbepoetin or C.E.R.A. once or twice a month is also sufficient to achieve serum hemoglobin target levels, [135] making the treatment safer and more comfortable both for the patients and the personnel. These synthetic erythropoietin receptor stimulating molecules, along with recombinant human erythropoietin, are together called "Erythropoiesis Stimulating Agents". The recombinant human erythropoietins and allied proteins (epoetin-alfa, attempted copies and biosimilar variants of epoetin-alfa, epoetin beta, epoetin delta, epoetin zeta, epoetin theta, epoetin omega, darbepoetin-alfa, and methoxy-polyethylene glycol-epoetin beta) are among the most successful and earliest examples of biotechnologically manufactured products to be used in clinical medicine (Table 2) [136].

| AVALAIBLE ESAs | DOSE REGIMEN |
|---|---|
| **Prototype** | |
| epoetin-alfa* | Correction phase:<br>50 IU/kg, 3 times per week.<br>When a dose adjustment is necessary, this should be done in steps of at least four weeks. At each step, the increase or reduction in dose should be of 25 IU/kg, 3 times per week.<br>Maintenance phase:<br>Dosage adjustment in order to maintain haemoglobin values at the desired level: Hb between 10 and 12 g/dl (6.2 - 7.5 mmol/l).<br>The recommended total weekly dose is between 75 and 300 IU/kg. |
| epoetin beta* | 1. Correction phase<br>- Subcutaneous administration:<br>- The initial dosage is 3 x 20 IU/kg body weight per week. The dosage may be increased every 4 weeks by 3 x 20 IU/kg and week if the increase of Hb is not adequate (< 0.25 g/dl per week). |

| AVALAIBLE ESAs | DOSE REGIMEN |
|---|---|
| | - The weekly dose can also be divided into daily doses.<br>- Intravenous administration:<br>The initial dosage is 3 x 40 IU/kg per week. The dosage may be raised after 4 weeks to 80 IU/kg three times per week - and by further increments of 20 IU/kg if needed, three times per week, at monthly intervals.<br>For both routes of administration, the maximum dose should not exceed 720 IU/kg per week.<br>2. Maintenance phase<br>To maintain an Hb of between 10 and 12 g/dl, the dosage is initially reduced to half of the previously administered amount. Subsequently, the dose is adjusted at intervals of one or two weeks individually for the patient (maintenance dose). |
| darbepoetin-alfa* | Correction phase:<br>The initial dose by subcutaneous or intravenous administration is 0.45 μg/kg body weight, as a single injection once weekly.<br>If the rise in haemoglobin is greater than 2 g/dl (1.25 mmol/l) in four weeks reduce the dose by approximately 25%.Dosing should be titrated as necessary to maintain the haemoglobin target.<br>If a dose adjustment is required to maintain haemoglobin at the desired level, it is recommended that the dose is adjusted by approximately 25% |
| Methoxy-polyethylene glycol-epoetin beta* | a starting dose of 0.6 microgram/kg bodyweight may be administered once every two weeks as a single intravenous or subcutaneous injection in patients on dialysis or not on dialysis. The dose may be increased by approximately 25% of the previous dose if the rate of rise in haemoglobin is less than 1.0 g/dl (0.621 mmol/l) over a month. Further increases of approximately 25% may be made at monthly intervals until the individual target haemoglobin level is obtained. |
| **Biosimilar** | |
| epoetin zeta* | 1. Correction phase:<br>50 IU/kg 3 times per week. When a dose adjustment is necessary, this should be done in steps of at least four weeks. At each step, the increase or reduction in dose should be of 25 IU/kg 3 times per week<br>2. Maintenance phase:<br>Dose adjustment in order to maintain haemoglobin (Hb) values at the desired level: Hb between 10 and 12 g/dl (6.2-7.5 mmol/l). The recommended total weekly dose is between 75 and 300 IU/kg. |
| epoetin delta** | For Epoetin delta it is recommended to adjust the dose individually to maintain the target haemoglobin in the range 10 to 12 g/dl. A starting dose is recommended of 50 IU/kg three times a week if given intravenously or twice a week if given subcutaneously |

| AVALAIBLE ESAs | DOSE REGIMEN |
|---|---|
| epoetin omega*** | Starting with 20 to 50 IU / kg three times a week, with a gradual increase in dose or frequency of issuance before the impact. Beyond hemoglobin levels to 12 g / m and Hematocrit-35 %. Dose reduction or no treatment. If there Effect dose increase to 40 to 55 IU / kg three times a week for two weeks, if necessary, until 60-75 IU / kg The course continues until the level Hematocrit (35 vol. %) And hemoglobin (12 g / m); Total weekly dose should not exceed 225 IU / kg supporting-60 IU / kg per week for 2-3 reception |
| epoetin theta** | Correction phase<br>Subcutaneous administration: The initial posology is 20 IU/kg body weight 3 times per week. The dose may be increased after 4 weeks to 40 IU/kg, 3 times per week, if the increase in haemoglobin is not adequate (< 1 g/dl [0.62 mmol/l] within 4 weeks). Further increases of 25% of the previous dose may be made at monthly intervals until the individual target haemoglobin level is obtained.<br>Intravenous administration: The initial posology is 40 IU/kg body weight 3 times per week. The dose may be increased after 4 weeks to 80 IU/kg, 3 times per week, and by further increases of 25% of the previous dose at monthly intervals, if needed.<br>For both routes of administration, the maximum dose should not exceed 700 IU/kg body weight per week.<br>Maintenance phase<br>The dose should be adjusted as necessary to maintain the individual target haemoglobin level between 10 g/dl (6.21 mmol/l) to 12 g/dl (7.45 mmol/l), whereby a haemoglobin level of 12 g/dl (7.45 mmol/l) should not be exceeded. If a dose adjustment is required to maintain the desired haemoglobin level, it is recommended that the dose be adjusted by approximately 25%. Subcutaneous administration: The weekly dose can be given as one injection per week or three times per week.<br>Intravenous administration: Patients who are stable on a three times weekly dosing regimen may be switched to twice-weekly administration.<br>If the frequency of administration is changed, haemoglobin level should be monitored closely and dose adjustments may be necessary.<br>The maximum dose should not exceed 700 IU/kg body weight per week |

**Table 2.** Available ESAs worldwide. *: ww.medicines.org.uk, **: www.ema.europa.eu, ***: www.pharmabook.net

In hemodialysed patients the intravenous route is preferred, but the subcutaneous administration can substantially reduce dose requirements [137-139]. However, there are studies according to which conversion from SC to IV epoetin administration did not result in changes in Hb levels or epoetin dosage requirements in iron-replete hemodialysis patients, [140] but it seems that SC route of administration was associated with modestly higher hemoglobin variability [138].

There are ongoing clinical trials with erythropoiesis stimulating molecules that can be administered by inhalation or per os [137]. It is also known from other studies that some comorbidities like antecedents of malignant neoplasm are associated with EPO responsiveness [141]. In a pre-dialysis population, female gender, cardiovascular disease, malnutrition and inflammation are associated with ESA hyporesponsiveness [142]. EPO resistance in a pediatric dialysis cohort was predicted by nutritional deficits, inflammation, poor dialysis, and hyperparathyroidism, while iron and folic acid deficits were the major determinants in adults. Although confounded by the pattern of EPO prescription, neither age nor gender was predictive of EPO resistance in the two study groups [143]. Additionally delivered dialysis (Kt/ V(urea)) does not seem to be a significant predictor of erythropoietin responsiveness [144]. It also seems that there is difference in EPO hyporesponsiveness prevalence among different countries and different modalities [145]. The proportion of age has a limited influence on the level of anemia in pre-dialysis patients and is similar in both genders [146] There are, although, studies according to which there is higher proportion of anemia in female patients [147]. In a multicenter study with 8154 dialysis patients, females, blacks, patients between 18 and44 years old on hemodialysis less than six months exhibited significantly lower mean hemoglobin values despite being prescribed, on average, significantly higher epoetin alfa doses than males, whites and older patients, on hemodialysis more than six months. A significant regional variation in the prescribing patterns for s.c. epoetin alfa and i.v. iron has been described in this study [148]. Comparisons between patients from western and from eastern/central Europe show that patients from eastern/central Europe are less likely to receive epoetin treatment before starting dialysis, and have lower Hb concentrations at the start of epoetin treatment as well as at the start of dialysis [149]. In another multicenter study by Nissenson et al. there were wide variations in hemoglobin response rate among patients on hemodialysis, hemofiltration and hemodiafiltration [150].

Other factors such as cytokines like IL6 are induced by malignant tumors and may impair erythropoiesis. Also, TNF-$\alpha$ is known to inhibit this pathway [151]. Low ESA responsiveness was associated with higher mortality in both HD and PD patients [152]. In patients with persistently low Hb levels, mortality risk is strongly associated with the patient's ability to achieve a hematopoietic response rather than the magnitude of EPO dose titrations [153]. ESA dosing may be directly associated with risk of death, but the nature of the association likely varies according to hemoglobin concentration. Small doses with hemoglobin ≤12 g/dl and large doses with hemoglobin ≥10 g/dl may both be associated with poor outcomes [154].

Serum albumin concentration is an important predictor of both baseline Hb and EPO sensitivity in chronic hemodialysis patients. Factors that improve serum albumin may also improve Hb in hemodialysis patients [155]. Hyperleptinemia reflects better nutritional status and rHuEPO response in long-term HD patients. Increasing energy intake improves erythropoiesis, which may be mediated in part by an increase in serum leptin levels [156, 157]. Statin therapy may improve responsiveness to erythropoietin-stimulating agents in patients with end-stage renal disease, increasing erythropoiesis by targeting hepcidin and iron regulatory pathways, independent of erythropoietin [158, 159]. The initial and sustained erythropoietic responses are independent from each other and are associated with different factors. Treatment focusing on these factors may improve the response [160]. A pleiotropic effect of EPO has been shown in the kidney, the central nervous system, and the cardiovascular system, [161] such as significant slowing of progression and substantial retardation of maintenance dialysis [162, 163].

Although ESA use in patients with chronic kidney disease or/and on dialysis were studied extensively, the optimal target hemoglobin concentration as well as the required ESA dose and dosing interval to achieve this concentrations remain elusive (NHS, CREATE, CHOIR and TREAT) [164-167]. Hb can be increased with erythropoiesis-stimulating proteins (ESPs); however, 5-10% of patients respond poorly. The patient incidence of hyporesponse seems to be around 14%, and a mean 9% of patients is hyporesponsive at any given time. The most common potential causes of hyporesponse is iron deficiency (being reported in 39% of hyporesponse events), medication (immunosuppressive agents, ACE inhibitors), secondary hyperparathyroidism [168] and inflammation/malnutrition [169]. The safety profile of epoetin-alfa and darbepoetin-alfa are similar, but the longer half-life of darbepoetin-alfa permits administration on a once a week or once-monthly basis in patients with CKD and anemia. Extended dosing of CERA also appears safe and effective on dialysis patients with CKD [81].

*Epoetin alfa:* is a recombinant form of erythropoietin, a glycoprotein hormone which stimulates red blood cell production by stimulating the activity of erythroid progenitor cells. Intravenous and subcutaneous therapy with epoetin alfa raises hematocrit and hemoglobin levels, and reduces transfusion requirements, in anemic patients with end-stage renal failure undergoing hemodialysis. The drug is also effective in the correction of anemia on patients with chronic renal failure not yet requiring dialysis and does not appear to affect renal hemodynamics adversely or to precipitate the onset of end-stage renal failure. Epoetin alfa does not appear to exert any direct cerebrovascular adverse effects [170]. Administration of epoetin alfa at once weekly and fortnightly intervals are potential alternatives to three times per week dosing for the treatment of anemia [171-173].

*Epoetin beta:* is a recombinant form of erythropoietin. The drug binds to and activates receptors on erythroid progenitor cells which then develop into mature erythrocytes. Epoetin beta increases reticulocyte counts, hemoglobin levels and hematocrit in a dose-proportional manner. Increases of 15 to 54% in hemoglobin levels and 17 to 60% in hematocrit were reported after subcutaneous or intravenous epoetin beta therapy in studies of 8 weeks' to 12 months' duration. Comparative data indicate that dosage reductions of approximately 30% compared with intravenous therapy are possible when subcutaneous administration of epoetin beta is used. Hematocrit increased more rapidly in 5 multicenter studies on patients who received epoetin beta subcutaneously than on those who received the same dosage intravenously. It also causes significant improvements on quality of life, exercise capacity and overall well-being. Results of clinical studies indicate that subcutaneous administration is desirable where possible in the majority of patients [174].

*Darboepoetin-alfa:* It is a hyperglycosylated analog of recombinant human erythropoietin with the same mechanism of action as erythropoietin, but with a three-fold longer terminal half-life after intravenous administration than recombinant human erythropoietin and the native hormone both in animal models and in humans. It is administered less frequently (once weekly or every other week) [175, 176]. The recommended starting dose in chronic renal failure patients is 0.45mcg/kg once weekly for both intravenous and subcutaneous administration, with subsequent titration based on the hemoglobin concentration. The adverse event profile of darbepoetin-alfa is similar to that of recombinant human erythropoietin in both settings, [177, 178] and effectively maintains hemoglobin in the target range in dialysis patients with renal anemia [179]. It also has been shown to be effective when administered once/week and once every 2, 3, or 4 weeks [180]. There are no reports of antibody formation associated with darbepoetin-alfa on chronic renal failure patients, and three cases of antibody formation, with neutralizing activity in one of the cases, reported on cancer patients [181-184].

*Cera:* Methoxy polyethylene glycol-epoetin beta (MPG-EPO; Mircera®, Roche, Basel, witzerland) is an agent that has a different interaction with the erythropoietin receptor than previous agents and has a long elimination half-life (approximately 130 hours) [185]. MPG-EPO is the only ESA generated by chemical modification of glycosylated erythropoietin, by the integration of one specific, long, linear chain of polyethylene glycol. The resultant molecule has a molecular weight of approximately 60 kDa, which is twice that of epoetin. The methoxy polyethylene glycol polymer chain is integrated through amide bonds between the N-terminal amino group or the ε-amino group (predominantly lysine-52 or lysine-45) with a single butanoic acid linker [186]. In ESA-naïve patients, the recommended starting dose is 0.6 μg/kg administered once every 2 weeks as a subcutaneous or intravenous injection, in order to reach a hemoglobin level of.11 g/dL. The dose may be increased by approximately 25% if hemoglobin levels increase by, 1.0 g/dL over a month. Further increases of approximately 25% may be made once per month until the individual target hemoglobin level is reached. If a hemoglobin level of.11 g/dL is reached for an individual patient, MPG-EPO may be continued once per month using a dose equal to twice the previous dose once every 2 weeks. Patients currently being treated with ESA can be directly converted to MPG-EPO administered once per month as a single intravenous or subcutaneous injection. The starting dose of this agent is based on the calculated weekly equivalent dose of DA or epoetin at the time of conversion [187]. The first injection of MPG-EPO should start at the next scheduled dose of the previously administered DA or epoetin dose. On patients receiving treatment with ESA and those naive to ESA, the MPG-EPO dose should be reduced by approximately 25% if the hemoglobin level increases by more than 2 g/dL in 1 month or if the hemoglobin level approaches 12 g/dL. If hemoglobin levels continue to increase, MPG-EPO administration should be interrupted until these levels begin to decrease (a decrease of approximately 0.35 g/dL per week is expected). Therapy should then be resumed at a dose approximately 25% less than the previously administered dose. Dose adjustments should not be made more frequently than once per month [17, 188]. Once-monthly CERA therapy maintains stable Hb values with low intra-individual variability and few dose adaptations in hemodialysis patients when administered entirely according to local practice, and the regimen is well-tolerated [189]. C.E.R.A. can be administered to patients at any time during hemodialysis or hemofiltration without appreciable loss in the extracorporeal circuit [190].

*Peginesatide (formerly known as Hematide™):* is a synthetic, peptide-based erythropoiesis-stimulating agent linked to polyethylene glycol. Based on extensive preclinical and clinical data substantiating the efficacy and safety of this agent, it was approved in the U.S. in March 2012 for the treatment of anemia due to chronic kidney disease in adult patients on dialysis. Peginesatide (Omontys®) was launched in the U.S. in April 2012 [191, 192]. A drug capable of stimulating erythropoiesis is the first ESA that bears no structural similarity to rhuEPO. Peginesatide is a synthetic, dimeric peptide that is covalently linked to polyethylene glycol (PEG). Peginesatide binds to and activates the human EPO receptor, stimulating the proliferation and differentiation of human red cell precursors in vitro in a manner similar to ESAs [193]. Peginesatide administered once monthly was as effective as epoetin alfa given thrice weekly (dialysis patients) or darbepoetin given once weekly (nondialysis patients), in correcting anemia of chronic kidney disease as well as maintaining hemoglobin within the desired target range [194-196].

### 4.4. Biosimilar

*Epoetin zeta:* Epoetin zeta is therapeutically equivalent to epoetin alfa in the maintenance of target Hb levels on patients with renal anemia. No unexpected adverse effects were seen [197-201].

*Epoetin theta:* Has efficacy comparable with epoetin beta (s.c.) in pre-dialysis patients with renal anemia based on Hb changes from baseline to end of treatment (non-inferiority). The safety profile was also comparable. Patients could be switched from maintenance treatment with epoetin beta to epoetin theta without relevant dose changes [202].

*Epoetin omega:* Epoetin-omega is a sialoglycoprotein with smaller amounts of O-bound sugars, less acidic and with different hydrophylity than the other 2 epoetins. The initial weekly dose of epoetin-omega was 90 units per kg of body weight (b.w.) divided in 3 equal portions and administered subcutaneously after each dialysis session. After correction of the hemoglobin, the dose of rHuEPO was individualized to keep Hb within target limits of 100-120 g/l. The mean dose of epoetin-omega during the correction period never exceeded 100 U/kg b.w. per week and the average maintenance dose between 50-60 U/kg b.w. per week [203, 204].

*HX575:* Is a biosimilar version of epoetin-$\alpha$ that is approved for the treatment of anemia associated with chronic kidney disease (CKD) using the intravenous route of administration [205, 206]. In a study for S.C. use two patients developed neutralizing antibodies (NAbs) to erythropoietin, which resulted in the study being terminated prematurely [207].

### 4.5. Adverse effects of EPO therapy

Adverse effects of EPO therapy are uncommon, apart from a moderate increase in blood pressure and an increased rate of vascular access thrombosis. In spite of the fact that, these effects are probably dependent to a large degree on the increase in Hb concentrations, there are some concerns that ESA therapy may enhance thrombogenicity and tumor growth on patients with malignant disease as well as exacerbate vascular events in CKD independently of Hb concentrations [208]. In treatment with epoetin alfa hypertension occurs in 30 to 35% of patients with end-stage renal failure, but this can be managed successfully with correction of fluid status and antihypertensive medication where necessary, and is minimized by avoiding rapid increases in hematocrit. Although vascular access thrombosis has not been conclusively linked to therapy with the drug, increased heparinisation may be required when it is administered to patients on hemodialysis [170]. On patients who receive epoetin beta, hypertension may occur but may be minimized by avoiding rapid increases in hematocrit (> 0.5%/week), and is managed in most cases with control of fluid status and antihypertensive medication. Although clotting of the vascular access has not been conclusively linked to epoetin beta, caution is recommended on patients undergoing hemodialysis. Increased heparinisation is recommended to prevent clotting in dialysis equipment [174]. Before 1998, EPO alfa in Europe was formulated with human serum albumin, but because of a change in European regulations, this was replaced with polysorbate 80. EPO beta is formulated with polysorbate 20, along with urea, calcium chloride, and five amino acids as excipients. The importance of the formulation of the EPO products was highlighted in 2002 with an upsurge in cases of antibody-mediated pure red cell aplasia in association with the subcutaneous use of EPO alfa after its change for indicate mulation. Patients affected by this complication develop neutralizing antibodies against both rhuEPO and the endogenous hormone, which result in severe anemia and transfusion dependence [209, 210]. The cause of this serious complication in which there is a break in B-cell tolerance remains obscure, although it seems likely that factors such as a breach of the cold storage chain were relevant, and the subcutaneous application route was a prerequisite; circumstantial evidence also suggested that rubber stoppers of prefilled syringes used in one of the albumin-free EPO alfa formulations may have released organic compounds that acted as immunologic adjuvants [211].

### 4.6. Which target is the best for the correction of anemia on hemodialysis patients?

There has been considerable debate in recent times about the optimal target range of Hb in CKD patients [133]. The improvement in quality of life with increasing Hb concentrations supports a level above 10 to 11 g/dl in all CKD patients, [16, 17] but some studies have indicated increased risks associated with attempts to completely correct anemia. No survival benefit is evident at a higher level of anemia correction, [13, 164, 165, 167] although quality of life and exercise capacity may be greater. Thus, there is a possible tradeoff between improved quality of life and increased cost and risk for harm, so that a target level of Hb above 13 g/dl should be avoided [16]. Clinical trials of erythropoiesis-stimulating agents indicate that targeting the complete correction of anemia in patients with chronic kidney disease results in a greater risk of morbidity and mortality despite improved hemoglobin and quality of life [59, 164, 212]. Although there are studies that state the opposite [213, 214]. Relationships between hemoglobin concentration and mortality differed between African Americans and whites. Additionally, the relationship of lower mortality with greater achieved hemoglobin concentration seen in white patients was observed for all-cause, but not cardiovascular mortality [215]. Erythropoiesis-stimulating agents should be used to target hemoglobin 11-12 g/dl on patients with chronic kidney disease. However, a risk-benefit evaluation is warranted in individual patients, and high ESA doses driven by hyporesponsiveness should be avoided [216]. Intravenous iron may be beneficial for patients with hemoglobin less than

11 g/dl and transferrin saturation less than 25% despite elevated ferritin (500-1200 ng/ml) [217, 218]. TREAT and other large randomized, controlled trials of ESA treatment on patients with CKD have not demonstrated a clinical benefit in terms of mortality, morbidity, or quality of life improvement of targeting Hb levels greater than 12-13 g/dl. Some of these studies have demonstrated increased risk of stroke, vascular access thrombosis, hypertension, and other events [219]. The European Renal Best Practice (ERBP), which are issued by ERA-EDTA, are suggestions for clinical practice in areas in which evidence is lacking or weak, together with position statements on published randomized controlled trials, or on existing guidelines and recommendations. In 2009, the Anemia Working Group of ERBP published its first position statement about the hemoglobin target to aim for with erythropoietin-stimulating agents (ESA) and on issues that were not covered by K-DOQI in 2006-07. Following the findings of the TREAT study, the Anemia Working Group of ERBP maintains its view that 'Hb values of 11-12 g/dL should be generally sought in the CKD population without intentionally exceeding 13 g/dL and that the doses of ESA therapy to achieve the target hemoglobin should also be considered. More caution is suggested when treating anemia with ESA therapy on patients with type 2 diabetes not undergoing dialysis (and probably in diabetics at all CKD stages). To those with ischemic heart disease or with a previous history of stroke, possible benefits should be weighed up against an increased risk of stroke recurrence, when deciding which Hb level to aim for. These recommendations are not intended to represent a new guideline as they are not the result of a systematic review of evidence [220]. The National Kidney Foundation (NKF) and the Food and Drug Administration (FDA) recommend different target levels for hemoglobin in patients with terminal kidney disease treated by hemodialysis [79, 221]. The NKF recognizes also the importance of individualizing the treatment of anemia. The optimal range of target hemoglobin levels in Kainz et al analysis of hemodialysis patients was 11 g/day. Furthermore, ESA hypo-responders showed an increased risk of mortality with higher hemoglobin levels, and ESA responders actually exhibited a decreased risk [222]. A corrected weekly ESA dose up to 16 000 units with achieved hemoglobin levels ~11 g/dL exhibited the lowest mortality risk. Hemoglobin variability as well as ESA hypo-response causing low hemoglobin levels was associated with a numerically increased risk of mortality compared with patients with stable hemoglobin levels between 10 and 12 g/dL. Furthermore, ESA response requiring more than 16 000 units per week was also associated with an increased risk of death in ESA responders [222]. The Japanese Society for Dialysis Therapy (JSDT) guideline committee presents the Japanese guidelines entitled "Guidelines for Renal Anemia in Chronic Kidney Disease." These guidelines replace the "2004 JSDT Guidelines for Renal Anemia in Chronic Hemodialysis Patients," and contain new, additional guidelines for peritoneal dialysis (PD), non-dialysis (ND), and pediatric CKD patients [223]. Values for diagnosing anemia are based on the most recent epidemiological data from the general Japanese population. To both men and women, Hb levels decrease along with an increase in age and the level for diagnosing anemia has been set at <13.5 g/dL on males and <11.5 g/dL on females. Renal anemia is identified as an "endocrine disease." It is believed that in this way defining renal anemia will be extremely beneficial for ND patients exhibiting renal anemia despite having a high GFR. We have also emphasized that renal anemia may not only be treated with ESA therapy but also with ap-

propriate iron supplementation and the improvement of anemia associated with chronic disease, which is associated with inflammation, and inadequate dialysis, another major cause of renal anemia. In Japanese HD patients, Hb levels following hemodialysis rise considerably above their previous levels because of ultrafiltration-induced hemoconcentration; and (ii) as noted in the 2004 guidelines, although 10 to 11 g/dL was optimal for long-term prognosis if the Hb level prior to the hemodialysis session in an HD patient had been established at the target level, it has been reported that, based on data accumulated on Japanese PD and ND patients, higher levels have a cardiac or renal function protective effect, on patients without serious cardiovascular disease,without any safety issues.. Accordingly, the guidelines establish a target Hb level in PD and ND patients of 11 g/dL or more, and recommend 13 g/dL as the criterion for dose reduction/withdrawal. If the serum ferritin is <100 ng/mL and the transferrin saturation rate (TSAT) is <20%, then the criteria for iron supplementation will be met; if only one of these criteria is met, then iron supplementation should be considered unnecessary [223]. Italian Society of Nephrology in its guidelines for the treatment of anemia in chronic renal failure supports that before beginning epoetin treatment, it is essential to evaluate the level of anemia by the measuring Hb concentration, Red blood cell indices (MCV, MCH, MCHC), Reticulocyte count, Iron stores and availability and C-reactive protein (CRP). The minimum target Hb concentration to be attained is 11 g/dL. The upper limit is established individually on a clinical basis. Pending further data, it is advisable to maintain and not exceed 12 g/dL for patients with cardiovascular disease, diabetes, and graft access. In the presence of adequate reserves of iron the need for higher dosages of epoetin define a state of resistance [224].

Iron deficiency (60%) measured by ferritin levels and TSAT at start of dialysis was found in Predialysis Survey on Anemia Management (21 European countries, Israel and South Africa) despite the majority of patients under nephrologist's care for more than twelve months. Only 27% of patients had started epoetin treatment before dialysis therapy. Thirteen percent had started dialysis therapy first, 33% had started epoetin and dialysis therapy simultaneously, and 28% had not been administered epoetin at any time (total n = 4,095).

[225] Difference in hemoglobin levels was found in DOPPS study and mean Hgb levels were 12 g/dL in Sweden; 11.6 to 11.7 g/dL in the United States, Spain, Belgium, and Canada; 11.1 to 11.5 g/dL in Australia/New Zealand, Germany, Italy, the United Kingdom, and France; and 10.1 g/dL in Japan. Hgb levels were substantially lower for new patients with end-stage renal disease, and EPO use before ESRD ranged from 27% (United States) to 65% (Sweden) [21].

At present, there is a "grey zone" also between the intervention threshold of Hb< 9 g/dl and an Hb level > 13 g/dl, at which CKD is associated with a higher risk of cardiovascular events. It seems to be clearly evident that ESA activate platelets directly and indirectly, and that pathologically extended bleeding time is normalized when an Hb level of 10 g/dl is reached; from the hemostaseological perspective, a threshold level for treatment of renal anemia with ESA is thus defined. According to the present state of knowledge, an Hb target range of 10-11 g/dl seems reasonable for renal anemia; this is also compatible with current recommendations by ESA producers and the Food and Drug Administration (FDA) [226]. This target range avoids the upper and lower risk levels for Hb, and probably ensures a positive ESA effect on quality of life; it is much more cost-efficient than the target range of 11-12 g/dl recommended by the Kidney Disease Outcomes Quality Initiative (KDOQI) in 2007 [227]. ESA treatment for renal anemia should be aimed at reducing transfusion risk, with a treatment target in most patients of 10-12 g/dl; therapy should be individualized, rapid increases in Hb level should probably be avoided, and lowest appropriate ESA doses should be used. Temptation to increase ESA doses to very high levels in an attempt to overcome ESA hypo responsiveness should be resisted [219]. It seems that greater hemoglobin variability is independently associated with higher mortality [228]. Variability caused by laboratory assays, biological factors, and therapeutic response determines patient Hb level variability. Improving factors that can be manipulated (e.g., standardizing EPO and iron algorithms) and adjustment of the target Hb level range, specifically, by increasing the upper bound, likely will decrease the observed variability and further enhance the quality of anemia management [229, 230].

## 5. Conclusion

It is obvious that renal anemia in hemodialysis patients remain a serious problem. This was greater before EPO era, when blood transfusion was the only therapeutic approach. Insufficiency of iron and EPO are the most important causes of this anemia. Nowadays with the availability of new I.V. iron supplementation and ESAs this problem became more manageable. The high cost of the EPO treatment makes the iron therapy essential in order to maximize EPO administration result with the lower dose. The ideal hemoglobin target has to be established despite the numerous trials worldwide, and the treatment has to be individualized.

## Author details

Konstantinos Pantelias[1*] and Eirini Grapsa[2]

*Address all correspondence to: drkpantelias@yahoo.com

1 Nephrology Department, Aretaieio University Hospital, Greece

2 Athens Medical School, Nephrology Department, Aretaieio University Hospital, Greece

## References

[1] Nutritional anaemias. (1968). Report of a WHO scientific group. *World Health Organ Tech Rep Ser*, 405, 5-37, PMID: 4975372].

[2] Robinson, B. E. (2006). Epidemiology of chronic kidney disease and anemia. J Am Med Dir Assoc 9 quiz S17-21 [PMID: 17098633 S1525-8610(06)00457-9 [pii]10.1016/j.jamda.2006.09.004 , 7, 3-6.

[3] Macdougall, C. (2010). Iain EK-U. Anemia in Chronic Kidney Disease. *In: Jurgen Floege RJ, John Feehally, editor Comprehensive Clinical Nephrology. Fourth ed. St. Louis, Missouri: Elsevier Saunders*, 951-958.

[4] Valderrabano, F., Jofre, R., & Lopez-Gomez, J. M. (2001). Quality of life in end-stage renal disease patients. *Am J Kidney Dis*, 38(3), 443-464, PMID: 11532675, S0272638601973688.

[5] Obrador, G. T, & Pereira, B. J. (2002). Anaemia of chronic kidney disease: an under-recognized and under-treated problem. *Nephrol Dial Transplant*, 11(17), 44-46, PMID: 12386258].

[6] Merkus, M. P., Jager, K. J., Dekker, F. W., Boeschoten, E. W., Stevens, P., & Krediet, R. T. (1997). Quality of life in patients on chronic dialysis: self-assessment 3 months after the start of treatment. The Necosad Study Group. *Am J Kidney Dis*, 29(4), 584-592, PMID: 9100049, S0272638697000747.

[7] Locatelli, F., Pisoni, R. L., Combe, C., Bommer, J., Andreucci, V. E., Piera, L., Greenwood, R., Feldman, H. I., Port, F. K., & Held, P. J. (2004). Anaemia in haemodialysis patients of five European countries: association with morbidity and mortality in the Dialysis Outcomes and Practice Patterns Study (DOPPS). *Nephrol Dial Transplant*, 19(1), 121-132, PMID: 14671047].

[8] Astor, B. C., Coresh, J., Heiss, G, Pettitt, D., & Sarnak, M. J. (2006). Kidney function and anemia as risk factors for coronary heart disease and mortality: the Atherosclerosis Risk in Communities (ARIC) Study. *Am Heart J*, S0002-8703(05)00358-3, [PMID: 16442920, 151(2), 492-500, [pii]10.1016/j.ahj.2005.03.055.

[9] Dhingra, R., Gaziano, J. M., & Djousse, L. (2011). Chronic kidney disease and the risk of heart failure in men. *Circ Heart Fail*, 4(2), 138-144, PMID: 21216838 PMCID: 3059366, 10.1161/CIRCHEARTFAILURE.109.899070.

[10] Taddei, S., Nami, R., Bruno, R. M., Quatrini, I., & Nuti, R. (2011). Hypertension, left ventricular hypertrophy and chronic kidney disease. *Heart Fail Rev*, 16(6), 615-620, PMID: 21116711, s10741-010-9197-z.

[11] Vlagopoulos, P. T., Tighiouart, H., Weiner, D. E., Griffith, J., Pettitt, D., Salem, D. N., Levey, A. S., & Sarnak, M. J. (2005). Anemia as a risk factor for cardiovascular disease and all-cause mortality in diabetes: the impact of chronic kidney disease. *J Am Soc Nephrol*, 16(11), 3403-3410, PMID: 16162813, 10.1681/ASN.2005030226.

[12] Parfrey, P. (2001). Anaemia in chronic renal disease: lessons learned since Seville 1994. *Nephrol Dial Transplant*, 7(16), 41-45, PMID: 11590256].

[13] Madore, F., Lowrie, E. G., Brugnara, C., Lew, N. L., Lazarus, J.M, Bridges, K., & Owen, W. F. (1997). Anemia in hemodialysis patients: variables affecting this outcome predictor. *J Am Soc Nephrol*, PMID: 9402095, 8(12), 1921-1929.

[14] Astor, B. C., Muntner, P., Levin, A., Eustace, J. A., & Coresh, J. (2002). Association of kidney function with anemia: the Third National Health and Nutrition Examination Survey (1988-1994). *Arch Intern Med*, 162(12), 1401-1408, PMID: 12076240, ioi10526.

[15] Mc Clellan, W., Aronoff, S. L., Bolton, W. K., Hood, S., Lorber, D. L., Tang, K. L., Tse, T. F., Wasserman, B., & Leiserowitz, M. (2004). The prevalence of anemia in patients with chronic kidney disease. *Curr Med Res Opin*, 20(9), 1501-1510, PMID: 15383200, X2763.

[16] KDOQI. (2006). Clinical Practice Guidelines and Clinical Practice Recommendations for Anemia in Chronic Kidney Disease. *Am J Kidney Dis*, S0272-6386(06)00454-9, 47(5, 3), PMID: 16678659, S11-145, [pii] 10.1053/j.ajkd.2006.03.010.

[17] Locatelli, F., Aljama, P., Barany, P., Canaud, B., Carrera, F., Eckardt, K. U., Horl, W. H., Macdougal, I. C., Macleod, A., Wiecek, A., & Cameron, S. (2004). Revised European best practice guidelines for the management of anaemia in patients with chronic renal failure. *Nephrol Dial Transplant*, 19(2), 1-47, PMID: 15206425].

[18] New, J. P., Aung, T., Baker, P. G., Yongsheng, G., Pylypczuk, R., Houghton, J., Rudenski, A., New, R. P., Hegarty, J., Gibson, J. M., O'Donoghue, D. J., & Buchan, I. E. (2008). The high prevalence of unrecognized anaemia in patients with diabetes and chronic kidney disease: a population-based study. *Diabet Med*, DME2424, 25(5), 564-569, PMID: 18445169 [pii]10.1111/j.1464-5491.2008.02424.x.

[19] Eckardt, K. U. (1994). Erythropoietin: oxygen-dependent control of erythropoiesis and its failure in renal disease. *Nephron*, 67(1), 7-23, PMID: 8052371.

[20] Dowling, T. C. (2007). Prevalence, etiology, and consequences of anemia and clinical and economic benefits of anemia correction in patients with chronic kidney disease: an overview. *Am J Health Syst Pharm*, 64/13_Supplement_8/S3, 64(13, 8), 3-7, quiz S23-25 [PMID: 17591994[pii]10.2146/ajhp070181.

[21] Pisoni, R. L., Bragg-Gresham, J. L., Young, E. W., Akizawa, T., Asano, Y., Locatelli, F., Bommer, J., Cruz, J. M., Kerr, P. G., Mendelssohn, D. C., Held, P. J., & Port, F. K. (2004). Anemia management and outcomes from 12 countries in the Dialysis Outcomes and Practice Patterns Study (DOPPS). *Am J Kidney Dis*, 44(1), 94-111, PMID: 15211443, S0272638604005062.

[22] Agarwal, A. K. (2006 ). Practical approach to the diagnosis and treatment of anemia associated with CKD in elderly. *J Am Med Dir Assoc*, S1525-8610(06)00458-0, S7-S12, (9), quiz S17-21 [PMID: 17098634 [pii]10.1016/j.jamda.2006.09.005.

[23] Eschbach, J. W., Varma, A., & Stivelman, J. C. (2002). Is it time for a paradigm shift? Is erythropoietin deficiency still the main cause of renal anaemia? *Nephrol Dial Transplant*, 5(17), 2-7, PMID: 12091599].

[24] Adamson, J. W, & Eschbach, J. W. (1998). Erythropoietin for end-stage renal disease. *N Engl J Med*, 339(9), 625-627, PMID: 9718384, NEJM199808273390910.

[25] McCarthy, J. T. (1999). A practical approach to the management of patients with chronic renal failure. *Mayo Clin Proc*, 74(3), 269-273, PMID: 10089997, S0025-6196(11)63864-0, [pii]10.4065/74.3.269].

[26] Vigano, S. M., Filippo, S. D., Milia, V. L., Pontoriero, G., & Locatelli, F. (2012). Prospective randomized pilot study on the effects of two synthetic high-flux dialyzers on dialysis patient anemia. *Int J Artif Organs*, 35(5), 346-351, PMID: 22684617, ijao. 5000101EF9F6237-7BE3-43EB-840A-53B42D6E016A.

[27] Ayli, D., Ayli, M., Azak, A., Yuksel, C., Kosmaz, G. P., Atilgan, G., Dede, F., Abayli, E., & Camlibel, M. (2004). The effect of high-flux hemodialysis on renal anemia. *J Nephrol*, 17(5), 701-706, PMID: 15593038].

[28] Locatelli, F., Del Vecchio, L., Pozzoni, P., & Andrulli, S. (2006). Dialysis adequacy and response to erythropoiesis-stimulating agents: what is the evidence base? *Semin Nephrol*, 26(4), 269-274, [PMID: 16949464 DOI:, S0270-9295(06)00068-4, [pii]10.1016/ j.semnephrol.2006.05.002].

[29] Locatelli, F., Manzoni, C., Del Vecchio, L., Di Filippo, S., Pontoriero, G., & Cavalli, A. (2011). Management of anemia by convective treatments. *Contrib Nephrol*, 168, 162-172, PMID: 20938137, 10.1159/000321757.

[30] Ifudu, O., Feldman, J., & Friedman, E. A. (1996). The intensity of hemodialysis and the response to erythropoietin in patients with end-stage renal disease. *N Engl J Med*, 334(7), 420-425, PMID: 8552143, NEJM199602153340702.

[31] Wang, A. Y, & Lai, K. N. (2006). The importance of residual renal function in dialysis patients. *Kidney Int*, 69(10), 1726-1732, PMID: 16612329, 10.1038/sj.ki.5000382.

[32] Penne, E. L., van der Weerd, N. C., Grooteman, M. P., Mazairac, A. H., van den Dorpel, M. A., Nube, M. J., Bots, M. L., Levesque, R., Ter Wee, P. M., & Blankestijn, P. J. (2011). Role of residual renal function in phosphate control and anemia management in chronic hemodialysis patients. Clin J Am Soc Nephrol CJN.04480510 PMID: 21030579 PMCID: 3052217 [pii]10.2215/CJN.04480510 , 6(2), 281-289.

[33] Onoyama, K., Sanai, T., Motomura, K., & Fujishima, M. (1989). Worsening of anemia by angiotensin converting enzyme inhibitors and its prevention by antiestrogenic steroid in chronic hemodialysis patients. *J Cardiovasc Pharmacol*, 13(3), 27-30, PMID: 2474097].

[34] Mohanram, A., Zhang, Z., Shahinfar, S., Lyle, P. A., & Toto, R. D. (2008). The effect of losartan on hemoglobin concentration and renal outcome in diabetic nephropathy of type 2 diabetes. *Kidney Int*, 73(5), 630-636, PMID: 18094675, 10.1038/sj.ki.5002746.

[35] Kamper, A. L., & Nielsen, O. J. (1990). Effect of enalapril on haemoglobin and serum erythropoietin in patients with chronic nephropathy. *Scand J Clin Lab Invest*, 50(6), 611-618, PMID: 2247767, 10.3109/00365519009089178.

[36] Hirakata, H., Onoyama, K., Iseki, K., Kumagai, H., Fujimi, S., & Omae, T. (1984). Worsening of anemia induced by long-term use of captopril in hemodialysis patients. *Am J Nephrol*, 4(6), 355-360, PMID: 6393769].

[37] Hirakata, H., Onoyama, K., Hori, K., & Fujishima, M. (1986). Participation of the renin-angiotensin system in the captopril-induced worsening of anemia in chronic hemodialysis patients. *Clin Nephrol*, 26(1), 27-32, PMID: 3524928].

[38] Mpio, I., Boumendjel, N., Karaaslan, H., Arkouche, W., Lenz, A., Cardozo, C., Cardozo, J., Pastural-Thaunat, M., Fouque, D., Silou, J., Attaf, D., & Laville, M. (2011). Secondary hyperparathyroidism and anemia. Effects of a calcimimetic on the control of anemia in chronic hemodialysed patients. Pilot Study. *Nephrol Ther*, S1769-7255(11)00044-7, 7(4), 229-236, PMID: 21353659 [pii]10.1016/j.nephro.2011.01.008.

[39] Oshiro, Y., Tanaka, H., & Okimoto, N. (2011). A patient undergoing chronic dialysis whose renal anemia was successfully corrected by treatment with cinacalcet. *Clin Exp Nephrol*, 15(4), 607-610, PMID: 21455660, s10157-011-0433-1.

[40] Battistella, M., Richardson, R. M., Bargman, J. M., & Chan, C. T. (2011). Improved parathyroid hormone control by cinacalcet is associated with reduction in darbepoetin requirement in patients with end-stage renal disease. *Clin Nephrol*, 76(2), 99-103, PMID: 21762640, 8739.

[41] Drueke, T. B., & Eckardt, K. U. (2002). Role of secondary hyperparathyroidism in erythropoietin resistance of chronic renal failure patients. *Nephrol Dial Transplant*, 5(17), 28-31, PMID: 12091604].

[42] Chow, T. L., Chan, T. T., Ho, Y. W., & Lam, S. H. (2007). Improvement of anemia after parathyroidectomy in Chinese patients with renal failure undergoing long-term dialysis. Arch Surg PMID: 17638802 142/7/644pii]10.1001/archsurg.142.7.644], 142(7), 644-648.

[43] Lin, C. L., Hung, C. C., Yang, C. T., & Huang, C. C. (2004). Improved anemia and reduced erythropoietin need by medical or surgical intervention of secondary hyperparathyroidism in hemodialysis patients. *Ren Fail*, 26(3), 289-295, PMID: 15354979].

[44] Lee, G.H, Benner, D, Regidor, D.L, & Kalantar-Zadeh, K. (2007). Impact of kidney bone disease and its management on survival of patients on dialysis. J Ren Nutr S1051-2276(06)00160-9[pii]10.1053/j.jrn.2006.07.006 PMID: 17198930 , 17(1), 38-44.

[45] Kalantar-Zadeh, K., Lee, G. H., Miller, J. E., Streja, E., Jing, J., Robertson, J. A., & Kovesdy, C. P. (2009). Predictors of hyporesponsiveness to erythropoiesis-stimulating agents in hemodialysis patients. Am J Kidney Dis PMID: 19339087 PMCID: 2691452 S0272-6386(09)00403-X [pii]10.1053/j.ajkd.2008.12.040, 53(5), 823-834.

[46] De Francisco, A. L., & Pinera, C. (2011). Anemia trials in CKD and clinical practice: refining the approach to erythropoiesis-stimulating agents. Contrib Nephrol PMID: 21625120 000327173pii]10.1159/000327173], 171, 248-254.

[47] Bellizzi, V., Minutolo, R., Terracciano, V., Iodice, C., Giannattasio, P., De Nicola, L., Conte, G., & Di Iorio, B. R. (2002). Influence of the cyclic variation of hydration status on hemoglobin levels in hemodialysis patients. Am J Kidney Dis PMID: 12200807 S0272-6386(02)00080-X[pii]10.1053/ajkd.2002.34913 , 40(3), 549-555.

[48] Nissenson, A. R. (1992). Erythropoietin and peritoneal dialysis: the efficacy of intra-peritoneal dosing. *Perit Dial Int*, 12(4), 350-352, PMID: 1420491].

[49] David Barth, J. V. H. (2007). Anemia. *In: Douglas C. Tkachuk JVH, editor Wintrobe's Atlas of Clinical Hematology. Philadelphia, USA: Lippincott Williams and Wilkins*, 1-47.

[50] Locatelli, F., & Del Vecchio, L. (2003). Dialysis adequacy and response to erythropoietic agents: what is the evidence base? *Nephrol Dial Transplant*, 18(8), 29-35, PMID: 14607998].

[51] Locatelli, F., Pozzoni, P., & Del Vecchio, L. (2005). Anemia and heart failure in chronic kidney disease. Semin Nephrol PMID: 16298261 S0270-9295(05)00103-8[pii]10.1016/j.semnephrol.2005.05.008 , 25(6), 392-396.

[52] Cole, J., Ertoy, D., Lin, H., Sutliff, R. L., Ezan, E., Guyene, T. T., Capecchi, M., Corvol, P., & Bernstein, K. E. (2000). Lack of angiotensin II-facilitated erythropoiesis causes anemia in angiotensin-converting enzyme-deficient mice. *J Clin Invest*, 106(11), 1391-1398, PMID: 11104792 PMCID: 381466, JCI10557.

[53] Le Meur, Y., Lorgeot, V., Comte, L., Szelag, J. C., Aldigier, J. C., Leroux-Robert, C., & Praloran, V. (2001). Plasma levels and metabolism of AcSDKP in patients with chronic renal failure: relationship with erythropoietin requirements. *Am J Kidney Dis*, 38(3), 510-517, PMID: 11532682, S0272638601352332.

[54] Clark, A. L. (2011). The origins of anaemia in patients with chronic heart failure. *Br J Cardiol*, 18(2), 15.

[55] Winkelmayer, W. C., Kewalramani, R., Rutstein, M., Gabardi, S., Vonvisger, T., & Chandraker, A. (2004). Pharmacoepidemiology of anemia in kidney transplant recipients. *J Am Soc Nephrol*, 15(5), 1347-1352, PMID: 15100376].

[56] Weatherall, D. J. (2003). Anaemia: pathophysiology, classification, and clinical features. *In: David A. Warrell TMC, John D. Firth, Edward J. Benz, J R., editor Oxford Textbook of Medicine. 4th ed: OUP Oxford*, 2916-2919.

[57] Macdougall, I. C., Lewis, N. P., Saunders, M. J., Cochlin, D. L., Davies, M. E., Hutton, R. D., Fox, K. A., Coles, G. A., & Williams, J. D. (1990). Long-term cardiorespiratory effects of amelioration of renal anaemia by erythropoietin. *Lancet*, 335(8688), 489-493, PMID: 1968526, 0140-6736(90)90733-L.

[58] Parfrey, P.S., Foley, R.N., Wittreich, B. H., Sullivan, D. J., Zagari, M. J., & Frei, D. (2005). Double-blind comparison of full and partial anemia correction in incident hemodialysis patients without symptomatic heart disease. J Am Soc Nephrol PMID: 15901766 ASN.2004121039[pii]10.1681/ASN.2004121039 , 16(7), 2180-2189.

[59] Foley, R. N., Parfrey, P. S., Morgan, J., Barre, P. E., Campbell, P., Cartier, P., Coyle, D., Fine, A., Handa, P., Kingma, I., Lau, C. Y., Levin, A., Mendelssohn, D., Muirhead, N., Murphy, B., Plante, R. K., Posen, G., & Wells, G. A. (2000). Effect of hemoglobin levels in hemodialysis patients with asymptomatic cardiomyopathy. Kidney Int PMID: 10972697 kid289[pii]10.1046/j.1523-1755.2000.00289.x , 58(3), 1325-1335.

[60] Weisbord, S. D., & Kimmel, P. L. (2008). Health-related quality of life in the era of erythropoietin. Hemodial Int PMID: 18271834 HDI233[pii]10.1111/j.1542-4758.2008.00233.x , 12(1), 6-15.

[61] Kimmel, P. L., Cohen, S. D., & Weisbord, S. D. (2008). Quality of life in patients with end-stage renal disease treated with hemodialysis: survival is not enough! J Nephrol 13 PMID: 18446733], 21, S54-S58.

[62] Levin, N. W. (1992). Quality of life and hematocrit level. *Am J Kidney Dis*, 20(1, 1), 16-20, [PMID: 1626552].

[63] Nissenson, A. R. (1989). Recombinant human erythropoietin: impact on brain and cognitive function, exercise tolerance, sexual potency, and quality of life. *Semin Nephrol*, 9(1, 2), 25-31, [PMID: 2669083].

[64] Auer, J., Oliver, D. O., & Winearls, C. G. (1990). The quality of life of dialysis patients treated with recombinant human erythropoietin. *Scand J Urol Nephrol Suppl*, 131, 61-65, PMID: 2075472].

[65] Barany, P., Pettersson, E., & Bergstrom, J. (1990). Erythropoietin treatment improves quality of life in hemodialysis patients. *Scand J Urol Nephrol Suppl*, 131, 55-60, PMID: 2075471].

[66] Barany, P., Pettersson, E., & Konarski-Svensson, J. K. (1993). Long-term effects on quality of life in haemodialysis patients of correction of anaemia with erythropoietin. *Nephrol Dial Transplant*, 8(5), 426-432, PMID: 8393547].

[67] Lankhorst, C. E., & Wish, J. B. (2010). Anemia in renal disease: diagnosis and management. *Blood Rev*, S0268-960X(09)00054-X, 24(1), 39-47, PMID: 19833421 [pii]10.1016/j.blre.2009.09.001.

[68] Macdougall, I. C. (1994). Monitoring of iron status and iron supplementation in patients treated with erythropoietin. Curr Opin Nephrol Hypertens PMID: 7881986], 3(6), 620-625.

[69] Conditions, R., Co, P. L. N. C., & Cf, C. (2006). Anaemia management in chronic kidney disease: national clinical guideline for management in adults and children.

[70] Funk, F., Ryle, P., Canclini, C., Neiser, S., & Geisser, P. (2010). The new generation of intravenous iron: chemistry, pharmacology, and toxicology of ferric carboxymaltose. *Arzneimittelforschung*, 60(6a), 345-353, PMID: 20648926, s-0031-1296299.

[71] Organization, W. H. (1998). Iron Deficiency Anemia: Assessment, Prevention and Control. *Report of a Joint WHO/UNICEF/UNU Consultation 1998*.

[72] Jacobs, A., & Worwood, M. (1975). Ferritin in serum. Clinical and biochemical implications. *N Engl J Med*, 292(18), 951-956, PMID: 1090831, NEJM197505012921805.

[73] Bainton, D. F., & Finch, C. A. (1964). The Diagnosis of Iron Deficiency Anemia. *Am J Med*, 37, 62-70, PMID: 14181150].

[74] Eschbach, J. W., Egrie, J. C., Downing, M. R., Browne, J. K., & Adamson, J. W. (1987). Correction of the anemia of end-stage renal disease with recombinant human erythropoietin. Results of a combined phase I and II clinical trial. *N Engl J Med*, 316(2), 73-78, PMID: 3537801, NEJM198701083160203.

[75] Fishbane, S., & Lynn, R. I. (1995). The efficacy of iron dextran for the treatment of iron deficiency in hemodialysis patients. *Clin Nephrol*, 44(4), 238-240, PMID: 8575123].

[76] Fishbane, S., & Maesaka, J. K. (1997). Iron management in end-stage renal disease. *Am J Kidney Dis*, 29(3), 319-333, PMID: 9041207, S0272-6386(97)90192-X.

[77] Taylor, J. E., Peat, N., Porter, C., & Morgan, A. G. (1996). Regular low-dose intravenous iron therapy improves response to erythropoietin in haemodialysis patients. *Nephrol Dial Transplant*, 11(6), 1079-1083, PMID: 8671972].

[78] Coyne, D. (2006). Challenging the boundaries of anemia management: a balanced approach to i.v. iron and EPO therapy. *Kidney Int Suppl* [101], S 1-S3, PMID: 16830698].

[79] KDOQI (2007). Clinical Practice Guideline and Clinical Practice Recommendations for anemia in chronic kidney disease: 2007 update of hemoglobin target. Am J Kidney Dis S0272-6386(07)00934-1 [pii]10.1053/j.ajkd.2007.06.008 PMID: 17720528 , 50(3), 471-530.

[80] Fishbane, S., Frei, G. L., & Maesaka, J. (1995). Reduction in recombinant human erythropoietin doses by the use of chronic intravenous iron supplementation. *Am J Kidney Dis*, 26(1), 41-46, PMID: 7611266, 0272-6386(95)90151-5.

[81] Grabe, D. W. (2007). Update on clinical practice recommendations and new therapeutic modalities for treating anemia in patients with chronic kidney disease. Am J Health Syst Pharm 8 64/13_Supplement_8/S8 quiz S23-15 [PMID: 17591995 [pii]10.2146/ajhp070182, 64(13), S8-14.

[82] Johnson, D. W., Herzig, K. A., Gissane, R., Campbell, S. B., Hawley, C. M., & Isbel, N. M. (2001). A prospective crossover trial comparing intermittent intravenous and continuous oral iron supplements in peritoneal dialysis patients. *Nephrol Dial Transplant*, 16(9), 1879-1884, PMID: 11522873.

[83] Ahsan, N. (1998). Intravenous infusion of total dose iron is superior to oral iron in treatment of anemia in peritoneal dialysis patients: a single center comparative study. *J Am Soc Nephrol*, 9(4), 664-668, PMID: 9555669].

[84] Kalantar-Zadeh, K., Streja, E., Miller, J. E., & Nissenson, A. R. (2009). Intravenous iron versus erythropoiesis-stimulating agents: friends or foes in treating chronic kid-

ney disease anemia? Adv Chronic Kidney Dis [PMID: 19233073 S1548-5595(08)00215-2 [pii]10.1053/j.ackd.2008.12.008], 16(2), 143-151.

[85] Mircescu, G., Garneata, L., Capusa, C., & Ursea, N. (2006). Intravenous iron supplementation for the treatment of anaemia in pre-dialyzed chronic renal failure patients. *Nephrol Dial Transplant*, 21(1), 120-124, PMID: 16144853, 10.1093/ndt/gfi087.

[86] Uehata, T., Tomosugi, N., Shoji, T., Sakaguchi, Y., Suzuki, A., Kaneko, T., Okada, N., Yamamoto, R., Nagasawa, Y., Kato, K., Isaka, Y., Rakugi, H., & Tsubakihara, Y. (2012). Serum hepcidin-25 levels and anemia in non-dialysis chronic kidney disease patients: a cross-sectional study. *Nephrol Dial Transplant*, 27(3), 1076-1083, PMID: 21799206, 10.1093/ndt/gfr431.

[87] Ganz, T., & Nemeth, E. (2012). Hepcidin and iron homeostasis. Biochim Biophys Acta PMID: 22306005 S0167-4889(12)00016-X[pii]10.1016/j.bbamcr.2012.01.014

[88] Means, R. T. Jr. (2012). Hepcidin and Iron Regulation in Health and Disease. *Am J Med Sci*, [PMID: 22627267, MAJ.0b013e318253caf1.

[89] Mastrogiannaki, M., Matak, P., Mathieu, J. R., Delga, S., Mayeux, P., Vaulont, S., & Peyssonnaux, C. (2012). Hepatic hypoxia-inducible factor-2 down-regulates hepcidin expression in mice through an erythropoietin-mediated increase in erythropoiesis. Haematologica PMID: 22207682 PMCID: 3366646 haematol.2011.056119[pii]10.3324/haematol.2011.056119 , 97(6), 827-834.

[90] Ganz, T. (2007). Molecular control of iron transport. J Am Soc Nephrol PMID: 17229910 ASN.2006070802 [pii]10.1681/ASN.2006070802], 18(2), 394-400.

[91] Verga Falzacappa, M. V., & Muckenthaler, M. U. (2005). Hepcidin: iron-hormone and anti-microbial peptide. Gene PMID: 16203112 S0378-1119(05)00438-5[pii]10.1016/j.gene.2005.07.020 , 364, 37-44.

[92] Martinez-Ruiz, A., Tornel-Osorio, P. L., Sanchez-Mas, J., Perez-Fornieles, J., Vilchez, J. A., Martinez-Hernandez, P., & Pascual-Figal, D. A. (2012). Soluble TNFalpha receptor type I and hepcidin as determinants of development of anemia in the long-term follow-up of heart failure patients. Clin Biochem [PMID: 22609894 S0009-9120(12)00244-5 [pii]10.1016/j.clinbiochem.2012.05.011]

[93] Maruyama, Y., Yokoyama, K., Yamamoto, H., Nakayama, M., & Hosoya, T. (2012). Do serum hepcidin-25 levels correlate with oxidative stress in patients with chronic kidney disease not receiving dialysis? *Clin Nephrol*, [PMID: 22541685, CN1074249647.

[94] Park, C. H., Valore, E. V., Waring, A. J., & Ganz, T. (2001). Hepcidin, a urinary antimicrobial peptide synthesized in the liver. *J Biol Chem*, 276(11), 7806-7810, PMID: 11113131, jbc.M008922200M008922200.

[95] Swinkels, D. W., Girelli, D., Laarakkers, C., Kroot, J., Campostrini, N., Kemna, E. H., & Tjalsma, H. (2008). Advances in quantitative hepcidin measurements by time-of-flight mass spectrometry. PLoS One; [PMID: 18628991 PMCID: 2442656 journal.pone.0002706 , 3(7), e2706.

[96] Nemeth, E., Valore, E. V., Territo, M., Schiller, G., Lichtenstein, A., & Ganz, T. (2003). Hepcidin, a putative mediator of anemia of inflammation, is a type II acute-phase protein. *Blood,* 101(7), 2461-2463, [PMID: 12433676, 10.1182/blood-2002-10-32352002-10-3235.

[97] Nicolas, G., Chauvet, C., Viatte, L., Danan, J. L., Bigard, X., Devaux, I., Beaumont, C., Kahn, A., & Vaulont, S. (2002). The gene encoding the iron regulatory peptide hepcidin is regulated by anemia, hypoxia, and inflammation. *J Clin Invest,* 110(7), 1037-1044, PMID: 12370282 PMCID: 151151, JCI15686.

[98] Nemeth, E., Rivera, S., Gabayan, V., Keller, C., Taudorf, S., Pedersen, B. K., & Ganz, T. (2004). IL-6 mediates hypoferremia of inflammation by inducing the synthesis of the iron regulatory hormone hepcidin. *J Clin Invest,* 113(9), 1271-1276, PMID: 15124018 PMCID: 398432, JCI20945.

[99] Weiss, G., & Goodnough, L. T. (2005). Anemia of chronic disease. *N Engl J Med,* 352(10), 1011-1023, PMID: 15758012, 10.1056/NEJMra041809.

[100] Kato, A., Tsuji, T., Luo, J., Sakao, Y., Yasuda, H., & Hishida, A. (2008). Association of prohepcidin and hepcidin-25 with erythropoietin response and ferritin in hemodialysis patients. *Am J Nephrol,* 28(1), 115-121, PMID: 17943020, 10.1159/000109968.

[101] Taes, Y. E., Wuyts, B., Boelaert, J. R., De Vriese, A. S., & Delanghe, J. R. (2004). Prohepcidin accumulates in renal insufficiency. *Clin Chem Lab Med,* 42(4), 387-389, [PMID: 15147148, 10.1515/CCLM.2004.069.

[102] Mahdavi, M. R., Makhlough, A., Kosaryan, M., & Roshan, P. (2011). Credibility of the measurement of serum ferritin and transferrin receptor as indicators of iron deficiency anemia in hemodialysis patients. *Eur Rev Med Pharmacol Sci,* 15(10), 1158-1162, PMID: 22165676].

[103] Hudson, J. Q., & Comstock, T. J. (2001). Considerations for optimal iron use for anemia due to chronic kidney disease. *Clin Ther,* 23(10), 1637-1671, [PMID: 11726002 DOI:, S0149-2918(01)80135-1.

[104] Spiegel, D. M., & Chertow, G. M. (2009). Lost without directions: lessons from the anemia debate and the drive study. Clin J Am Soc Nephrol [PMID: 19357246 10.2215/CJN.00270109], 4(5), 1009-1010.

[105] Coyne, D. W. (2010). It's time to compare anemia management strategies in hemodialysis. *Clin J Am Soc Nephrol,* 5(4), 740-742, [PMID: 20299363, 10.2215/CJN.02490409.

[106] Aronoff, G. R., Bennett, W. M., Blumenthal, S., Charytan, C., Pennell, J. P., Reed, J., Rothstein, M., Strom, J., Wolfe, A., Van Wyck, D., & Yee, J. (2004). Iron sucrose in hemodialysis patients: safety of replacement and maintenance regimens. *Kidney Int,* 66(3), 1193-1198, [PMID: 15327417, 10.1111/j.1523-1755.2004.00872.xKID872.

[107] Atalay, H., Solak, Y., Acar, K., Govec, N., & Turk, S. (2011). Safety profiles of total dose infusion of low-molecular-weight iron dextran and high-dose iron sucrose in re-

nal patients. *Hemodial Int*, 15(3), 374-378, [PMID: 21564503, 10.1111/j.1542-4758.2011.00550.x.

[108] Coppol, E., Shelly, J., Cheng, S., Kaakeh, Y., & Shepler, B. (2011). A Comparative Look at the Safety Profiles of Intravenous Iron Products Used in the Hemodialysis Population (February). *Ann Pharmacother*, [PMID: 21304025, 10.1345/aph.1P466.

[109] Kes, P., Basic-Jukici, N., & Juric, I. (2009). How do we need to maintain the iron status in dialyzed patients treated with erythropoesis stimulating agents. *Acta Med Croatica*, 63(1), 54-61, PMID: 20232552].

[110] Siga, E., Aiziczon, D., & Diaz, G. (2011). Optimizing iron therapy in hemodialysis: a prospective long term clinical study. *Medicina (B Aires)*, 71(1), 9-14, PMID: 21296714].

[111] Covic, A., & Mircescu, G. (2010). The safety and efficacy of intravenous ferric carboxymaltose in anaemic patients undergoing haemodialysis: a multi-centre, open-label, clinical study. *Nephrol Dial Transplant*, 25(8), 2722-2730, PMID: 20190247 PMCID: 2905444, 10.1093/ndt/gfq069.

[112] Michael, B., Coyne, D. W., Fishbane, S., Folkert, V., Lynn, R., Nissenson, A. R., Agarwal, R., Eschbach, J. W., Fadem, S. Z., Trout, J. R., Strobos, J., & Warnock, D. G. (2002). Sodium ferric gluconate complex in hemodialysis patients: adverse reactions compared to placebo and iron dextran. *Kidney Int*, 61(5), 830-839, [PMID: 11967034, 10.1046/j.1523-1755.2002.00314.x.

[113] Fishbane, S. (2003). Safety in iron management. *Am J Kidney Dis*, 41(5), 18-26, PMID: 12776310, S0272638603003731.

[114] Bregman, D. (2009). Important Drug Warning for Dexferrum® (iron dextran injection, USP). *Shirley New York*.

[115] Bailie, G. R., Clark, J. A., Lane, C. E., & Lane, P. L. (2005). Hypersensitivity reactions and deaths associated with intravenous iron preparations. *Nephrol Dial Transplant*, 20(7), 1443-1449, [PMID: 15855210, 10.1093/ndt/gfh820.

[116] Locatelli, F., & Del Vecchio, L. (2011). New erythropoiesis-stimulating agents and new iron formulations. *Contrib Nephrol*, 171, 255-260, PMID: 21625121, 10.1159/000327328.

[117] Geisser, P., Baer, M., & Schaub, E. (1992). Structure/histotoxicity relationship of parenteral iron preparations. *Arzneimittelforschung*, 42(12), 1439-1452, PMID: 1288508].

[118] Qunibi, W.Y. (2010). The efficacy and safety of current intravenous iron preparations for the management of iron-deficiency anaemia: a review. *Arzneimittelforschung*, 60(6a), 399-412, PMID: 20648931, s-0031-1296304.

[119] Bailie, G.R. (2010). Efficacy and safety of ferric carboxymaltose in correcting iron-deficiency anemia: a review of randomized controlled trials across different indications. *Arzneimittelforschung*, 60(6a), 386-398, PMID: 20648930, s-0031-1296303.

[120] Lyseng-Williamson, K. A., & Keating, G. M. (2009). Ferric carboxymaltose: a review of its use in iron-deficiency anaemia. *Drugs*, 69(6), 739-756, [PMID: 19405553, 10.2165/00003495-200969060-000077.

[121] Fragoulakis, V., Kourlaba, G., Goumenos, D., Konstantoulakis, M., & Maniadakis, N. (2012). Economic evaluation of intravenous iron treatments in the management of anemia patients in Greece. *Clinicoecon Outcomes Res*, 4, 127-134, [PMID: 22629113 PMCID: 3358814, 10.2147/CEOR.S30514ceor-4-127.

[122] Gutzwiller, F. S., Schwenkglenks, M., Blank, P. R., Braunhofer, P. G., Mori, C., Szucs, T. D., Ponikowski, P., & Anker, S. D. (2012). Health economic assessment of ferric carboxymaltose in patients with iron deficiency and chronic heart failure based on the FAIR-HF trial: an analysis for the UK. *Eur J Heart Fail*, 14(7), 782-790, PMID: 22689292 PMCID: 3380546, 10.1093/eurjhf/hfs083.

[123] Gentile, M. G., Manna, G. M., D'Amico, G., Testolin, G., Porrini, M., & Simonetti, P. (1988). Vitamin nutrition in patients with chronic renal failure and dietary manipulation. Contrib Nephrol PMID: 3168460], 65, 43-50.

[124] Pietrzak, I. (1995). Vitamin disturbances in chronic renal insufficiency. I. Water soluble vitamins. *Przegl Lek*, 52(10), 522-525, PMID: 8834846].

[125] Stein, G., Sperschneider, H., & Koppe, S. (1985). Vitamin levels in chronic renal failure and need for supplementation. *Blood Purif*, 3(1-3), 52-62, [PMID: 4096835].

[126] Deved, V., Poyah, P., James, M. T., Tonelli, M., Manns, B. J., Walsh, M., & Hemmelgarn, B. R. (2009). Ascorbic acid for anemia management in hemodialysis patients: a systematic review and meta-analysis. *Am J Kidney Dis*, 54(6), 1089-1097, [PMID: 19783342, S0272-6386(09)00988-3, [pii]10.1053/j.ajkd.2009.06.040].

[127] Emami, Naini. A., Moradi, M., Mortazavi, M., Amini, Harandi. A., Hadizadeh, M., Shirani, F., Basir, Ghafoori. H., & Emami, Naini. P. (2012). Effects of Oral L-Carnitine Supplementation on Lipid Profile, Anemia, and Quality of Life in Chronic Renal Disease Patients under Hemodialysis: A Randomized, Double-Blinded, Placebo-Controlled Trial. J Nutr Metab; [PMID: 22720143 PMCID: 3374945 10.1155/2012/510483] , 510483.

[128] Dimkovic, N. (2001). Erythropoietin beta in the treatment of anemia in patients with chronic renal insufficiency. *Med Pregl*, 54(5-6), 235-240, [PMID: 11759218].

[129] Mydlik, M., & Derzsiova, K. (1999). Vitamin levels in the serum and erythrocytes during erythropoietin therapy in hemodialyzed patients. *Bratisl Lek Listy*, 100(8), 426-431, PMID: 10645030].

[130] Jelkmann, W. (2004). Molecular biology of erythropoietin. *Intern Med*, 43(8), 649-659, PMID: 15468961].

[131] Mikhail, A., Covic, A., & Goldsmith, D. (2008). Stimulating erythropoiesis: future perspectives. *Kidney Blood Press Res*, 31(4), 234-246, PMID: 18587242, 10.1159/000141928.

[132] Cody, J., Daly, C., Campbell, M., Donaldson, C., Grant, A., Khan, I., Vale, L., Wallace, S., & Mac, Leod. A. (2002). Frequency of administration of recombinant human erythropoietin for anaemia of end-stage renal disease in dialysis patients. *Cochrane Database Syst Rev* [4], [PMID: 12519614, CD003895.

[133] Berns, J. S. (2005). Should the target hemoglobin for patients with chronic kidney disease treated with erythropoietic replacement therapy be changed? *Semin Dial*, 18(1), 22-29, [PMID: 15663760, 10.1111/j.1525-139X.2005.18105.x.

[134] Mohini, R. (1989). Clinical efficacy of recombinant human erythropoietin in hemodialysis patients. *Semin Nephrol*, 9(1, 1), 16-21, [PMID: 2648516].

[135] Carrera, F., Lok, C. E., de Francisco, A., Locatelli, F., Mann, J. F., Canaud, B., Kerr, P. G., Macdougall, I. C., Besarab, A., Villa, G., Kazes, I., Van Vlem, B., Jolly, S., Beyer, U., & Dougherty, F. C. (2010). Maintenance treatment of renal anaemia in haemodialysis patients with methoxy polyethylene glycol-epoetin beta versus darbepoetin alfa administered monthly: a randomized comparative trial. *Nephrol Dial Transplant*, 25(12), 4009-4017, PMID: 20522670 PMCID: 2989790, 10.1093/ndt/gfq305.

[136] Goldsmith, D. (2009). a requiem for rHuEPOs--but should we nail down the coffin in 2010? *Clin J Am Soc Nephrol 2010*, 5(5), 929-935, [PMID: 20413441, 10.2215/CJN.09131209.

[137] Zakar, G. (2007). Current issues in erythropoietin therapy of renal anemia. *Lege Artis Med*, 17(10), 667-673, PMID: 19227596].

[138] Patel, T., Hirter, A., Kaufman, J., Keithi-Reddy, S. R., Reda, D., & Singh, A. (2009). Route of epoetin administration influences hemoglobin variability in hemodialysis patients. *Am J Nephrol*, 29(6), 532-537, PMID: 19088467 PMCID: 2818471, 10.1159/000187649.

[139] Besarab, A. (1993). Optimizing epoetin therapy in end-stage renal disease: the case for subcutaneous administration. *Am J Kidney Dis*, 22(2, 1), 13-22, [PMID: 8352267, S0272638693001751.

[140] Pizzarelli, F., David, S., Sala, P., Icardi, A., & Casani, A. (2006). Iron-replete hemodialysis patients do not require higher EPO dosages when converting from subcutaneous to intravenous administration: results of the Italian Study on Erythropoietin Converting (ISEC). *Am J Kidney Dis*, 47(6), 1027-1035, [PMID: 16731298, S0272-6386(06)00380-5, [pii]10.1053/j.ajkd.2006.02.176].

[141] Lopez-Gomez, J. M., Portoles, J. M., & Aljama, P. (2008). Factors that condition the response to erythropoietin in patients on hemodialysis and their relation to mortality. *Kidney Int*, (111), S75-81, [PMID: 19034333, 10.1038/ki.2008.523.

[142] de Lurdes, Agostinho., Cabrita, A., Pinho, A., Malho, A., Morgado, E., Faisca, M., Carrasqueira, H., Silva, A. P., & Neves, P. L. (2011). Risk factors for high erythropoiesis stimulating agent resistance index in pre-dialysis chronic kidney disease patients, stages 4 and 5. *Int Urol Nephrol*, 43(3), 835-840, PMID: 20640598, s11255-010-9805-9.

[143] Bamgbola, O. F., Kaskel, F. J., & Coco, M. (2009). Analyses of age, gender and other risk factors of erythropoietin resistance in pediatric and adult dialysis cohorts. *Pediatr Nephrol*, 24(3), 571-579, PMID: 18800231, s00467-008-0954-3.

[144] Tonelli, M., Blake, P. G., & Muirhead, N. (2001). Predictors of erythropoietin responsiveness in chronic hemodialysis patients. *ASAIO J*, 47(1), 82-85, PMID: 11199321].

[145] Greenwood, R. N., Ronco, C., Gastaldon, F., Brendolan, A., Homel, P., Usvyat, L., Bruno, L., Carter, M., & Levin, N. W. (2003). Erythropoeitin dose variation in different facilities in different countries and its relationship to drug resistance. *Kidney Int Suppl* [87], S78-86, PMID: 14531778].

[146] Jungers, P. Y., Robino, C., Choukroun, G., Nguyen-Khoa, T., Massy, Z. A., & Jungers, P. (2002). Incidence of anaemia, and use of epoetin therapy in pre-dialysis patients: a prospective study in 403 patients. *Nephrol Dial Transplant*, 17(9), 1621-1627, PMID: 12198213].

[147] Excerpts from United States Renal Data System. (1999). Annual Data Report. *Am J Kidney Dis*, 34(2, 1), S1-176, PMID: 10447494].

[148] Frankenfield, D. L, & Johnson, C. A. (2002). Current management of anemia in adult hemodialysis patients with end-stage renal disease. *Am J Health Syst Pharm*, 59(5), 429-435, PMID: 11887409].

[149] Valderrabano, F., Horl, W. H., Macdougall, I. C., Rossert, J., Rutkowski, B., & Wauters, J. P. (2003). PRE-dialysis survey on anaemia management. *Nephrol Dial Transplant*, 18(1), 89-100, PMID: 12480965].

[150] Nissenson, A. R., Swan, S. K., Lindberg, J. S., Soroka, S. D., Beatey, R., Wang, C., Picarello, N., Mc Dermott-Vitak, A., & Maroni, B. J. (2002). Randomized, controlled trial of darbepoetin alfa for the treatment of anemia in hemodialysis patients. *Am J Kidney Dis*, 40(1), 110-118, [PMID: 12087568, S0272-6386(02)00014-8, [pii]10.1053/ajkd.2002.33919].

[151] Miller, C. B., Jones, R. J., Piantadosi, S., Abeloff, M. D., & Spivak, J. L. (1990). Decreased erythropoietin response in patients with the anemia of cancer. *N Engl J Med*, 322(24), 1689-1692, PMID: 2342534, NEJM199006143222401.

[152] Duong, U., Kalantar-Zadeh, K., Molnar, M. Z., Zaritsky, J. J., Teitelbaum, I., Kovesdy, C. P., & Mehrotra, R. (2012). Mortality associated with dose response of erythropoiesis-stimulating agents in hemodialysis versus peritoneal dialysis patients. *Am J Nephrol*, 35(2), 198-208, PMID: 22286821 PMCID: 3326284, 10.1159/000335685.

[153] Bradbury, B. D., Danese, M. D., Gleeson, M., & Critchlow, C. W. (2009). Effect of Epoetin alfa dose changes on hemoglobin and mortality in hemodialysis patients with hemoglobin levels persistently below 11 g/dL. *Clin J Am Soc Nephrol*, 4(3), 630-637, [PMID: 19261826 PMCID: 2653654, 10.2215/CJN.03580708.

[154] Weinhandl, E. D, Gilbertson, D. T, & Collins, A. J. (2011). Association of mean weekly epoetin alfa dose with mortality risk in a retrospective cohort study of Medicare hemodialysis patients. *Am J Nephrol*, 34(4), 298-308, PMID: 21829009, 10.1159/000330693.

[155] Agarwal, R., Davis, J. L., & Smith, L. (2008). Serum albumin is strongly associated with erythropoietin sensitivity in hemodialysis patients. Clin J Am Soc Nephrol [PMID: 18045859 PMCID: 2390989 10.2215/CJN.03330807], 3(1), 98-104.

[156] Hung, S. C., Tung, T. Y., Yang, C. S., & Tarng, D. C. (2005). High-calorie supplementation increases serum leptin levels and improves response to rHuEPO in long-term hemodialysis patients. *Am J Kidney Dis*, 45(6), 1073-1083, PMID: 15957137, S0272638605002921.

[157] Axelsson, J., Qureshi, A. R., Heimburger, O., Lindholm, B., Stenvinkel, P., & Barany, P. (2005). Body fat mass and serum leptin levels influence epoetin sensitivity in patients with ESRD. Am J Kidney Dis [PMID: 16183417 S0272-6386(05)00793-6 [pii]10.1053/j.ajkd.2005.06.004] , 46(4), 628-634.

[158] Chang, C. C., Chiu, P. F., Chen, H. L., Chang, T. L., Chang, Y. J., & Huang, C. H. (2012). Simvastatin downregulates the expression of hepcidin and erythropoietin in HepG2 cells. *Hemodial Int*, [PMID: 22716163, 10.1111/j.1542-4758.2012.00716.x.

[159] Park, S. J., & Shin, J. I. (2012). The beneficial effect of statins on renal anemia in hemodialysis patients: another point of view. *Hemodial Int*, 16(2), 322-323, [PMID: 22100011, 10.1111/j.1542-4758.2011.00631.x.

[160] Liu, W. S., Wu, Y. L., Li, S. Y., Yang, W. C., Chen, T. W., & Lin, C. C. (2012). The waveform fluctuation and the clinical factors of the initial and sustained erythropoietic response to continuous erythropoietin receptor activator in hemodialysis patients. *Scientific World Journal*, 157437, [PMID: 22619601 PMCID: 3349104, 10.1100/2012/157437.

[161] Kes, P., & Basic-Jukic, N. (2009). Erythropoesis-stimulating agents: past, present and future. *Acta Med Croatica*, 63(1), 3-6, PMID: 20235351].

[162] Jungers, P., Choukroun, G., Oualim, Z., Robino, C., Nguyen, A. T., & Man, N. K. (2001). Beneficial influence of recombinant human erythropoietin therapy on the rate of progression of chronic renal failure in predialysis patients. *Nephrol Dial Transplant*, 16(2), 307-312, PMID: 11158405].

[163] Iseki, K., & Kohagura, K. (2007). Anemia as a risk factor for chronic kidney disease. *Kidney Int Suppl* [107], S4-9, PMID: 17943141, 10.1038/sj.ki.5002481.

[164] Besarab, A., Bolton, W. K., Browne, J. K., Egrie, J. C., Nissenson, A. R., Okamoto, D. M., Schwab, S. J., & Goodkin, D. A. (1998). The effects of normal as compared with low hematocrit values in patients with cardiac disease who are receiving hemodialysis and epoetin. *N Engl J Med*, 339(9), 584-590, PMID: 9718377, NEJM199808273390903.

[165] Drueke, T. B., Locatelli, F., Clyne, N., Eckardt, K. U., Macdougall, I. C., Tsakiris, D., Burger, H. U., & Scherhag, A. (2006). Normalization of hemoglobin level in patients with chronic kidney disease and anemia. *N Engl J Med*, 355(20), 2071-2084, [PMID: 17108342 DOI: 355/20/2071 [pii], 10.1056/NEJMoa062276.

[166] Pfeffer, M. A., Burdmann, E. A., Chen, C. Y., Cooper, M. E., de Zeeuw, D., Eckardt, K. U., Feyzi, J. M., Ivanovich, P., Kewalramani, R., Levey, A. S., Lewis, E. F., Mc Gill, J. B., Mc Murray, J. J., Parfrey, P., Parving, H. H., Remuzzi, G., Singh, A. K., Solomon, S. D., & Toto, R. (2009). A trial of darbepoetin alfa in type 2 diabetes and chronic kidney disease. N Engl J Med [PMID: 19880844 10.1056/NEJMoa0907845], 361(21), 2019-2032.

[167] Singh, A. K., Szczech, L., Tang, K. L., Barnhart, H., Sapp, S., Wolfson, M., & Reddan, D. (2006). Correction of anemia with epoetin alfa in chronic kidney disease. *N Engl J Med*, 355(20), 2085-2098, [PMID: 17108343, 355/20/2085, [pii]10.1056/NEJMoa065485].

[168] Kiss, Z., Ambrus, C., Almasi, C., Berta, K., Deak, G., Horonyi, P., Kiss, I., Lakatos, P., Marton, A., Molnar, M. Z., Nemeth, Z., Szabo, A., & Mucsi, I. (2011). Serum 25(OH)-cholecalciferol concentration is associated with hemoglobin level and erythropoietin resistance in patients on maintenance hemodialysis. *Nephron Clin Pract*, 117(4), c373-378, PMID: 21071961, 10.1159/000321521.

[169] Waterschoot, M. (2007). Evaluation of response to various erythropoiesis--stimulating proteins using anemia management software. J Ren Care PMID: 17702511], 33(2), 78-82.

[170] Dunn, C. J, & Wagstaff, A. J. (1995). Epoetin alfa. A review of its clinical efficacy in the management of anaemia associated with renal failure and chronic disease and its use in surgical patients. *Drugs Aging*, 7(2), 131-156, PMID: 7579784].

[171] Pergola, P. E., Gartenberg, G., Fu, M., Wolfson, M., Rao, S., & Bowers, P. (2009). A randomized controlled study of weekly and biweekly dosing of epoetin alfa in CKD Patients with anemia. *Clin J Am Soc Nephrol*, 4(11), 1731-1740, [PMID: 19808215 PMCID: 2774960, 10.2215/CJN.03470509.

[172] Lee, Y. K., Kim, S. G., Seo, J. W., Oh, J. E., Yoon, J. W., Koo, J. R., Kim, H. J., & Noh, J. W. (2008). A comparison between once-weekly and twice- or thrice-weekly subcutaneous injection of epoetin alfa: results from a randomized controlled multicentre study. *Nephrol Dial Transplant*, 23(10), 3240-3246, PMID: 18469158, 10.1093/ndt/gfn255.

[173] Barre, P., Reichel, H., Suranyi, M. G., & Barth, C. (2004). Efficacy of once-weekly epoetin alfa. *Clin Nephrol*, 62(6), 440-448, PMID: 15630903].

[174] Dunn, C. J., & Markham, A. (1996). Epoetin beta. A review of its pharmacological properties and clinical use in the management of anaemia associated with chronic renal failure. *Drugs*, 51(2), 299-318, PMID: 8808169].

[175] Macdougall, I. C. (2002). Optimizing the use of erythropoietic agents-- pharmacokinetic and pharmacodynamic considerations. *Nephrol Dial Transplant,* 17(5), 66-70, PMID: 12091611].

[176] Macdougall, I. C., Padhi, D., & Jang, G. (2007). Pharmacology of darbepoetin alfa. Nephrol Dial Transplant 4 iv9 [PMID: 17526547 suppl_4/iv2 [pii]10.1093/ndt/gfm160] , 22, 2.

[177] Martinez Castelao, A., Reyes, A., Valdes, F., Otero, A., Lopez de Novales, E., Pallardo, L., Tabernero, J. M., Hernandez, Jaras. J., & Llados, F. (2003). Multicenter study of darbepoetin alfa in the treatment of anemia secondary to chronic renal insufficiency on dialysis. *Nefrologia,* 23(2), 114-124, PMID: 12778875].

[178] Ibbotson, T., & Goa, K. L. (2001). Darbepoetin alfa. *Drugs,* 61(14), 2097-2104, discussion 2105-2096 [PMID: 11735636, 611407.

[179] Kessler, M., Hannedouche, T., Fitte, H., Cayotte, J. L., Urena, P., & Reglier, J. C. (2006). Darbepoetin-alfa treatment of anemia secondary to chronic renal failure in dialysis patients: Results of a French multicenter study. Nephrol Ther [PMID: 16966064 S1769-7255(06)00090-3 [pii]10.1016/j.nephro.2006.06.004] , 2(4), 191-199.

[180] Hudson, J. Q., & Sameri, R. M. (2002). Darbepoetin alfa, a new therapy for the management of anemia of chronic kidney disease. *Pharmacotherapy,* 22(9pt2), 141S-149S, [PMID: 12222584].

[181] Cases, A. (2003). Darbepoetin alfa: a novel erythropoiesis-stimulating protein. *Drugs Today (Barc),* 39(7), 477-495, PMID: 12973399, 799441.

[182] Locatelli, F., Canaud, B., Giacardy, F., Martin-Malo, A., Baker, N., & Wilson, J. (2003). Treatment of anaemia in dialysis patients with unit dosing of darbepoetin alfa at a reduced dose frequency relative to recombinant human erythropoietin (rHuEpo). *Nephrol Dial Transplant,* 18(2), 362-369, PMID: 12543893].

[183] Macdougall, I. C. (2002). Darbepoetin alfa: a new therapeutic agent for renal anemia. *Kidney Int Suppl* [80], 55-61, [PMID: 11982814, kid011.

[184] Macdougall, I. C., Matcham, J., & Gray, S. J. (2003). Correction of anaemia with darbepoetin alfa in patients with chronic kidney disease receiving dialysis. *Nephrol Dial Transplant,* 18(3), 576-581, PMID: 12584282].

[185] Macdougall, I. C., Robson, R., Opatrna, S., Liogier, X., Pannier, A., Jordan, P., Dougherty, F. C., & Reigner, B. (2006). Pharmacokinetics and pharmacodynamics of intravenous and subcutaneous continuous erythropoietin receptor activator (C.E.R.A.) in patients with chronic kidney disease. *Clin J Am Soc Nephrol,* 1(6), 1211-1215, [PMID: 17699350, 10.2215/CJN.00730306.

[186] Macdougall, I. C., & Eckardt, K. U. (2006). Novel strategies for stimulating erythropoiesis and potential new treatments for anaemia. *Lancet,* 368(9539), 947-953, PMID: 16962885, 10.1016/S0140-6736(06)69120-4.

[187] Ohashi, N., Sakao, Y., Yasuda, H., Kato, A., & Fujigaki, Y. (2012). Methoxy polyethylene glycol-epoetin beta for anemia with chronic kidney disease. *Int J Nephrol Renovasc Dis*, 5, 53-60, [PMID: 22536082 PMCID: 3333806, 10.2147/IJNRD.S23447ijnrd-5-053.

[188] Micera, Roche. (2012). ®solution for injection in pre-filled syringe [summary of product characteristics. *Welwyn Garden City*.

[189] Weinreich, T., Leistikow, F., Hartmann, H. G., Vollgraf, G., & Dellanna, F. (2012). Monthly continuous erythropoietin receptor activator treatment maintains stable hemoglobin levels in routine clinical management of hemodialysis patients. *Hemodial Int*, 16(1), 11-19, [PMID: 22098689, 10.1111/j.1542-4758.2011.00608.x.

[190] Leypoldt, J. K., Loghman-Adham, M., Jordan, P., & Reigner, B. (2012). Effect of hemodialysis and hemofiltration on plasma C.E.R.A. concentrations. *Hemodial Int*, 16(1), 20-30, [PMID: 22098670, 10.1111/j.1542-4758.2011.00634.x.

[191] Graul, A. I. (2012). Peginesatide for the treatment of anemia in the nephrology setting. *Drugs Today (Barc)*, 48(6), 395-403, [PMID: 22745925, 10.1358/dot.2012.48.6.1825620.

[192] Neumann, M. E. (2012). FDA approval of Omontys changes the ESA playing field. *Nephrol News* [26], PMID: 22690453].

[193] Green, J. M., Leu, K., Worth, A., Mortensen, R. B., Martinez, D. K., Schatz, P. J., Wojchowski, D. M., & Young, P. R. (2012). Peginesatide and erythropoietin stimulate similar erythropoietin receptor-mediated signal transduction and gene induction events. Exp Hematol [PMID: 22406924 S0301-472X(12)00087-2 [pii]10.1016/j.exphem.2012.02.007] , 40(7), 575-587.

[194] Mikhail, A. (2012). Profile of peginesatide and its potential for the treatment of anemia in adults with chronic kidney disease who are on dialysis. *J Blood Med*, 3, 25-31, [PMID: 22719216 PMCID: 3377433, 10.2147/JBM.S23270jbm-3-025.

[195] Macdougall, I. C., Wiecek, A., Tucker, B., Yaqoob, M., Mikhail, A., Nowicki, M., Mac Phee. I., Mysliwiec, M., Smolenski, O., Sulowicz, W., Mayo, M., Francisco, C., Polu, K. R., Schatz, P. J., & Duliege, A. M. (2011). Dose finding study of peginesatide for anemia correction in chronic kidney disease patients. *Clin J Am Soc Nephrol*, 6(11), 2579-2586, [PMID: 21940838 PMCID: 3359570, 10.2215/CJN.10831210.

[196] Doss, S., & Schiller, B. (2010). Peginesatide: a potential erythropoiesis stimulating agent for the treatment of anemia of chronic renal failure. *Nephrol Nurs J*, 37(6), 617-626, PMID: 21290916].

[197] Wizemann, V., Rutkowski, B., Baldamus, C., Scigalla, P., & Koytchev, R. (2008). Comparison of the therapeutic effects of epoetin zeta to epoetin alfa in the maintenance phase of renal anaemia treatment. *Curr Med Res Opin*, 24(3), 625-637, PMID: 18208642, X273264.

[198] Krivoshiev, S., Wizemann, V., Czekalski, S., Schiller, A., Pljesa, S., Wolf-Pflugmann, M., Siebert-Weigel, M., Koytchev, R., & Bronn, A. (2010). Therapeutic equivalence of epoetin zeta and alfa, administered subcutaneously, for maintenance treatment of renal anemia. *Adv Ther*, 27(2), 105-117, PMID: 20369312, s12325-010-0012-y.

[199] Krivoshiev, S., Todorov, V. V., Manitius, J., Czekalski, S., Scigalla, P., & Koytchev, R. (2008). Comparison of the therapeutic effects of epoetin zeta and epoetin alpha in the correction of renal anaemia. *Curr Med Res Opin*, 24(5), 1407-1415, PMID: 18394266, 10.1185/030079908X297402.

[200] Baldamus, C., Krivoshiev, S., Wolf-Pflugmann, M., Siebert-Weigel, M., Koytchev, R., & Bronn, A. (2008). Long-term safety and tolerability of epoetin zeta, administered intravenously, for maintenance treatment of renal anemia. *Adv Ther*, 25(11), 1215-1228, PMID: 18931828, s12325-008-0111-1.

[201] Lonnemann, G., & Wrenger, E. (2011). Biosimilar epoetin zeta in nephrology- a single-dialysis center experience. *Clin Nephrol*, 75(1), 59-62, PMID: 21176751, 8251.

[202] Gertz, B., Kes, P., Essaian, A., Bias, P., Buchner, A., & Zellner, D. (2012). Epoetin theta: efficacy and safety of subcutaneous administration in anemic pre-dialysis patients in the maintenance phase in comparison to epoetin beta. *Curr Med Res Opin*, 28(7), 1101-1110, [PMID: 22533679, 10.1185/03007995.2012.688736.

[203] Sikole, A., Spasovski, G., Zafirov, D., & Polenakovic, M. (2002). Epoetin omega for treatment of anemia in maintenance hemodialysis patients. *Clin Nephrol*, 57(3), 237-245, PMID: 11924756].

[204] Bren, A., Kandus, A., Varl, J., Buturovic, J., Ponikvar, R., Kveder, R., Primozic, S., & Ivanovich, P. (2002). A comparison between epoetin omega and epoetin alfa in the correction of anemia in hemodialysis patients: a prospective, controlled crossover study. *Artif Organs*, 26(2), 91-97, PMID: 11879235].

[205] Haag-Weber, M., Vetter, A., & Thyroff-Friesinger, U. (2009). Therapeutic equivalence, long-term efficacy and safety of HX575 in the treatment of anemia in chronic renal failure patients receiving hemodialysis. *Clin Nephrol*, 72(5), 380-390, PMID: 19863881, 6742.

[206] Horl, W. H., Locatelli, F., Haag-Weber, M., Ode, M., & Roth, K. (2012). Prospective multicenter study of HX575 (biosimilar epoetin-alpha) in patients with chronic kidney disease applying a target hemoglobin of 10--12 g/dl. *Clin Nephrol*, 78(1), 24-32, PMID: 22732334, 9782.

[207] Haag-Weber, M., Eckardt, K. U., Horl, W. H., Roger, S. D., Vetter, A., & Roth, K. (2012). Safety, immunogenicity and efficacy of subcutaneous biosimilar epoetin-alpha (HX575) in non-dialysis patients with renal anemia: a multi-center, randomized, double-blind study. *Clin Nephrol*, 77(1), 8-17, PMID: 22185963, 9283.

[208] Kaufman, J. S., Reda, D. J., Fye, C. L., Goldfarb, D. S., Henderson, W. G., Kleinman, J. G., Vaamonde, C., & A.19, . C.A.(1998). Subcutaneous compared with intravenous

epoetin in patients receiving hemodialysis. Department of Veterans Affairs Cooperative Study Group on Erythropoietin in Hemodialysis Patients. N Engl J Med PMID: 9718376 NEJM199808273390902 , 339(9), 578-583.

[209] Rossert, J., Casadevall, N., & Eckardt, K. U. (2004). Anti-erythropoietin antibodies and pure red cell aplasia. *J Am Soc Nephrol*, 15(2), 398-406, PMID: 14747386].

[210] Pljesa, S. (2004). Possible complications of erythropoietin therapy in patients with chronic renal failure. *Med Pregl*, 57(5-6), 254-257.

[211] Boven, K., Stryker, S., Knight, J., Thomas, A., van Regenmortel, M., Kemeny, D. M., Power, D., Rossert, J., & Casadevall, N. (2005). The increased incidence of pure red cell aplasia with an Eprex formulation in uncoated rubber stopper syringes. *Kidney Int*, 67(6), 2346-2353, [PMID: 15882278, KID340, [pii]10.1111/j.1523-1755.2005.00340.x].

[212] Littlewood, T. J. (2009). Is normalising haemoglobin in patients with CKD harmful and if so, why? *J Ren Care*, 35(2), 25-28, [PMID: 19891682, JORC123, [pii]10.1111/j.1755-6686.2009.00123.x].

[213] Ofsthun, N., Labrecque, J., Lacson, E., Keen, M., & Lazarus, J. M. (2003). The effects of higher hemoglobin levels on mortality and hospitalization in hemodialysis patients. Kidney Int [PMID: 12675871 kid937 [pii]10.1046/j.1523-1755.2003.00937.x] , 63(5), 1908-1914.

[214] Avram, M. M., Blaustein, D., Fein, P. A., Goel, N., Chattopadhyay, J., & Mittman, N. (2003). Hemoglobin predicts long-term survival in dialysis patients: a 15-year single-center longitudinal study and a correlation trend between prealbumin and hemoglobin. *Kidney Int Suppl* [87], S6-11, [PMID: 14531767].

[215] Servilla, K. S., Singh, A. K., Hunt, W. C., Harford, A. M., Miskulin, D., Meyer, K. B., Bedrick, E. J., Rohrscheib, M. R., Tzamaloukas, A. H., Johnson, H. K., & Zager, P. G. (2009). Anemia management and association of race with mortality and hospitalization in a large not-for-profit dialysis organization. *Am J Kidney Dis*, 54(3), 498-510, [PMID: 19628315, S0272-6386(09)00772-0, [pii]10.1053/j.ajkd.2009.05.007].

[216] Locatelli, F., & Del Vecchio, L. (2011). Erythropoiesis-stimulating agents in renal medicine. *Oncologist*, 16(3), 19-24, [PMID: 21930831, 10.1634/theoncologist.2011-S3-19.

[217] Novak, J. E, & Szczech, L. A. (2008). Triumph and tragedy: anemia management in chronic kidney disease. *Curr Opin Nephrol Hypertens*, 17(6), 580-588, PMID: 18941350, MNH.0b013e32830c488d00041552-200811000-00006.

[218] Kapoian, T. (2008). Challenge of effectively using erythropoiesis-stimulating agents and intravenous iron. *Am J Kidney Dis*, 52(6), S21-28, [PMID: 19010258, S0272-6386(08)01300-0, [pii]10.1053/j.ajkd.2008.09.004].

[219] Berns, J. S. (2010). Are there implications from the Trial to Reduce Cardiovascular Events with Aranesp Therapy study for anemia management in dialysis patients? *Curr Opin Nephrol Hypertens*, 19(6), 567-572, PMID: 20601876, MNH.0b013e32833c3cc7.

[220] Locatelli, F., Aljama, P., Canaud, B., Covic, A., De Francisco, A., Macdougall, I. C., Wiecek, A., & Vanholder, R. (2010). Target haemoglobin to aim for with erythropoiesis-stimulating agents: a position statement by ERBP following publication of the Trial to reduce cardiovascular events with Aranesp therapy (TREAT) study. *Nephrol Dial Transplant*, 25(9), 2846-2850, PMID: 20591813, 10.1093/ndt/gfq336.

[221] Erythropoiesis-stimulating agents (ESAs). (2009). Epoetin alfa (marketedas Procrit and Epogen). *Darbepoetin alfa (marketed as Aranesp).*

[222] Kainz, A., Mayer, B., Kramar, R., & Oberbauer, R. (2010). Association of ESA hyporesponsiveness and haemoglobin variability with mortality in haemodialysis patients. *Nephrol Dial Transplant*, 25(11), 3701-3706, PMID: 20507852 PMCID: 3360143, 10.1093/ndt/gfq287.

[223] Tsubakihara, Y., Nishi, S., Akiba, T., Hirakata, H., Iseki, K., Kubota, M., Kuriyama, S., Komatsu, Y., Suzuki, M., Nakai, S., Hattori, M., Babazono, T., Hiramatsu, M., Yamamoto, H., Bessho, M., & Akizawa, T. (2008). Japanese Society for Dialysis Therapy: guidelines for renal anemia in chronic kidney disease. Ther Apher Dial 2010 [PMID: 20609178 TAP836 [pii]10.1111/j.1744-9987.2010.00836.x] , 14(3), 240-275.

[224] Triolo, G. (2003). Guidelines for the treatment of anemia in chronic renal failure. *G Ital Nefrol*, 20(24), S61-82, PMID: 14666504].

[225] Horl, W. H., Macdougall, I. C., Rossert, J., Rutkowski, B., Wauters, J. P., & Valderrabano, F. (2003). Predialysis Survey on Anemia Management: patient referral. *Am J Kidney Dis*, 41(1), 49-61, [PMID: 12500221, 10.1053/ajkd.2003.50018S0272638602691206.

[226] Manns, B. J., & Tonelli, M. (2012). The new FDA labeling for ESA--implications for patients and providers. *Clin J Am Soc Nephrol*, 7(2), 348-353, [PMID: 22266575 PMCID: 3280029, 10.2215/CJN.09960911.

[227] Maurin, N. (2008). Regarding the optimal hemoglobin target range in renal anemia. *Med Klin (Munich)*, 103(9), 633-637, PMID: 18813886, s00063-008-1102-3.

[228] Yang, W., Israni, R. K., Brunelli, S. M., Joffe, M. M., Fishbane, S., & Feldman, H. I. (2007). Hemoglobin variability and mortality in ESRD. *J Am Soc Nephrol*, 18(12), 3164-3170, PMID: 18003781, 10.1681/ASN.2007010058.

[229] Lacson, E. Jr, Ofsthun, N., & Lazarus, J. M. (2003). Effect of variability in anemia management on hemoglobin outcomes in ESRD. *Am J Kidney Dis*, 41(1), 111-124, [PMID: 12500228, 10.1053/ajkd.2003.50030S0272638602691322.

[230] Kalantar-Zadeh, K., & Aronoff, G. R. (2009). Hemoglobin variability in anemia of chronic kidney disease. *J Am Soc Nephrol*, 20(3), 479-487, PMID: 19211716, 10.1681/ASN.2007070728.

Chapter 3

# rhEPO for the Treatment of Erythropoietin Resistant Anemia in Hemodialysis Patients – Risks and Benefits

Sandra Ribeiro, Elísio Costa, Luís Belo,
Flávio Reis and Alice Santos-Silva

Additional information is available at the end of the chapter

## 1. Introduction

Anemia is a common complication in hemodialysis (HD) patients, mainly due to the insufficient production of erythropoietin (EPO) by the failing kidneys [1]. Anemia itself can worsens cardiac function, cognitive function, exercise capacity and quality of life, and it has been independently associated with increased mortality and progression of renal disease [2, 3]. A successful management of anemia is, therefore, crucial, as it may improve clinical outcome. The introduction of recombinant human EPO (rhEPO) therapy to treat anemia of chronic kidney disease (CKD) patients reduced anemia, improving patients' quality of life [3]. There is, however, a marked variability in the response to this therapy and 5-10% of patients develop resistance to rhEPO therapy [4]. Resistance to rhEPO therapy has been associated to inflammation, oxidative stress and "functional" iron deficiency, as major causes.

EPO presents also an important protective role in other tissues, outside of the erythropoietic system. Actually, a biological response to EPO and the expression of EPO receptors, have been observed in many different cells, namely, in endothelial, neural and cardiac cells. However, HD patients requiring high rhEPO doses present an increased risk of death [5]. Recently, randomized controlled trials showed no benefit, or even increased risk of mortality and/or cardiovascular complications, in HD patients with hemoglobin (Hb) concentration higher than the target levels [6].

In this book chapter, a review of the etiological mechanisms associated with the development of EPO resistant anemia, in HD patients, will be performed. We also intend to review also the risk-benefits associated with high rhEPO doses used to achieve the target Hb levels.

## 2. Anemia of chronic kidney disease

CKD is a pathological condition that results from a gradual, permanent loss of kidney function over time, usually, months to years. CKD can result from primary diseases of the kidneys. However, diabetic nephropathy and hypertension have been considered as the main causes of CKD [1]. Anemia is a common complication of CKD that develops early in the course of the disease increasing its frequency with the decline of renal function. The incidence of anemia is less than 2 % in CKD stages 1 and 2, about 5% in CKD stage 3, 44% in CKD stage 4 and more than 70% in the end-stage renal disease (ESRD) [7]. This condition is associated with a decreased quality of life [3], increased hospitalization [2, 8], cardiovascular complications - angina, left ventricular hypertrophy (LVH) and chronic heart failure – and mortality [9-12].

The European Best Practice Guidelines for the management of anemia in patients with CKD recommends that a diagnosis of anemia in these patients should be considered when Hb concentration falls below 11.5 g/dL in women, 13.5 g/dL in adult men and 12.0 g/dL in men older than age 70 [13].

The anemia of these patients is, mainly, due to decreased kidney's secretion of EPO. In CKD patients there is a failure in increasing the EPO levels in response to hypoxia, as occurs in others types of anemia. These patients present an EPO deficiency, rather than an absolute lack, as EPO remains detectable even in the most advanced stages of CKD [14]. However, other factors contribute to the anemia in these patients, as reduced red blood cell (RBC) life span, iron deficiency, uremic toxins, HD procedure, blood loss and inflammation.

## 3. Erythropoiesis-stimulating agents

The correction of anemia in CKD patients needs pharmaceutical intervention with erythropoiesis-stimulating agents (ESAs). An intravenous (i.v.) iron supplementation, as adjuvant therapy, should be administrated to prevent iron deficiency and minimize the dose of ESA needed to achieve the target-range of Hb levels [4, 13]. However, recently, some concerns about this treatment of the anemia were raised and questioned in several studies, namely, the need to define Hb targets, safety, benefits and costs of ESA treatments.

### 3.1. Pharmacology of erythropoiesis- stimulating agents

The introduction of ESAs revolutionized the treatment of anemia in CKD patients. After cloning of the EPO gene, the recombinant human technology allowed the production of ESAs that present the physiological role of EPO. Epoetin beta was the first ESA to be used. It was presented in 1987 [15] and approved by the Food and Drug Administration (FDA) in 1989. Since then, other ESAs appeared, with similar actions, differing in their half-life. Consequently, they were divided in "short-acting" and "long-acting" ESAs (Table 1). The frequency of administration and route of administration (usually, the intravenous (i.v.) administration is more convenient for HD patients) is, therefore, conditioned by their half-life.

In humans, it seems that the rhEPO treatment increases Hb concentration, and, thus, arterial oxygen content, by increasing red cell volume and depressing plasma volume, probably through a mechanism involving the reduction of the renin–angiotensin–aldosterone axis activity [16].

The mechanisms for ESAs elimination are not well elucidated, and several hypotheses have been considered [17, 18]:

- ESAs are primarily cleared by a hepatic pathway;
- Clearance of ESAs occurs through the kidneys;
- ESAs may be cleared via EPO receptor-mediated endocytosis and subsequent intracellular degradation.

However, other mechanisms, not yet elucidated can be responsible for ESAs elimination.

| ESA | Approval | | Characteristics | Half-life | Frequency administration |
|---|---|---|---|---|---|
| | FDA | EMA | | | |
| **Short-acting** | | | | | |
| **Epoetin beta** | | 1989 | Identical a.a. and carbohydrate composition to EPO | i.v. 4 - 12 h<br>s.c. 12 – 28 h | 3 times/week |
| **Epoetin alpha** | 1989 | 1989 | Identical a.a. and carbohydrate composition to EPO | i.v. ≈ 5h<br>s.c. ≈ 24h | 3 times/week |
| Epoetin zeta (biosimilar medicine) | | 2007 | Identical a.a. and carbohydrate composition to EPO | i.v. ≈ 5h<br>s.c. ≈ 24h | 3 times/week |
| Epoetin theta (biosimilar medicine) | | 2009 | Identical a.a. and carbohydrate composition to EPO | i.v.≈ 4h<br>s.c. ≈ 34h | 3 times/week |
| **Long-acting** | | | | | |
| **Darbopoetin alpha** | 2001 | 2001 | 2 additional N-linked carbohydrate chains compared to EPO | i.v. 21 hours<br>s.c. 73 hours | once/week |
| **Methoxy polyethylene glycol-epoetin beta** | 2007 | 2007 | continuous erythropoietin receptor activator | i.v. 134 hours<br>s.c. 139 hours | once/month |
| **Peginesatide** | 2012 | | PEGylated, homodimeric peptide with no sequence homology to rhEPO | | once/month |

Abbreviations: FDA – Food and Drug Administration; EMA – European Medicines Agency; a.a. – amino acid; i.v. – intravenous; s.c. – subcutaneous. rhEPO – recombinant human erythropoietin. Adapted from Food and Drug Administration (2012) [19], European Medecines Agency (2012) [20] and Green et al. (2012) [21].

**Table 1.** Erythropoiesis – stimulating agents.

### 3.2. Non-hematopoietic actions of erythropoietin and erythropoiesis- stimulating agents

ESAs are designed to treat anemia, but recent evidences points to other non-hematopoietic actions of EPO and ESAs [22]. Several pleiotropic effects have been attributed to EPO, such as cytoprotective, antiapoptotic, anti-inflammatory and angiogenic capacities.

The erythropoietic and non-erythropoietic effects of EPO appear to result from the existence of two different receptors with different affinities for EPO [23].

In erythroid cells, picomolar concentrations of EPO bind to the EPOR homodimers, whereas on other cells and tissues EPO binds to an heterodimer receptor, constituted by EPOR and CD131 (beta common receptor – βcR), and, high local EPO concentrations are needed to exert its action [23-25]. The EPO variants, including asialo-EPO, carbamylated EPO (CEPO) or carbamylated darbopoetin alpha (C-darbe), that present the protective effects of EPO in non-haematopoietic tissues, but no hematopoietic activity [26-28], suggested the presence of two types of receptors. EPOR are present in several cells and tissues, as brain (neurons, astrocytes, and microglia) [29, 30], kidney [31], female reproductive system [32], vascular endothelial cells [33], cardiomyocytes [34], lymphocytes and monocytes [35], among others.

Some of the non-hematopoietic effects of EPO are summarized:

- Cardioprotection: several studies showed that ESAs promote cardioprotection through the inhibition of cardiomyocyte apoptosis, reduction of inflammation and oxidative stress, and induction of angiogenesis [22-24, 34, 36].
- Anti-inflammatory properties: EPO and its derivates reduce the production of pro-inflammatory cytokines, such as TNF-α, IL-6 and IL-1β, and NO (nitric oxide) via inducible NO synthase (iNOS) through the inhibition of NF-κB pathway [23, 24, 37].
- Neuroprotection: EPO seems to be important for the neural development, as it stimulates the differentiation of neural progenitor cells [29], but it also promotes angiogenesis and reduces inflammation, oxidative stress and neuronal apoptosis in some conditions, as hypoxia-ischemia (HI), stroke and neurotoxicity of glutamate [22-24, 29].
- Angiogenesis: EPO increases the number of functionally active endothelial progenitor cells (EPCs), enhancing angiogenesis, and seems to be dependent on functional endothelial NO synthase (eNOS) [24, 38]. EPO plays an important role in uterine angiogenesis, through EPOR expressed by endometrial vascular endothelial cells [33].
- Immunomodulation: EPO may have effects on dendritic cells [potent antigen presenting cells (APCs) that possess the ability to stimulate naïve T cells], presenting effects in innate immunity [39].
- Renoprotection: several studies on acute kidney injury reported that a single dose of rHuEPO reduces kidney dysfunction through an antiapoptotic mechanism, and increased NO production, but only in intact vessels [31]. However, it appears that this renoprotection is achieved only with low doses of EPO, non-hematopoietic doses, as high EPO doses cause an increase in hematocrit that is accompanied with changes in hemorheology, activation of thrombocytes and increased platelet adhesion to injured endothelium [31].

### 3.3. Benefits of erythropoiesis-stimulating agents

ESAs have beneficial effects by correcting anemia and their associated symptons (fatigue, dizziness, shortness of breath, among others), improving the quality of life of these patients [40-42]. ESAs also reduce the need for transfusions, thereby reducing transfusion reactions (immunological sensitization), transmission of infectious agents and iron overload [43].

The anemia of CKD is associated with cardiovascular complications, due to increasing blood pressure and LVH. Indeed, LVH is present in many patients with CKD, even in the earlier stages of the disease (75% of patients who start HD have LVH) and may lead to heart failure, cardiac arrhythmia or both, that are considered as major causes of cardiac-related deaths in this population [44, 45]. LVH is a physiological adaption that results from long-term increase of myocardial work, from high-pressure or volume overload, which can lead to major cardiac events. Volume overload can result from anemia, as hypoxia and the decreased blood viscosity contribute to decrease peripheral resistance, and from increased venous return, both of which increase cardiac output [44, 46]. LVH is also a risk factor for the development of uremic cardiomyopathy, which is defined as congestive heart failure due to a primary disorder of the heart muscle in uremic patients, and is characterized by profound systolic dysfunction and cardiac fibrosis; however, increased sympathetic activity in response to anemia also appears to be a factor for this condition [47, 48].

Several studies report the synergy between anemia and LVH and that the use of ESAs for anemia correction (Hb target of approximately 11 g/dL) is associated with an improvement in heart failure symptoms and with a reduction in LVH [45, 49].

The effects of ESAs on the progression of renal function are controversial. Some studies demonstrated that following ESA initiation renal function declines at a slower rate and delays the dialysis initiation in pre-dialysis patients [50-52], while other studies reported that ESAs do not significantly slow renal function decline [53, 54].

### 3.4. Risks associated with erythropoiesis-stimulating agents

As referred, ESAs have several benefits beyond the treatment of anemia; however, its administration seems to associate some risks. Cardiovascular and thromboembolic events have been described. Some of the protective effects of EPO and ESAs, as described above, occurs upon the activation of the heterodimeric EPOR; however, as the affinity of EPO for this receptor is low, higher doses of EPO are needed to reach these effects.

One of the most described effects of ESAs is hypertension. Several mechanisms can explain the rise in blood pressure (BP) mediated by ESAs. Renal anemia is a factor predisposing to increase BP, due to the increased sympathetic activity and impaired NO availability [55]. ESAs impair the balance between vasodilating and vasoconstrictor factors, since it induces the production of vasoconstrictors as endothelin-1 (ET-1), thromboxane (TXB2) and prostaglandin $2\alpha$ (PGF$2\alpha$), and reduces the production of the vasodilatory prostacyclin (PGI2) [56, 57]. Chronic treatment with ESAs appears to impair the vasodilatory capacity of endothelial NO, through an increase in the asymmetrical dimethylarginine (ADMA), an inhibitor of eNOS [57]. ESAs seem to induce hypersensitivity to angiotensin II, a recognized vasoconstrictor [56, 57].

An increase in noradrenaline concentration and hypersensitivity - a vasoactive substance - may contribute also to hypertension during ESA therapy [56, 57].

Treatment with ESAs is associated with an increase in the incidence of thrombotic events [58]. EPO has the capacity of stimulating thrombopoiesis, increasing platelet count; however, EPO also increases platelet reactivity (especially on the newly synthesized ones) promoting a prothrombic effect [59]. Some other hemostatic disturbances have been described, as an increased expression in E selectin, P selectin, von Willebrand factor and plasminogen activator inhibitor-1, which may favor bleeding episodes, and increase the risk of thrombosis and thromboembolism, as occlusion of the vascular access [57].

An uncommon but serious complication associated with ESAs administration is pure red blood cell aplasia, an immunogenic side effect that results from the production of antiEPO antibodies induced by ESAs administration [60-62]. Indeed, the method used to produce ESAs may not eliminate impurities or aggregated protein that may trigger the immune response in patients [62]. Immunoprecipitation assays have shown that antiEPO antibodies are directed against the protein moiety of the molecule [61].

ESAs are also indicated in the treatment of symptomatic anemia in adult cancer patients with non-myeloid malignancies receiving chemotherapy. However, some evidences point that these agents can accelerate tumor growth, but data are controversial. High doses of EPO can stimulate endothelial and vascular smooth muscle cell proliferation and promote angiogenesis. The antiapoptotic pleiotropic effect of EPO can also contribute to tumor progression [57, 63].

## 4. Resistance to erythropoieses-stimulating agents

Although the majority of CKD patients respond adequately to ESAs, 10% of these patients develops resistance to this therapy [4]. According to the European best practice guidelines for the management of anemia in patients with chronic renal failure [13] resistance to ESAs is defined as a failure to achieve target Hb levels (11– 12 g/dl) with doses lower than 300 IU/kg/ week of epoetin or 1.5 μg/kg/ week of darbopoietin-α. For the National Kidney Foundation Disease Outcomes Quality Initiative (NKF KDOQI) guidelines [4], hyporesponsiveness to ESAs therapy is defined by, at least, one of these situations: a significant increase in the ESA dose required to maintain a certain Hb level, a significant decrease in Hb level at a constant ESA dose or a failure to increase the Hb level to higher values than 11 g/dL, despite the administration of an ESA dose equivalent to epoetin higher than 500 IU/kg/week.

ESAs resistance is associated with poor outcome, increasing the risk of mortality [5, 64, 65]. Hyporesponsiveness to ESAs therapy can have many underlying causes. The most common causes are iron deficiency (absolute or functional), and inflammation.

### 4.1. Iron deficiency

Iron-restricted erythropoiesis is frequent in CKD patients and is due to absolute or functional iron deficiency. The latter seems to be the most common cause of hyporesponsiveness to ESAs in HD patients [66, 67]. About 25-37% of CKD patients with anemia present with iron deficiency [66]. Iron therapy is recommended, and i.v. iron supplementation is more effective than oral supplementation in HD patients [67]. It is important to distinguish between absolute and functional iron deficiency. Indeed, there is a controversy about iron supplementation when transferring saturation is lower than 20% and ferritin is higher than 500ng/mL (functional deficiency) [67, 68]. In this situation, probably associated with an inflammatory response, an excess of iron can be potentially harmful to these patients.

### 4.2. Chronic blood loss

Blood loss is frequent in patients undergoing HD and could be a cause to an inadequate ESA response. This condition should always be suspected in several conditions, namely, in patients who need a higher dose of ESA to maintain a stable Hb concentration, in patients whose Hb concentration is falling, and in patients who fail to increase iron stores, even after i.v. iron supplementation [13].

### 4.3. Inflammation

The anemia of CKD is often referred as an inflammatory anemia. Indeed, inflammation is a common feature in CKD patients, mainly, in those under HD. Inflammation is recognized as one cause to hyporesponsiveness to ESA therapy, and several studies reported an association between high levels of inflammatory markers and ESA resistance in CKD patients [5, 69-72]. Usually, HD patients present with high levels of inflammatory markers, namely, IL-6, CRP, TNF-$\alpha$, INF-$\gamma$, and with lower serum levels of albumin [69-71].

A week response to ESA also appears to be associated with enhanced T cell capacity to express IFN-$\gamma$, TNF-$\alpha$, IL-10, and IL-13 [70, 73]. Costa et al. [71] also reported a significant rise in neutrophil count in non-responder patients. They also found positive correlations between CRP and elastase and between elastase and rhEPO doses, suggesting that elastase, a neutrophil protease released by degranulation, could be a good marker of resistance to rhEPO therapy in HD patients under hemodialysis. Inflammation contributes to anemia through several ways:

- suppression of erythropoiesis: **directly**, by the inhibitory effects of pro-inflammatory cytokines: IL-1$\beta$ and TNF-$\alpha$ stimulate the growth of early progenitors BFU-E, but suppresses the growth of the later stages, inducing apoptosis in CFU-E [74]; **indirectly** as IL-1$\beta$ and TNF-$\alpha$ stimulate the production of INF-$\gamma$ [75], known to mediate erythropoiesis suppression.

- accelerated destruction of erythrocytes (as referred above in the uremic toxins section) by the reticulo-endothelial macrophages activated by the inflammatory state [76];

- reduction of EPO production: in hypoxic conditions, IL-1$\beta$ and TNF-$\alpha$ increase the expression GATA and NF-$\kappa$B, both inhibitory of the transcriptional factors of EPO gene [77];

- impaired iron availability for erythropoiesis: transferrin receptors in erythroid and non erythroid cells can be down-regulated by inflammatory cytokines reducing iron uptake [76]; they can also increase the expression of lactoferrin receptors and reduce the expression of ferroportin in macrophages, increasing the iron storage in these cells and reducing the iron availability [76, 78]; inflammation is responsible for the increase of hepcidin expression, a regulatory peptide in the iron cycling that reduces iron absorption and mobilization.

Recently, it was reported the existence of a soluble form of the EPOR (sEPOR) [79, 80]. Although this soluble receptor is able to bind to EPO, the role of these circulating sEPOR in humans remains largely unknown. sEPOR seems to be increased in patients receiving high ESA doses [79, 80], and the pro-inflammatory cytokines IL-6 and TNF-$\alpha$ can be responsible for this increment [79]. sEPOR could, therefore, be associated with ESA resistance through the inhibition of EPO effectiveness.

### 4.4. Decreased hepcidin excretion

In the last years hepcidin emerged as a key regulator of iron metabolism. Hepcidin is a peptide (25 aminoacids) produced, mainly, in hepatocytes, although other sites of production have been described, such as kidney [81], adipose tissue [82], brain [83] and heart [84, 85]. Hepcidin expression is regulated by the *HAMP* gene located in the long arm of chromosome 19 [86].

An increase of hepcidin levels leads to a decrease in iron absorption (hepcidin inhibits DMT1 transcription [87] or promotes an ubiquitin-dependent proteasome degradation of DMT1 [88]) and an inhibition of iron release from its storages (macrophages and hepatocytes) as hepcidin binds to ferroportin (the only known iron exporter in the cells) promoting its internalization and degradation in lysosomes (Fig. 1) [89, 90].

Hepcidin is increased in HD patients [91, 92], and it is regulated by inflammation [93] and linked to ESA resistance. Hepcidin correlates with IL-6, the cytokine that stimulate its production [94, 95], and with ferritin reflecting high inflammation and high levels of iron stores [96]. Some authors point that hepcidin could be a marker of functional iron deficiency [86] and that ESA therapy can decrease hepcidin levels [72, 96].

The kidney appears to play a role in the excretion of hepcidin, as this peptide is found in urine [97]. Hepcidin levels are increased in HD patients, and its levels appears to be reduced after HD procedure, supporting the role of kidneys in the excretion of this peptide [91, 92].

### 4.5. Secondary hyperparathyroidism

The parathyroid hormone (PTH) is considered by EUTox Work Group [98] as a middle molecule uremic toxin with some biological effects. Secondary hyperparathyroidism is a condition resulting from the deregulation of calcium and phosphorus homeostasis in the kidney. It seems that PTH could be a marker of hyporesponsiveness to ESAs in dialysis patients [99, 100].

Several mechanisms have been proposed as interference with RBC production as PTH causes bone marrow fibrosis, has an inhibitory effect on BFU-E and interferes with EPO endogenous

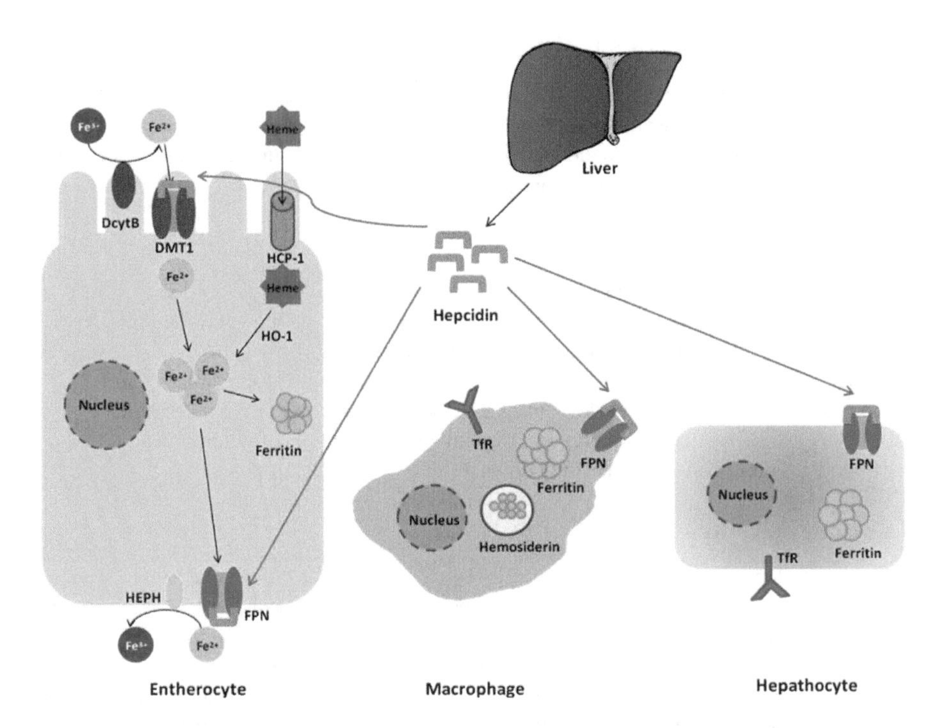


**Figure 1.** Iron metabolism and hepcidin. The iron is present in the diet as either heme iron ($Fe^{2+}$) or nonheme iron ($Fe^{3+}$). Nonheme iron must first be reduced to $Fe^{2+}$, by duodenal cytochrome B (DcytB), before it can be transported by the divalent metal iron transporter 1 (DMT1). Once inside the enterocyte, the newly absorbed iron enters the intracellular iron pool. If the iron is not required by the body, it is loaded onto the iron storage protein ferritin. Iron required by the body is transferred across the basolateral membrane by ferroportin (FPN). The export of iron also requires the ferroxidase hephaestin (HEPH). Heme carrier protein (HCP1) can transport heme; the enzyme heme-oxigenase 1 (HO-1) is required for releasing iron from heme. Hepcidin expression in the liver inhibits iron absorption from the diet and the release of iron from its storage.

production [99, 101-103]; interference with RBC survival as PTH increases osmotic fragility of erythrocytes [102, 103].

### 4.6. Aluminium toxicity

Although the recent progresses in the dialysis procedures, some patients present high levels of aluminium (Al) [104]. Usually, high levels of Al cause a microcytic, hypochromic or normochromic anemia that is hyporesponsive to ESA therapy, as it interferes with the enzymes necessary for the heme synthesis [67, 105]. The sources for the increase in plasma Al levels seems to be the water used for dialysis [105], medications given i.v. [104] and infections [106].

### 4.7. Vitamin deficiencies (e.g. folate or vitamin B12 deficiency)

The deficiency of folate or vitamine B12 is not very common in dialysis patients, but as these nutrients are water soluble and can be easily loss during dialysis, they can become a cause of ESA resistance, especially in patients with malnutrition. The supplementation of these nutrients seems to overcome ESA hyporesponsiveness [66, 67].

### 4.8. Malnutrition

Low body mass index (BMI) and low levels of cholesterol are related to poor outcomes in dialysis patients, increasing the risk of mortality [107]. This phenomenon, called as "reverse epidemiology", is based on the malnutrition-inflammatory complex [108]. These patients present a decreased nutritional reserve, reducing its capacity to overcome inflammation; they also present a reduced protein-calorie intake, chronic acidosis and failure of vascular access [108]. A diminished nutritional status and the enhancement of inflammation could be responsible for the requirement of higher EPO doses [69, 108].

### 4.9. Inadequate dialysis

Intensity or adequacy of dialysis (measured by Kt/V) is a factor that can modulate the response to ESA therapy. Inadequate dialysis is associated with the need for higher ESA doses. Some studies showed that convective treatments present benefits in ESA response, as compared with other treatments [109]. High flux HD (HF-HD) and online hemodialfiltration (OL-HDF) improve the response to ESAs, as compared to low flux HD (LF-HD), probably due to a better removal of middle and large molecules that impair erythropoiesis [67, 92, 109]. However, some studies failed to reach to these conclusions [110].

### 4.10. Angiotensin-converting enzyme inhibitors and angiotensin receptors blockers

These drugs, used for hypertension control, can be associated with ESA hyporesponsiveness due to its effects on angiotensin II. They can act through several mechanisms, not well understood, including inhibition of angiotensin-induced EPO release and increased plasma levels of N-acetyl-serylaspartyl-lysil-proline that impairs the recruitment of pluripotent hemopoietic stem cells [66, 67].

### 4.11. Testosterone deficiency

It appears that low testosterone levels may contribute to anemia in men with CKD and to ESA resistance. Testosterone stimulates erythropoiesis through the production of hematopoietic growth factors and possible improvement of iron bioavailability [111, 112].

## 5. Controversies in the treatment of anemia in chronic kidney disease

Since the introduction of ESAs therapy a demand exists to define the better Hb target associated with lower CV risks. Indeed, recent studies reported increased CV risk and death in patients treated with high doses of EPO to achieve higher Hb levels, and this led to the controversy of what is the cause of these increased risk: higher doses of EPO or higher levels of Hb?

### 5.1. Clinical trials

The correction of anemia to higher target Hb levels with ESAs in CKD or ESRD patients merits attention, as it may be associated with increased risk of death or of CV events, namely, stroke, hypertension, and vascular access thrombosis [6].

Only four studies assessed properly the effect of higher Hb levels on the increased risk of CV events and/or death.

#### *5.1.1. Normal hematocrit trial (NHT) [113]*

This study included patients under HD with congestive heart failure or ischemic heart disease. They were randomized to one of two groups to receive epoetin alpha, aiming to achieve and maintain a target hematocrit (Ht) of 42% or 30%. Primary end points were the length of time to death or for the first nonfatal myocardial infarction (MI). The study was interrupted due to the increased number of deaths observed in the high-Ht group and that were nearing the boundary of statistical significance. An increased rate of incidence of vascular access thrombosis was also reported in the high-Ht group. The study failed to reach statistical difference between the two groups, however, it was concluded that a target Ht of 42% is not recommended in HD patients.

#### *5.1.2. Cardiovascular risk reduction by early anemia treatment with epoetin beta (CREATE) [53]*

This study included pre-dialysis patients in stage 3 or 4 with mild-to-moderate anemia. They were randomly assigned to normalization of Hb values (13.0-15.0g/dL) or to a partial correction of anemia (10.5-11.5 g/dL), in order to investigate the effect of Hb correction on complications from CV causes. The primary endpoint was the time for the first CV event. Secondary objectives included the investigation of the effects of these treatments on the left ventricular mass index, the progression of CKD, and the quality of life. They did not find a significant difference in the risk for a first CV event between the two groups. However, this study reported a higher incidence of hypertension and headaches, and a higher risk for starting dialysis in the group aiming normalization of Hb values. But they also reported significant benefits on the quality of life for the patients with higher Hb targets.

In conclusion, they found that in pre-dialysis patients with mild-to-moderate anemia, the normalization of Hb levels to 13.0 to 15.0 g/dL did not reduce CV events.

#### *5.1.3. Correction of hemoglobin and outcomes in renal insufficiency (CHOIR) [114]*

Non-dialysis patients with CKD were included and the effect of raising Hb concentration with epoetin alpha to a target Hb value of 13.5 g/dL or 11.3 g/dL was compared. The primary end point was the time of death, MI, hospitalization for congestive heart failure (excluding renal replacement therapy), or stroke.

An increased risk of the primary end point, for the high-Hb group, as compared with the low-Hb group was found. Death and hospitalization for congestive heart failure accounted for 74.8% of the events. An increased rate of thrombotic events was also reported in the group of high-Hb. Patients in the high-Hb group had a higher (but not significant) rate of both progression to renal replacement therapy and hospitalization for renal replacement therapy. They did not find any apparent additional benefit in quality of life. In conclusion, they recommended the use of a target Hb level of 11.0 to 12.0 g/dL rather than a level of 11.0 to 13.0 g/dL, because of the increased risk, increased costs, and no quality-of-life benefit.

*5.1.4. Trial to reduce cardiovascular events with aranesp therapy (TREAT) [115]*

In this trial patients with type 2 diabetes mellitus, CKD and anemia were enrolled. Patients were randomized to receive darbepoetin-alfa (in order to achieve a target Hb of 13.0 g/dL) or placebo (in this group were prescribed blinded "rescue" darbepoetin for Hb level < 9.0 g/dL). The primary end point was time to death or hospitalization for myocardial ischemia. A significantly higher rate of strokes in patients treated with darbepoetin was observed. A higher rate of both thromboembolism and cancer-related deaths among patients with a history of cancer in the treatment group was also reported in the treatment group.

Higher targets of Hb levels imply the use of higher ESA doses. Therefore, the increased risk for adverse CV outcomes could also result from the higher ESAs doses and not only from the normalization of Hb [116]. In this sense, a trial has been designed to identify the potential benefits and harms of different fixed doses of ESA. The Clinical Evaluation of the DOSe of Erythropoietins (C.E. DOSE) trial [117] enrolled HD patients that were randomized 1:1 to 4000 IU/week *versus* 18000 IU/week of i.v. epoietin alfa or beta, or of any other ESA in equivalent doses. The primary outcome was death, non fatal stroke, non fatal MI and hospitalization for CV causes.

Several potential mechanisms for harm with higher Hb targets have been proposed and revised by Fishbane et al. [118]. The hypothesis is that increased viscosity and hemoconcentration, the increased BP, the toxic effect of iron and unphysiological doses of ESAs contribute to ESAs toxicity. The rise in Ht results in a higher viscosity and, consequently, higher risk of thomboembolism. It also favors platelet activation by increasing the interaction between the endothelial cells and platelets in blood vessels. Hemoconcentration is a phenomenon observed in these patients after a dialysis session that results from the removal of large amounts of fluids.

### 5.2. Safety advisories

Considering the results of these studies, in 2007 the FDA launched a safety advisory, recommending that patients do not exceed the Hb level of 12g/dL [119]. At the same time, the NKF KDOQI made an update on its guidelines, recommending that the selected Hb target should generally be in the range of 11.0 to 12.0 g/dL, but should not be greater than 13.0 g/dL [120].

In 2010, the European Best Practice Guidelines Work Group published the recommendation that "Hb values of 11-12 g/dL should be generally sought in the CKD population without intentionally exceeding 13 g/dL" [121]. In 2011, the FDA introduced warnings in the ESA label giving the recommendations "for more conservative dosing of Erythropoiesis-Stimulating Agents (ESAs) in patients with chronic kidney disease (CKD) to improve the safe use of these drugs" [122].

### 5.3. Hemoglobin variability

In conjugation with the optimal Hb target and ESA dose, there is a study of Hb variability (Hb-var). It was noted that during the treatment of HD patients with ESAs the level of Hb have a great fluctuation, that is, the Hb levels tends to rise or fall in a cyclic pattern, that is different for each patient [123]. However, the impact of this Hb-var is not still elucidated. Some studies show that there is an association between Hb-var and increase of death [11, 64, 65], especially if this variability is greater than 1g/dL [11]. The main factor for this variability is ESA dose; however, other factors have been pointed, as i.v. iron and other biological factors (inflammation and nutritional status) [123].

Hb-var represents an important physiological stress, as the ESA treatment involves short, intermittent burst of plasma EPO availability that do not coincide, either temporally or in magnitude with its physiological action. Under physiological conditions EPO levels are maintained in a narrow range, through several mechanisms, in order to support a constant oxygen supply to the organs. The impact of Hb-var on the organism is not fully understood, but the myocardium may be one of the most affected organs, as it has to compensate with an increased output and cardiomyocytes proliferation during the periods of reduced oxygen availability, that occur when Hb reaches lower levels, before the new ESA administration. This might result in deregulation of cardiac growth signal, leading to left ventricular dilation and hypertrophy [11, 123]. The autonomic nervous system can also suffer from this Hb-var; actually, autonomic dysfunction occurs in other pathological conditions, where Hb-var also occurs, like sickle cell anemia [11]. Fishane et al. also [123] found that better responders to ESA tend to have a higher degree of Hb-var.

## 6. Conclusion

Despite all the technologic advances in HD procedure and medical support, the morbidity and mortality in CKD patients remains high, particularly in hyporesponsiveness patients to ESAs therapy. The clinical trials showed that a higher Hb target is associated with increased risk of cardiovascular complications and death; however, the impact of higher ESAs doses to achieve higher Hb targets remains unclear. Some evidence points that the pleiotropic effects of ESAs can contribute to the ESAs toxicity observed with higher doses. Meanwhile, the recommendations to target Hb to a range of 11 – 12 g/dL, without exceeding the 13g/dL, with the lower doses of ESAs to accomplish this goal, can reduce the risks associated with higher Hb target and higher ESAs doses in CKD patients. More studies are needed on this field to evaluate the impact of the linkage anemia/high sustained ESAs therapeutic doses in CKD that might explain the high mortality in hyporesponsiveness patients. To accomplish these goals blood, cellular and tissue studies are need that cannot be performed in humans; therefore, the use of appropriate animal models could be useful to understand whether the association of moderate anemia and high sustained therapeutic doses of ESAs in non-responders is beneficial or an increasing risk; to clarify the underlying mechanisms and, eventually, to propose new therapeutic strategies to reduce mortality in HD patients.

## Acknowledgements

Portuguese Foundation for Science and Technology (FCT) and COMPETE, project PTDC/SAU-TOX/114253/2009.

## Author details

Sandra Ribeiro[1,2], Elísio Costa[1,2], Luís Belo[1,2], Flávio Reis[3] and Alice Santos-Silva[1,2]

1 Faculdade de Farmácia, Universidade do Porto, Portugal

2 Instituto de Biologia Molecular e Celular, Universidade do Porto, Portugal

3 Instituto de Farmacologia e Terapêutica Experimental, IBILI, Universidade de Coimbra, Portugal

## References

[1] Weiner, D. E. Causes and consequences of chronic kidney disease: implications for managed health care. Journal of managed care pharmacy : JMCP (2007). S, 1-9.

[2] Staples, A. O, Wong, C. S, Smith, J. M, et al. Anemia and risk of hospitalization in pediatric chronic kidney disease. Clin J Am Soc Nephrol (2009). , 4, 48-56.

[3] Weisbord, S. D, & Kimmel, P. L. Health-related quality of life in the era of erythropoietin. Hemodial Int (2008). , 12, 6-15.

[4] KDOQI Clinical Practice Guidelines and Clinical Practice Recommendations for Anemia in Chronic Kidney DiseaseAm J Kidney Dis (2006). S, 11-145.

[5] Panichi, V, Rosati, A, Bigazzi, R, et al. Anaemia and resistance to erythropoiesis-stimulating agents as prognostic factors in haemodialysis patients: results from the RISCAVID study. Nephrol Dial Transplant (2011). , 26, 2641-2648.

[6] Palmer, S. C, Navaneethan, S. D, Craig, J. C, et al. Meta-analysis: erythropoiesis-stimulating agents in patients with chronic kidney disease. Ann Intern Med (2010). , 153, 23-33.

[7] Astor, B. C, Muntner, P, Levin, A, Eustace, J. A, & Coresh, J. Association of kidney function with anemia: the Third National Health and Nutrition Examination Survey (1988-1994). Arch Intern Med (2002). , 162, 1401-1408.

[8] Liu, J, Guo, H, Gilbertson, D, Foley, R, & Collins, A. Associations of anemia persistency with medical expenditures in Medicare ESRD patients on dialysis. Ther Clin Risk Manag (2009). , 5, 319-330.

[9] Collins, A. J. Influence of target hemoglobin in dialysis patients on morbidity and mortality. Kidney Int Suppl (2002). , 2002, 44-48.

[10] Robinson, B. M, Joffe, M. M, Berns, J. S, Pisoni, R. L, Port, F. K, & Feldman, H. I. Anemia and mortality in hemodialysis patients: accounting for morbidity and treatment variables updated over time. Kidney Int (2005). , 68, 2323-2330.

[11] Yang, W, Israni, R. K, Brunelli, S. M, Joffe, M. M, Fishbane, S, & Feldman, H. I. Hemoglobin variability and mortality in ESRD. J Am Soc Nephrol (2007). , 18, 3164-3170.

[12] Locatelli, F, Pisoni, R. L, Combe, C, et al. Anaemia in haemodialysis patients of five European countries: association with morbidity and mortality in the Dialysis Outcomes and Practice Patterns Study (DOPPS). Nephrol Dial Transplant (2004). , 19, 121-132.

[13] Locatelli, F, Aljama, P, Barany, P, et al. Revised European best practice guidelines for the management of anaemia in patients with chronic renal failure. Nephrol Dial Transplant (2004). Suppl 2:ii, 1-47.

[14] Artunc, F, & Risler, T. Serum erythropoietin concentrations and responses to anaemia in patients with or without chronic kidney disease. Nephrol Dial Transplant (2007). , 22, 2900-2908.

[15] Eschbach, J. W, Egrie, J. C, Downing, M. R, Browne, J. K, & Adamson, J. W. Correction of the anemia of end-stage renal disease with recombinant human erythropoietin. Results of a combined phase I and II clinical trial. N Engl J Med (1987). , 316, 73-78.

[16] Lundby, C, Thomsen, J. J, Boushel, R, et al. Erythropoietin treatment elevates haemoglobin concentration by increasing red cell volume and depressing plasma volume. J Physiol (2007). , 578, 309-314.

[17] Gross, A. W, & Lodish, H. F. Cellular trafficking and degradation of erythropoietin and novel erythropoiesis stimulating protein (NESP). J Biol Chem (2006). , 281, 2024-2032.

[18] Agoram, B, Aoki, K, Doshi, S, et al. Investigation of the effects of altered receptor binding activity on the clearance of erythropoiesis-stimulating proteins: Nonerythropoietin receptor-mediated pathways may play a major role. J Pharm Sci (2009). , 98, 2198-2211.

[19] Food and Drug AdministrationFDA Approved Drug Products. http://www.accessdata.fda.gov/scripts/cder/drugsatfda/index.cfmaccessed 06 June (2012).

[20] European Medicines AgencySummary of Product Characteristics. http://www.ema.europa.eu/ema/index.jsp?curl=/pages/medicines/ landing/ epar_search.jsp&mid=WC0b01ac058001d124 (accessed 06 June (2012).

[21] Green, J. M, Leu, K, Worth, A, et al. Peginesatide and erythropoietin stimulate similar erythropoietin receptor-mediated signal transduction and gene induction events. Exp Hematol (2012).

[22] Arcasoy, M. O. The non-haematopoietic biological effects of erythropoietin. Br J Haematol (2008)., 141, 14-31.

[23] Nairz, M, Sonnweber, T, Schroll, A, Theurl, I, & Weiss, G. The pleiotropic effects of erythropoietin in infection and inflammation. Microbes Infect (2012)., 14, 238-246.

[24] Chateauvieux, S, Grigorakaki, C, Morceau, F, Dicato, M, & Diederich, M. Erythropoietin, erythropoiesis and beyond. Biochem Pharmacol (2011)., 82, 1291-1303.

[25] Brines, M, Grasso, G, Fiordaliso, F, et al. Erythropoietin mediates tissue protection through an erythropoietin and common beta-subunit heteroreceptor. Proc Natl Acad Sci U S A (2004)., 101, 14907-14912.

[26] Moon, C, Krawczyk, M, Paik, D, et al. Erythropoietin, modified to not stimulate red blood cell production, retains its cardioprotective properties. J Pharmacol Exp Ther (2006)., 316, 999-1005.

[27] Villa, P, Van Beek, J, Larsen, A. K, et al. Reduced functional deficits, neuroinflammation, and secondary tissue damage after treatment of stroke by nonerythropoietic erythropoietin derivatives. J Cereb Blood Flow Metab (2007)., 27, 552-563.

[28] Ramirez, R, Carracedo, J, Nogueras, S, et al. Carbamylated darbepoetin derivative prevents endothelial progenitor cell damage with no effect on angiogenesis. J Mol Cell Cardiol (2009)., 47, 781-788.

[29] Alnaeeli, M, Wang, L, Piknova, B, Rogers, H, Li, X, & Noguchi, C. T. Erythropoietin in brain development and beyond. Anat Res Int (2012).

[30] Nagai, A, Nakagawa, E, Choi, H. B, Hatori, K, Kobayashi, S, & Kim, S. U. Erythropoietin and erythropoietin receptors in human CNS neurons, astrocytes, microglia, and oligodendrocytes grown in culture. J Neuropathol Exp Neurol (2001). , 60, 386-392.

[31] Bahlmann, F. H, & Fliser, D. Erythropoietin and renoprotection. Curr Opin Nephrol Hypertens (2009)., 18, 15-20.

[32] Yokomizo, R, Matsuzaki, S, Uehara, S, Murakami, T, Yaegashi, N, & Okamura, K. Erythropoietin and erythropoietin receptor expression in human endometrium throughout the menstrual cycle. Mol Hum Reprod (2002)., 8, 441-446.

[33] Ribatti, D, Vacca, A, Roccaro, A. M, Crivellato, E, & Presta, M. Erythropoietin as an angiogenic factor. Eur J Clin Invest (2003). , 33, 891-896.

[34] Teixeira, M, Rodrigues-santos, P, Garrido, P, et al. Cardiac antiapoptotic and proproliferative effect of recombinant human erythropoietin in a moderate stage of chronic renal failure in the rat. J Pharm Bioallied Sci (2012). , 4, 76-83.

[35] Lisowska, K. A, Debska-slizien, A, Bryl, E, Rutkowski, B, & Witkowski, J. M. Erythropoietin receptor is expressed on human peripheral blood T and B lymphocytes and monocytes and is modulated by recombinant human erythropoietin treatment. Artif Organs (2010). , 34, 654-662.

[36] Noguchi, C. T, Wang, L, Rogers, H. M, Teng, R, & Jia, Y. Survival and proliferative roles of erythropoietin beyond the erythroid lineage. Expert Rev Mol Med (2008). e36.

[37] Tanaka, Y, Joki, N, Hase, H, et al. Effect of erythropoietin-stimulating agent on uremic inflammation. J Inflamm (Lond) (2012).

[38] Uscio, d, Smith, L. V, Santhanam, L. A, Richardson, A. V, Nath, D, & Katusic, K. A. ZS. Essential role of endothelial nitric oxide synthase in vascular effects of erythropoietin. Hypertension (2007). , 49, 1142-1148.

[39] Lifshitz, L, Prutchi-sagiv, S, Avneon, M, Gassmann, M, Mittelman, M, & Neumann, D. Non-erythroid activities of erythropoietin: Functional effects on murine dendritic cells. Mol Immunol (2009). , 46, 713-721.

[40] Finkelstein, F. O, Story, K, Firanek, C, et al. Health-related quality of life and hemoglobin levels in chronic kidney disease patients. Clin J Am Soc Nephrol (2009). , 4, 33-38.

[41] Foley, R. N, Curtis, B. M, & Parfrey, P. S. Erythropoietin therapy, hemoglobin targets, and quality of life in healthy hemodialysis patients: a randomized trial. Clin J Am Soc Nephrol (2009). , 4, 726-733.

[42] Johansen, K. L, Finkelstein, F. O, Revicki, D. A, et al. Systematic review of the impact of erythropoiesis-stimulating agents on fatigue in dialysis patients. Nephrol Dial Transplant (2012). , 27, 2418 2425.

[43] Ibrahim, H. N, Ishani, A, Guo, H, & Gilbertson, D. T. Blood transfusion use in non-dialysis-dependent chronic kidney disease patients aged 65 years and older. Nephrol Dial Transplant (2009). , 24, 3138-3143.

[44] Weiner, D. E, Tighiouart, H, Vlagopoulos, P. T, et al. Effects of anemia and left ventricular hypertrophy on cardiovascular disease in patients with chronic kidney disease. J Am Soc Nephrol (2005). , 16, 1803-1810.

[45] Foley, R. N, Curtis, B. M, Randell, E. W, & Parfrey, P. S. Left ventricular hypertrophy in new hemodialysis patients without symptomatic cardiac disease. Clin J Am Soc Nephrol (2010). , 5, 805-813.

[46] Astor, B. C, Coresh, J, Heiss, G, Pettitt, D, & Sarnak, M. J. Kidney function and anemia as risk factors for coronary heart disease and mortality: the Atherosclerosis Risk in Communities (ARIC) Study. Am Heart J (2006). , 151, 492-500.

[47] London, G. Pathophysiology of cardiovascular damage in the early renal population. Nephrol Dial Transplant (2001). Suppl , 2, 3-6.

[48] Gross, M. L, & Ritz, E. Hypertrophy and fibrosis in the cardiomyopathy of uremia--beyond coronary heart disease. Semin Dial (2008). , 21, 308-318.

[49] Parfrey, P. S, Lauve, M, Latremouille-viau, D, & Lefebvre, P. Erythropoietin therapy and left ventricular mass index in CKD and ESRD patients: a meta-analysis. Clin J Am Soc Nephrol (2009). , 4, 755-762.

[50] Gouva, C, Nikolopoulos, P, Ioannidis, J. P, & Siamopoulos, K. C. Treating anemia early in renal failure patients slows the decline of renal function: a randomized controlled trial. Kidney Int (2004). , 66, 753-760.

[51] Dean, B. B, Dylan, M, & Gano, A. Jr., Knight K, Ofman JJ, Levine BS. Erythropoiesis-stimulating protein therapy and the decline of renal function: a retrospective analysis of patients with chronic kidney disease. Curr Med Res Opin (2005). , 21, 981-987.

[52] Palazzuoli, A, Silverberg, D, Iovine, F, et al. Erythropoietin improves anemia exercise tolerance and renal function and reduces B-type natriuretic peptide and hospitalization in patients with heart failure and anemia. Am Heart J (2006). e, 1099-1015.

[53] Drueke, T. B, Locatelli, F, Clyne, N, et al. Normalization of hemoglobin level in patients with chronic kidney disease and anemia. N Engl J Med (2006). , 355, 2071-2084.

[54] Villar, E, Lievre, M, Kessler, M, et al. Anemia normalization in patients with type 2 diabetes and chronic kidney disease: results of the NEPHRODIAB2 randomized trial. J Diabetes Complications (2011). , 25, 237-243.

[55] Baylis, C. Nitric oxide synthase derangements and hypertension in kidney disease. Curr Opin Nephrol Hypertens (2012). , 21, 1-6.

[56] Krapf, R, & Hulter, H. N. Arterial hypertension induced by erythropoietin and erythropoiesis-stimulating agents (ESA). Clin J Am Soc Nephrol (2009). , 4, 470-480.

[57] Vaziri, N. D, & Zhou, X. J. Potential mechanisms of adverse outcomes in trials of anemia correction with erythropoietin in chronic kidney disease. Nephrol Dial Transplant (2009). , 24, 1082-1088.

[58] Corwin, H. L, Gettinger, A, Fabian, T. C, et al. Efficacy and safety of epoetin alfa in critically ill patients. N Engl J Med (2007). , 357, 965-976.

[59] Stohlawetz, P. J, Dzirlo, L, Hergovich, N, et al. Effects of erythropoietin on platelet reactivity and thrombopoiesis in humans. Blood (2000). , 95, 2983-2989.

[60] Casadevall, N, Nataf, J, Viron, B, et al. Pure red-cell aplasia and antierythropoietin antibodies in patients treated with recombinant erythropoietin. N Engl J Med (2002). , 346, 469-475.

[61] Casadevall, N. Pure red cell aplasia and anti-erythropoietin antibodies in patients treated with epoetin. Nephrol Dial Transplant (2003). Suppl 8:viii, 37-41.

[62] Praditpornsilpa, K, Tiranathanagul, K, Kupatawintu, P, et al. Biosimilar recombinant human erythropoietin induces the production of neutralizing antibodies. Kidney Int (2011). , 80, 88-92.

[63] Aapro, M, Jelkmann, W, Constantinescu, S. N, & Leyland-jones, B. Effects of erythropoietin receptors and erythropoiesis-stimulating agents on disease progression in cancer. Br J Cancer (2012). , 106, 1249-1258.

[64] Regidor, D. L, Kopple, J. D, Kovesdy, C. P, et al. Associations between changes in hemoglobin and administered erythropoiesis-stimulating agent and survival in hemodialysis patients. J Am Soc Nephrol (2006). , 17, 1181-1191.

[65] Kainz, A, Mayer, B, Kramar, R, & Oberbauer, R. Association of ESA hypo-responsiveness and haemoglobin variability with mortality in haemodialysis patients. Nephrol Dial Transplant (2010). , 25, 3701-3706.

[66] Priyadarshi, A, & Shapiro, J. I. Erythropoietin resistance in the treatment of the anemia of chronic renal failure. Semin Dial (2006). , 19, 273-278.

[67] Johnson, D. W, Pollock, C. A, & Macdougall, I. C. Erythropoiesis-stimulating agent hyporesponsiveness. Nephrology (Carlton) (2007). , 12, 321-330.

[68] Horl, W. H. Iron therapy for renal anemia: how much needed, how much harmful? Pediatr Nephrol (2007). , 22, 480-489.

[69] de Lurdes Agostinho Cabrita APinho A, Malho A, et al. Risk factors for high erythropoiesis stimulating agent resistance index in pre-dialysis chronic kidney disease patients, stages 4 and 5. Int Urol Nephrol (2011). , 43, 835-840.

[70] Costa, E, Lima, M, Alves, J. M, et al. Inflammation, T-cell phenotype, and inflammatory cytokines in chronic kidney disease patients under hemodialysis and its relationship to resistance to recombinant human erythropoietin therapy. J Clin Immunol (2008). , 28, 268-275.

[71] Costa, E, Rocha, S, Rocha-pereira, P, et al. Neutrophil activation and resistance to recombinant human erythropoietin therapy in hemodialysis patients. Am J Nephrol (2008). , 28, 935-940.

[72] Won, H. S, Kim, H. G, Yun, Y. S, et al. IL-6 is an independent risk factor for resistance to erythropoiesis-stimulating agents in hemodialysis patients without iron deficiency. Hemodial Int (2012). , 16, 31-37.

[73] Cooper, A. C, Mikhail, A, Lethbridge, M. W, Kemeny, D. M, & Macdougall, I. C. Increased expression of erythropoiesis inhibiting cytokines (IFN-gamma, TNF-alpha, IL-10, and IL-13) by T cells in patients exhibiting a poor response to erythropoietin therapy. J Am Soc Nephrol (2003). , 14, 1776-1784.

[74] Jeong, J. Y, Silver, M, Parnes, A, Nikiforow, S, Berliner, N, & Vanasse, G. J. Resveratrol ameliorates TNFalpha-mediated suppression of erythropoiesis in human CD34(+) cells via modulation of NF-kappaB signalling. Br J Haematol (2011). , 155, 93-101.

[75] Thawani, N, Tam, M, Chang, K. H, & Stevenson, M. M. Interferon-gamma mediates suppression of erythropoiesis but not reduced red cell survival following CpG-ODN administration in vivo. Exp Hematol (2006). , 34, 1451-1461.

[76] Chawla, L. S, & Krishnan, M. Causes and consequences of inflammation on anemia management in hemodialysis patients. Hemodial Int (2009). , 13, 222-234.

[77] La Ferla KReimann C, Jelkmann W, Hellwig-Burgel T. Inhibition of erythropoietin gene expression signaling involves the transcription factors GATA-2 and NF-kappaB. FASEB J (2002). , 16, 1811-1813.

[78] Munoz, M, Villar, I, & Garcia-erce, J. A. An update on iron physiology. World J Gastroenterol (2009). , 15, 4617-4626.

[79] Khankin, E. V, Mutter, W. P, Tamez, H, Yuan, H. T, Karumanchi, S. A, & Thadhani, R. Soluble erythropoietin receptor contributes to erythropoietin resistance in end-stage renal disease. PLoS One (2010). e9246.

[80] Inrig, J. K, Bryskin, S. K, Patel, U. D, Arcasoy, M, & Szczech, L. A. Association between high-dose erythropoiesis-stimulating agents, inflammatory biomarkers, and soluble erythropoietin receptors. BMC Nephrol (2011).

[81] Kulaksiz, H, Theilig, F, Bachmann, S, et al. The iron-regulatory peptide hormone hepcidin: expression and cellular localization in the mammalian kidney. J Endocrinol (2005). , 184, 361-370.

[82] Vokurka, M, Lacinova, Z, Kremen, J, et al. Hepcidin expression in adipose tissue increases during cardiac surgery. Physiol Res (2010). , 59, 393-400.

[83] Hanninen, M. M, Haapasalo, J, Haapasalo, H, et al. Expression of iron-related genes in human brain and brain tumors. BMC Neurosci (2009).

[84] Merle, U, Fein, E, Gehrke, S. G, Stremmel, W, & Kulaksiz, H. The iron regulatory peptide hepcidin is expressed in the heart and regulated by hypoxia and inflammation. Endocrinology (2007). , 148, 2663-2668.

[85] Isoda, M, Hanawa, H, Watanabe, R, et al. Expression of the peptide hormone hepcidin increases in cardiomyocytes under myocarditis and myocardial infarction. J Nutr Biochem (2010). , 21, 749-756.

[86] Malyszko, J, & Mysliwiec, M. Hepcidin in anemia and inflammation in chronic kidney disease. Kidney Blood Press Res (2007). , 30, 15-30.

[87] Mena, N. P, Esparza, A, Tapia, V, Valdes, P, & Nunez, M. T. Hepcidin inhibits apical iron uptake in intestinal cells. Am J Physiol Gastrointest Liver Physiol (2008). G, 192-198.

[88] Brasse-lagnel, C, Karim, Z, Letteron, P, Bekri, S, Bado, A, & Beaumont, C. Intestinal DMT1 cotransporter is down-regulated by hepcidin via proteasome internalization and degradation. Gastroenterology (2011). e1261., 140, 1261-1271.

[89] De Domenico, I, Ward, D. M, Langelier, C, et al. The molecular mechanism of hepcidin-mediated ferroportin down-regulation. Mol Biol Cell (2007). , 18, 2569-2578.

[90] De Domenico, I, Lo, E, Yang, B, et al. The role of ubiquitination in hepcidin-independent and hepcidin-dependent degradation of ferroportin. Cell Metab (2011). , 14, 635-646.

[91] Zaritsky, J, Young, B, Gales, B, et al. Reduction of serum hepcidin by hemodialysis in pediatric and adult patients. Clin J Am Soc Nephrol (2010). , 5, 1010-1014.

[92] Stefansson, B. V, Abramson, M, Nilsson, U, & Haraldsson, B. Hemodiafiltration improves plasma 25-hepcidin levels: a prospective, randomized, blinded, cross-over study comparing hemodialysis and hemodiafiltration. Nephron Extra (2012). , 2, 55-65.

[93] Nemeth, E, Valore, E. V, Territo, M, Schiller, G, Lichtenstein, A, & Ganz, T. Hepcidin, a putative mediator of anemia of inflammation, is a type II acute-phase protein. Blood (2003). , 101, 2461-2463.

[94] Nemeth, E, Rivera, S, Gabayan, V, et al. IL-6 mediates hypoferremia of inflammation by inducing the synthesis of the iron regulatory hormone hepcidin. J Clin Invest (2004). , 113, 1271-1276.

[95] Song, S. N, Tomosugi, N, Kawabata, H, Ishikawa, T, Nishikawa, T, & Yoshizaki, K. Down-regulation of hepcidin resulting from long-term treatment with an anti-IL-6 receptor antibody (tocilizumab) improves anemia of inflammation in multicentric Castleman disease. Blood (2010). , 116, 3627-3634.

[96] Kato, A. Increased hepcidin-25 and erythropoietin responsiveness in patients with cardio-renal anemia syndrome. Future Cardiol (2010). , 6, 769-771.

[97] Park, C. H, Valore, E. V, Waring, A. J, & Ganz, T. Hepcidin, a urinary antimicrobial peptide synthesized in the liver. J Biol Chem (2001). , 276, 7806-7810.

[98] European Uremic Toxin (EUTox) Work Group of the ESAO and ERA-EDTAhttp:// www.uremic-toxins.org/accessed 19 June (2012).

[99] Al-hilali, N, Al-humoud, H, Ninan, V. T, Nampoory, M. R, Puliyclil, M. A, & Johny, K. V. Does parathyroid hormone affect erythropoietin therapy in dialysis patients? Med Princ Pract (2007). , 16, 63-67.

[100] Kalantar-zadeh, K, Lee, G. H, Miller, J. E, et al. Predictors of hyporesponsiveness to erythropoiesis-stimulating agents in hemodialysis patients. Am J Kidney Dis (2009). , 53, 823-834.

[101] Rao, D. S, Shih, M. S, & Mohini, R. Effect of serum parathyroid hormone and bone marrow fibrosis on the response to erythropoietin in uremia. N Engl J Med (1993). , 328, 171-175.

[102] Drueke, T. B, & Eckardt, K. U. Role of secondary hyperparathyroidism in erythropoietin resistance of chronic renal failure patients. Nephrol Dial Transplant (2002). Suppl , 5, 28-31.

[103] Brancaccio, D, Cozzolino, M, & Gallieni, M. Hyperparathyroidism and anemia in uremic subjects: a combined therapeutic approach. J Am Soc Nephrol (2004). Suppl 1:S, 21-24.

[104] Bohrer, D, Bertagnolli, D. C, De Oliveira, S. M, et al. Role of medication in the level of aluminium in the blood of chronic haemodialysis patients. Nephrol Dial Transplant (2009). , 24, 1277-1281.

[105] Yaqoob, M, Ahmad, R, Mcclelland, P, et al. Resistance to recombinant human erythropoietin due to aluminium overload and its reversal by low dose desferrioxamine therapy. Postgrad Med J (1993). , 69, 124-128.

[106] Fenwick, S, Roberts, E. A, Mahesh, B. S, & Roberts, N. B. In end-stage renal failure, does infection lead to elevated plasma aluminium and neurotoxicity? Implications for monitoring. Ann Clin Biochem (2005). , 42, 149-152.

[107] Yen, T. H, Lin, J. L, Lin-tan, D. T, & Hsu, C. W. Association between body mass and mortality in maintenance hemodialysis patients. Ther Apher Dial (2010). , 14, 400-408.

[108] Locatelli, F, Andrulli, S, Memoli, B, et al. Nutritional-inflammation status and resistance to erythropoietin therapy in haemodialysis patients. Nephrol Dial Transplant (2006). , 21, 991-998.

[109] Bowry, S. K, & Gatti, E. Impact of hemodialysis therapy on anemia of chronic kidney disease: the potential mechanisms. Blood Purif (2011). , 32, 210-219.

[110] Locatelli, F, Altieri, P, Andrulli, S, et al. Predictors of haemoglobin levels and resistance to erythropoiesis-stimulating agents in patients treated with low-flux haemo-

dialysis, haemofiltration and haemodiafiltration: results of a multicentre randomized and controlled trial. Nephrol Dial Transplant (2012).

[111] Carrero, J. J, Barany, P, Yilmaz, M. I, et al. Testosterone deficiency is a cause of anaemia and reduced responsiveness to erythropoiesis-stimulating agents in men with chronic kidney disease. Nephrol Dial Transplant (2012). , 27, 709-715.

[112] Stenvinkel, P, & Barany, P. Hypogonadism in males with chronic kidney disease: another cause of resistance to erythropoiesis-stimulating agents? Contrib Nephrol (2012). , 178, 35-39.

[113] Besarab, A, Bolton, W. K, Browne, J. K, et al. The effects of normal as compared with low hematocrit values in patients with cardiac disease who are receiving hemodialysis and epoetin. N Engl J Med (1998). , 339, 584-590.

[114] Singh, A. K, Szczech, L, Tang, K. L, et al. Correction of anemia with epoetin alfa in chronic kidney disease. N Engl J Med (2006). , 355, 2085-2098.

[115] Mcmurray, J. J, Uno, H, Jarolim, P, et al. Predictors of fatal and nonfatal cardiovascular events in patients with type 2 diabetes mellitus, chronic kidney disease, and anemia: an analysis of the Trial to Reduce cardiovascular Events with Aranesp (darbepoetin-alfa) Therapy (TREAT). Am Heart J (2011). e743., 162, 748-755.

[116] Santos, P. R, Melo, A. D, Lima, M. M, et al. Mortality risk in hemodialysis patients according to anemia control and erythropoietin dosing. Hemodial Int (2011). , 15, 493-500.

[117] Strippoli, G. F. Effects of the dose of erythropoiesis stimulating agents on cardiovascular events, quality of life, and health-related costs in hemodialysis patients: the clinical evaluation of the dose of erythropoietins (C.E. DOSE) trial protocol. Trials (2010).

[118] Fishbane, S, & Besarab, A. Mechanism of increased mortality risk with erythropoietin treatment to higher hemoglobin targets. Clin J Am Soc Nephrol (2007). , 2, 1274-1282.

[119] Food and Drug AdministrationImportant Safety Advisory on Procrit, Aranesp and Epogen. http://www.accessdata.fda.gov/scripts/cdrh/cfdocs/psn/printer.cfm?id=516accessed 06 June (2012).

[120] KDOQI Clinical Practice Guideline and Clinical Practice Recommendations for anemia in chronic kidney disease: 2007 update of hemoglobin targetAm J Kidney Dis (2007). , 50, 471-530.

[121] Locatelli, F, Aljama, P, Canaud, B, et al. Target haemoglobin to aim for with erythropoiesis-stimulating agents: a position statement by ERBP following publication of the Trial to reduce cardiovascular events with Aranesp therapy (TREAT) study. Nephrol Dial Transplant (2010). , 25, 2846-2850.

[122] Food and Drug AdministrationFDA Drug Safety Communication: Modified dosing recommendations to improve the safe use of Erythropoiesis-Stimulating Agents

(ESAs) in chronic kidney disease. http://www.fda.gov/Drugs/DrugSafety/ucm259639.htmaccessed 06 June (2012).

[123] Fishbane, S, & Berns, J. S. Hemoglobin cycling in hemodialysis patients treated with recombinant human erythropoietin. Kidney Int (2005). , 68, 1337-1343.

Section 2

# New Developments in Dialysis Focused on Methods and Instruments

Chapter 4

# Advances in Hemodialysis Techniques

Ayman Karkar

Additional information is available at the end of the chapter

## 1. Introduction

Hemodialysis (HD) is a technique that is used to achieve the extracorporeal removal of waste products such as urea and creatinine and excess water from the blood when the kidneys are in a state of renal failure. HD is the most prevalent modality of renal replacement therapy for patients with kidney failure followed by kidney transplantation and peritoneal dialysis.

Hemodialysis treatment is provided for critically ill patients with acute kidney injury as in-patient therapy. More commonly, HD is routinely provided for stable patients with end-stage renal failure (ESRF) as an outpatient therapy conducted in a dialysis outpatient facility, either a purpose built room in a hospital or a dedicated stand-alone clinic. Less frequently HD is done at home, where it can be self-initiated and managed or done jointly with the assistance of a trained helper who is usually a family member.

The principle of HD is the same as other methods of dialysis; it involves diffusion of solutes across a semipermeable membrane. HD utilizes counter current flow, where the dialysate is flowing in the opposite direction to blood flow in the extracorporeal circuit. Counter-current flow maintains the concentration gradient across the membrane at a maximum and increases the efficiency of the dialysis. Fluid removal (ultrafiltration) is achieved by altering the hydrostatic pressure of the dialysate compartment, causing free water and some dissolved solutes to move across the membrane along a created pressure gradient. Urea, creatinine and other waste products, potassium, and phosphate diffuse into the dialysis solution. However, concentrations of sodium and chloride in the dialysate solution are similar to those of normal plasma to prevent loss. Sodium bicarbonate is added into dialysate in a higher concentration than plasma to correct blood acidity. A small amount of glucose may also be added to dialysate solution [1].

This chapter will focus on the recent advances in HD techniques, and illustrate and compare the different HD modalities that can achieve a better quality of life than the conventional HD treatment.

## 2. Background

Conventional HD remains the main modality of renal replacement therapy for patients with end-stage renal disease (ESRD) worldwide [1-5]. The technique of conventional HD is based on the physiologic principle of *"diffusion"*, which means clearance or removal of high concentration of uremic toxins (in the blood) to the lower concentration solution (dialysate) through a semi-permeable membrane (the dialyzer or filter) [6]. Conventional HD is usually conducted over four hour duration three times per week for stable patients with ESRD. The dialyzer or filter used is usually of low-flux type, and the filtered molecules are water-soluble small-size (molecular weight< 500 Dalton) compounds.

Conventional HD treatment had over many years improved the survival rate of patients with ESRD [2] (figure 1a, 1b). However, this basic modality of dialysis is far from replacing the function of the normal kidneys. In fact, conventional HD prescription provides only about 10% of the clearance power of the natural kidneys [7]. Although it is capable of removing excess water and small size uremic toxins, yet conventional HD is not capable of removing middle and large size (>500 Dalton) and protein-bound toxic molecules [8]. These middle- and large-size molecules, which cannot be cleared and could be harmful, include $\beta_2$-microglobulin ($\beta_2$-M), which is strongly associated with carpal tunnel syndrome and dialysis-related amyloidosis [9], and pro-inflammatory cytokines and severe vasoactive molecules such as p-cresol and uridine adenosine tetraphosphate (table 1). The accumulation and retention of all types and sizes of uremic compounds (and excess water), which have concentration-dependent toxicity, leads to increased morbidity and mortality. Furthermore, the unphysiologic pattern of conventional intermittent HD (three times per week) with rapid change in fluid volume and electrolytes and uremic solutes serum concentrations results in permanent disequilibrium of internal milieu and inter and intra-dialysis complications [10].

Conventional HD has been associated with frequent intradialysis complications (hypotension, sickness and cramps) and post-dialysis complaints of headache, fatigue and inability to concentrate and function, which may impair significantly the quality of life, result in poor compliance, inconsistency in achieving HD prescription and inadequacy of HD sessions. Inadequate HD is mainly due to poor compliance and non-adherence to HD regimens (e.g. fluid restriction, regular attendance of dialysis sessions and adherence to four hours session) and the clearance limitations of the conventional HD technique. It has been shown that skipping at least one dialysis session is associated with a 25%-30% increase in the risk of death [4]. Moreover, even patients attending regular HD sessions are at increased risk of death, heart attacks and hospital admissions (for myocardial infarction, congestive heart failure, dysrhythmia and stroke) on the day after the two-day interval between HD treatments each week than at other times [11]. Inadequate HD delivery also has cost implications as a consequence of increased hospitalization rate; days stay at hospital and inpatient expenditures [12].

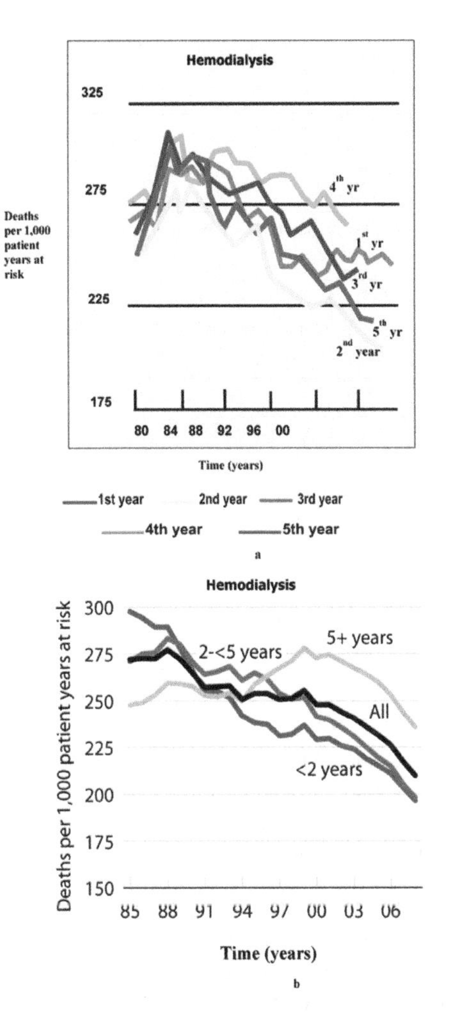


**Figure 1. a:** The undeniable clinical progress in hemodialysis reflected by the significant drop in mortality rates in incident ESRD patients from 1980-2010. *U.S. Renal Data System, the data supplied by the United States Renal Data System (USRDS): 2010 Annual Data Report: Atlas of End-Stage Renal Disease in the United States, National Institutes of Health, National Institute of Diabetes and Digestive and Kidney Diseases, Bethesda, MD, 2010.* **b:** The undeniable clinical progress in hemodialysis reflected by the significant drop in mortality rates in incident ESRD patients from 1980-2010. *U.S. Renal Data System, the data supplied by the United States Renal Data System (USRDS): 2010 Annual Data Report: Atlas of End-Stage Renal Disease in the United States, National Institutes of Health, National Institute of Diabetes and Digestive and Kidney Diseases, Bethesda, MD, 2010.*

| Small Water Soluble Molecules (MW <500 Daltons) | Middle Molecules (MW >500 Daltons) | Protein-Bound Molecules (MW >500 Daltons)* |
|---|---|---|
| Sodium (23) | Adrenomedullin (6032) (potent hypotensive peptide) | Hippuric acid (insulin resistance and glucose intolerance) |
| Phosphorus (31) | AGE* | Homocystein (atherogenecity and thrombogenecity) |
| Potassium (35) | AOP* | Indoxyl sulfate (pro-inflammatory effect & endothelial dysfunction) |
| Urea (60) | Vitamin B12 (1355) | - *p*-cresylsulfate – *p*-cresol (endothelial and pro-inflammatory) |
| Creatinine (113) | Endothelin (4238) (strong vasoconstrictor) | Polyamines (inhibit erythroid colony growth in a dose-dependent way) |
| Uric acid (168) | PTH (9225) | |
| Glucose (180) | $\beta_2$-M (11800) | |
| | Leptin (16000) | |
| | Cytokines (15000-30000) | |
| | Immunoglobulin LC (28000 – 56000 Da) | |
| | Uridine adenosine tetraphosphate (very strong vasoconstrictive) | |

**Table 1.** Examples of types and sizes of different uremic toxic molecules.

Patients managed with conventional HD are potentially exposed to hemodynamic instability, excessive intradialytic weight gain, anemia, mineral and bone metabolism disorder, inadequate nutrition, infection and sexual and psychosocial problems. The increased risks of fatal and non-fatal cardiovascular complications, which are the main cause of death in HD patients, continue to be much higher than in the general population. It has been reported that only 32% to 33% of patients on conventional HD survive to the fifth year of treatment [13]. In fact, the mortality rate in conventional HD ranges between 14-26% in Europe [14, 15] and 24% in USA [1, 2]. Actually, conventional HD does support life but has failed to restore the patient to full functional normality and longevity.

Quality management of dialysis patients is best achieved by implementation of "pre-dialysis care" [16], and care improvement at "post dialysis" stage [17]. Post-dialysis care should ensure strict control of infection [18, 19] and predominance of arterio-venous fistula (avoidance of indwelling catheters for vascular access) [20]. Furthermore, dialysis care should include (1) adequate control of body fluids (achievement of euvolemic status), where strict volume control has been shown to reduce both morbidity and mortality and dialysis adequacy outcomes [21, 22], (2) mitigation of left ventricular hypertrophy and fibrosis, and (3) efficient removal of all types and different sizes of retained uremic toxic solutes that would result in inflammation and exacerbation of cardiovascular damage [20]. Actually, improvement in quality HD care should achieve optimum HD rather than adequate HD.

The aim of HD technique has, and will always be, to simulate or reproduce the physiologic process of glomerular ultrafiltration. Conventional HD, which is performed over 4 hour duration and conducted three times per week, does not fulfill this criterion [1]. The major deficiencies of this technique are limited solute clearance and volume control, which have been associated with poor quality of life [23] and unacceptable high rates of morbidity and mortality [2, 14, 15, 24, 25].

Over the past four decades it has been suggested that the accumulation of various 'uremic toxins', and in particular middle-size and protein-bound molecules, contribute to this increased mortality. These toxins include urea, phosphorus, parathyroid hormone (PTH), $\beta_2$-microglobulin, homocysteine, leptin and a variety of esoteric molecules such as advanced glycation end products, asymmetric dimethylarginine and advanced oxidation protein products [8, 26, 27]. Furthermore, the persistence of increased interdialytic weight gains and the limited ability of conventional HD to maintain adequate homeostasis, without frequent episodes of hypotension and increased risk for cardiovascular and all-cause mortality [28], results in failure of many HD patients to achieve adequate volume control and remain permanently volume overloaded [21]. This has been associated with increased prevalence of hypertension, left ventricular hypertrophy and increased cardiovascular mortality, as a major cause of death, among patients treated with conventional HD [21, 29].

Observational studies [30-35] and randomized controlled trials [36, 37] of improving the efficiency of hemodialysis, by increasing frequency and duration of HD treatment, demonstrated better clearance efficiency of uremic toxins and volume control, and improved quality of life. However, the recent innovations in HD technologies paved the way for better quality HD. These include higher specifications of HD machines, creation and improvement in dialysis membranes with different transport (clearance) capabilities of middle, large and even protein-bound molecules by using all the available membrane separation phenomena: diffusion, convection and adsorption, and quality improvement in the technology of water treatment plants, with almost nil presence of bacteria growth and endotoxin concentration. Based on different observational studies and randomized clinical trials and new innovations, this chapter illustrates the possible and available options of different advances in HD techniques, their influence on improving the adequacy of HD, the patient's quality of life and the reduction in morbidity and mortality rates.

## 3. Adequacy of hemodialysis

The adequacy of HD is usually assessed and measured by Kt/V [38]. This represents the product of clearance (K) per time multiplied by the duration (t) and adjusted for body size by dividing this clearance by the distribution volume (V). Kt/V reflects the clearance of urea, as a surrogate marker for the clearance of small, but not middle or large-sized, uremic toxins. The single-pool Kt/V overestimates the delivered dose of dialysis, because it fails to account for blood urea rebound after dialysis. A more accurate measure of the dialysis dose, the equilibrated Kt/V, corrects for urea rebound and is usually 0.15 to 0.20 lower than the single-pool Kt/V. Ideally, single-pool Kt/V should not be below 1.4, as lower values have been associated with increased morbidity and costs [12], and reduction in survival rate [39-41]. The efficacy of HD, where low flux dialyzers are usually used, is limited by its inability to clear from circulation the middle or large-size or protein-bound toxic molecules. Increasing the dose of dialysis or using high-flux dialyzer membrane can help in ensuring optimal values of Kt/V. However, the hemodialyis (HEMO) Study, which was a randomized clinical trial, did not alter survival or morbidity by increasing the dose of dialysis or using a high-flux dialyzer membrane [42].

Adequacy and efficiency of HD can be increased by avoiding intradialytic hypotension episodes and frequent interruption of the 4 hours HD session. This can be achieved, in part, by controlling intradialytic weight gain (<4%) by fluid intake and sodium restriction and lowering dialysate sodium concentration [43], and avoiding rapid ultrafiltration (not to exceed 10 ml/Kg/hr), where exceeding this limit has been associated with increased risk for cardiovascular and all-cause mortality [28, 29]. The adequacy and efficiency of HD can also be improved by increasing the blood [44-47] and dialysate [48, 49] flow rates and the dialyzer size and surface area [50, 51]. However, recent improvements in dialyzers technology, such as hollow fiber undulations, spacer yarns and changes in fiber packing density [52], have led to improvement in dialysate flow distribution through the dialysate compartment (with improved urea clearance) and reduced the need of increasing dialysate flow rate from 600 ml/min to 800 ml/min; an achievement with important economic impact allowing a significant reduction (25%) in water consumption [53].

## 4. Efficient hemodialysis

The efficiency of HD is largely dependent on arterial blood flow rate from a well-preserved and functioning vascular access [44-47]. The vascular access is the life-line for end-stage renal disease patients on regular hemodialysis. There are three major types of vascular access: arterio-venous fistula (AVF), arterio-venous graft (AVG) and central venous catheter (CVC). The type of vascular access is associated with patient outcome. Despite the recent improvement and advanced technology of catheters, temporary and permanent catheters have been associated with increased incidence of luminal thrombosis, central venous stenosis, inadequate blood flow rate, inadequate dialysis, increased risk of infection, increased risk of hospitalization, increased risk of death and high cost [54-61]. AVG has also been associated with bleeding, infection and graft failure. The KDIGO guidelines published in 2001 [62] defined the ideal vascular access as that which (a) delivers a flow rate adequate for the dialysis prescription, (b) has a long use-life, and (c) has a low rate of complications (infection, stenosis, thrombosis, aneurysm and limb ischemia). Although none of the major types of vascular access fulfills all of these criteria, the native AVF is the closest to this definition [62].

The "Fistula First Breakthrough Initiative" [63] was established in 2003, where a goal set to have 40% AVF use in prevalent US hemodialysis patients. This goal was achieved in 2005. The bar was subsequently raised to 66% AVF use, a level which was comparable to that achieved in several European countries [64]. The current USA prevalent AVF use rate by network is about 60% but incident AVF use rate by network is still below 20% [65]. DOPPS 4 of 2010 Study showed Australia, New Zealand and some European countries (France, Italy and Germany) have achieved more than 70% AVF use compared with Japan who achieved more than 90% [65].

## 5. Compatible hemodialysis

Dialyzer membranes used to be made primarily of cellulose (derived from cotton linter). The surface of such membranes was not very biocompatible, because exposed hydroxyl groups would activate complement in the blood passing by the membrane. More recently, membranes have been made from synthetic materials, using polymers such as polyarylethersulfone, polyamide, polyvinylpyrrolidone, polycarbonate, and polyacrylonitrile [66]. These synthetic membranes activate complement to a lesser degree than unsubstituted cellulose membranes. Synthetic membranes can be made in either low- or high-flux configuration, but most are high-flux. Nanotechnology is being used in some of the most recent high-flux membranes to create a uniform pore size. These recent innovations in the technology of dialysis membranes have resulted in improvement of their biocompatibility and anti-thrombotic effect, as well as in their hydraulic and perm selective properties [67].

The contact and interaction of blood with artificial surfaces within the extracorporeal circuit (dialyzer, needles, catheters, tubing, and the arterial and venous bubble traps) induces profound activation of plasmatic coagulation [68]. Further risk factors for clotting of the extracorporeal circuit include slow/turbulent blood flow, excessive ultrafiltration (due to hemoconcentration), high hematocrit, and blood transfusions into the extracorporeal circuit [69]. This non-physiological environment leads to activation of platelets, leukocytes, and the coagulation cascade, resulting in fouling of the membrane and ultimately in clotting of fibers and the whole hemodialyzer. As hemodialysis requires access to the circulatory system and the passage of blood in the blood lines and the dialyzer, anticoagulation is vital to maintain the in- and outflow of blood through the extracorporeal circuit and dialyzer without clotting. There have been different anticoagulants used to prevent thrombosis in the blood circuit. These include unfractionated heparin, low molecular-weight heparin, natural and synthetic heparinoids, direct thrombin inhibitors, prostanoids, saline flushes and citrate infusion or citrate based dialysate [70]. Heparin has been the most commonly used anticoagulant as it is generally well tolerated, easily administered, low cost, short biological half-life, and can be quickly reversed with protamine sulfate [69]. However, long-term use of heparin can expose hemodialysis patients to thrombocytopenia, hypertriglyceridemia, osteoporosis, hypersensitivity, alopecia, metabolic disturbances, and hypotension [70]. Furthermore, there are some patients at high risk of bleeding, where heparin cannot be used. The recent improvement and innovation in dialysis membranes have yielded high-flux membranes grafted with unfractionated heparin that can be used to avoid or reduce the exposure to systemic heparin [71].

## 6. High-flux hemodialysis

The creation of larger pore size semipermeable membranes in compact cartridges (high-flux dialyzers), with variable sizes of these pores, enhanced their ability to remove small solutes and 'middle molecules' [66]. High-flux dialyzers allow the passage and removal of retained solutes of higher molecular weight than do low-flux membranes. Dialyzers are considered as high-flux type if their ultrafiltration coefficient (KUF) exceeds 15 ml/h/mmHg and their ability to clear $\beta_2$-M exceeds 20 ml/min (low-flux dialyzer clears KUF <15 ml/h/mmHg and $\beta_2$-M < 10 ml/min) [50]. However, the fluids (dialysate and water) used with these high-flux dialyzers should be sterile non-pyrogenic and endotoxin free in order to avoid reverse filtration of endotoxins and blood contamination [72]. Microbiological contamination of water is a serious health concern for patients on dialysis. Therefore, it is essential to regularly monitor both bacteria and endotoxin levels in the water used for dialysis especially with high-flux dialyzers and for patients treated with online hemofiltration or hemodiafiltration.

Conventional and high efficiency HD techniques, using low-flux dialyzers, are incapable of removing larger sized uremic toxins and/or protein-bound toxic molecules of > 500 Dalton (table 1). This would result in their accumulation in circulation where they can exert concentration-dependent toxicity, particularly on endothelium and cardiovascular system. Examples of these molecules include uridine adenosine tetraphosphate and endothelin [27], which exert vasoconstrictive effect, indoxyl sulfate and p-cresylsulfate – p-cresol, which has pro-inflammatory effect and cause endothelial dysfunction together with the pro-inflammatory cytokines, and has been associated with increased cardiovascular mortality [73]. Other retained molecules which are known to cause harmful effects include $\beta_2$-M, immunoglobulin light chains, parathyroid hormone, advanced glycation end products [74] and advanced oxidation products [27, 75, 76].

Beta 2-microglobulin, which is considered a surrogate marker of middle molecules, is strongly associated with carpal tunnel syndrome and dialysis-related amyloidosis [77]. Different studies have documented the efficiency of high-flux dialyzers in removing $\beta_2$-M from the circulation of patients on dialysis, which has been associated with clinical and radiological improvement of carpal tunnel syndrome and dialysis-related amyloidosis [78]. In addition, high-flux HD has been shown to be superior to peritoneal dialysis in clearing $\beta_2$-M and the protein-bound middle molecule p-cresol [71]. Furthermore, observational studies have documented the improvement of survival rates of patients on high-flux-dialyzers when compared with those on low-flux dialyzers [9, 79-82]. These findings have been confirmed by two large randomized clinical trials: the HEMO study and the MPO study. In the entire cohort in the HEMO Study the high-flux arm had no significant effect on the all-cause mortality rate or any of the four arm secondary outcomes. However, the high-flux HD provided significantly less cardiac and cerebrovascular mortality rates after 3.7 years HD than low-flux HD [42, 83, 84]. The Membrane Permeability Outcome (MPO) study, which was conducted in Europe, showed higher survival rate in high-flux HD patients with low serum albumin (≤ 4 g/dl) and diabetic patients [85]. Following these two major studies, the European Best Practice Guidelines have recommended the use of high-flux dialyzers in patients at high risk (serum albumin < 4 g/dl) and even in low-risk patients [86]. Ever since, high-flux dialysis has surpassed low-flux use worldwide [87].

## 7. Super high-flux hemodialysis

New 'super high-flux' membranes for hemodialysis have been developed with a high cut-off pore size allowing efficient removal of middle and large size uremic toxin molecules that cannot be removed by conventional dialysis membranes. The recent availability of a new generation of hemodialysis membranes with molecular weight cut-offs closer to that of the native kidney (65000 Dalton) has led to great benefits in several different clinical settings. These membranes have shown efficient removal of myoglobin in patients with rhabdomyolysis [88], efficient and direct removal of free light chains and other plasma components [89], and greater clearance of inflammatory cytokines than conventional high-flux membranes [90]. They also have a positive impact on restoration of immune cell function, attenuation of hemodynamic instability and decrease in plasma interleukin-6 levels in septic patients with acute kidney injury [91]. However, albumin loss may be a disadvantage of these membranes, though albumin losses can be replaced by infusion of human albumin solution [90].

## 8. Adsorption hemodialysis

Despite the efficiency of removing middle-size uremic toxin molecules by high-flux HD, yet this technique is still incapable of removing larger-size and, more importantly, the protein-bound uremic toxins. Protein-bound uremic toxins are, in fact, small in size but become larger molecular weight compounds (50,000 – 200,000 Dalton) once are bound to different types of proteins depending on their binding affinity. Protein-bound uremic toxins have been potentially involved in important uremia co-morbidities such as itching and altered immune response caused by the retained and deposited free molecules (κ-type and λ-type) of the immunoglobulin light chain in internal organs [92-95].

Removing protein-bound uremic toxins from the blood by means of diffusion and convection is virtually impracticable. The technology of dialysis membranes have yielded thicker type of membranes (more than conventional 1 micron thickness) that have a great affinity to stick larger size molecules to their surfaces, hence known as adsorptive membranes [96]. Adsorption can occur at the outer surface of the membrane when molecules cannot pass through the pores of the membrane and/or within the inner membrane matrix when the molecules can permeate the membrane [97]. Synthetic membrane micro porous zeolite silica lite (MFI) has been shown to be quite effective in adsorbing high levels of the protein-bound solute P-cresol [98], which is not eliminated efficiently by conventional HD. Furthermore, the synthetic thick polymethylmethacrylate (PMMA) membranes (30 micron thickness), which have good solute permeability and a high degree of biocompatibility, do have high adsorptive capacity reaching up to 160,000 Dalton [99].

Recent studies have shown a variety of efficient clinical implications for adsorption HD. The use of PMMA membranes has been shown to ameliorate the severity and frequency of pruritis [95] in HD patients due to adsorption of a 160,000 Dalton molecular weight molecule with stimulatory effect on mast cells [100]. PMMA membranes also efficiently adsorb $\beta_2$-M (representative of middle molecules), where they have been shown to improve carpal tunnel syndrome or total joint pain score in HD patients [99]. In addition, patients dialyzed with PMMA membrane have lower need for erythropoietin due to the elimination of an inhibitor of erythropoesis retrieved in the dialysate [101]. Furthermore, the free molecules ($\kappa$-type and $\lambda$-type) of the immunoglobulin light chain (Bence Jones protein), which accumulate at high levels in the blood of HD patients [102] may lead to various protein deposits in the internal organs and act as inhibitors of leukocyte and immune function in dialysis patients. These molecules, which usually exist as dimmers (56,000 Dalton) and not removed by high-flux HD, are significantly removed by HD with PMMA membrane [103] in patients with primary amyloidosis [104] and in patients on HD resulting in reduction in pain and frequency in analgesic treatment [105]. In addition, PMMA (BK-F) membranes have been shown to be quite effective in removing soluble CD40 from circulation of patients on HD. Soluble CD40, which mostly coexists as dimeric and even higher oligomerized forms of 50,000 and 150,000 Dalton, respectively [106], acts as natural antagonist of the CD40/CD40L contact [92, 106, 107] and have been associated with a lack of response to hepatitis B vaccination. The efficient removal of these molecules by PMMA membranes have been associated with improved response to hepatitis B immunization [94].

Finally, adsorption techniques have been used successfully, in conjunction with plasma filtration and hemofiltration, in clearing efficiently pro-inflammatory mediators in experimental animals [108] and in humans with acute kidney injury and sepsis [109]. This is known as "coupled plasma filtration adsorption" (CPFA) technique, where the treatment consists of the separation of plasma from the whole blood, using a plasma filter with high cutoff membrane of 800,000 Dalton, coupled with adsorption of the inflammatory mediators and cytokines from plasma, using a cartridge contains hydrophobic resins, followed by hemofiltration using a hemofilter.

## 9. Frequent hemodialysis

A significant improvement in efficiency of HD can be achieved by increasing the duration and frequency of dialysis sessions [110]. Different studies have confirmed that dialysis duration of less than 4 hours was associated with increased mortality rate by up to 42% [24, 25, 29]. By contrast, increasing the duration of dialysis, independent of blood or dialysate flow rates, to 8 hours has been associated with significant improvement in clearance of urea, creatinine, phosphorus, uric acid and even $\beta_2$-M, but not much of protein-bound toxic molecules [29, 111, 112].

Another approach to improve the efficiency of HD is by increasing the frequency of HD sessions. This can be achieved by avoiding the two days weekend gap and implementation of in-center every other day dialysis [11, 113]. A recent study of analyzing records of 32,000 people receiving dialysis three times a week from 2005 through 2008 found a 22% greater risk of death on the day after a long break, compared with other days. In particular, stroke and heart-related hospitalizations more than doubled on the days after the long break [11]. The efficiency of HD can also be improved by short daily dialysis [30, 34, 36, 111, 114], long slow nocturnal dialysis [32, 33] or home daily or nocturnal HD [35, 51], instead of three HD sessions per week.

Home, and in particular nocturnal, HD is probably the most convenient and efficient modality of HD. It can be performed on daily basis or at night at most suitable times, where the patient on nocturnal HD dialyzes for about twice the time (approximately eight hours per session) of conventional in-center HD sessions. This ensures a better chance that the patient will not be under-dialyzed; therefore, more toxins and fluids may be removed. Because this process occurs more slowly, there is less of a chance of cramping and hypotension episodes during dialysis [35]. Unlike conventional HD, patients on nocturnal HD do not report the "washed out" feeling after longer dialysis (no need to take a nap after treatment). Different studies have repeatedly confirmed the strong positive impact of nocturnal or more frequent dialysis on ultrafiltration rate (much better control of fluid excess), clearance of uremic toxins and adequacy of dialysis [36]. The better ultrafiltration rate has been associated with better control of blood pressure [33, 36, 37], where the majority of dialysis patients discontinued antihypertensive medications after 6-12 months of daily/nocturnal dialysis [30, 115]. Increasing dialysis frequency, and in particular nocturnal HD, has also been linked to significant improvement in renal anemia [31, 116] and reduction in erythropoietin dosage and iron supplements [115], significant reduction in left ventricular mass index [33, 36, 117], improvement in mineral metabolism and significant reduction in phosphorus binders [33, 36, 37, 114], improvement in nutritional status [30, 118], enhanced quality of life [33, 36, 119] and increased cumulative survival rate [34]. Moreover, patients on nocturnal HD have a similar survival rate as that in deceased kidney transplant recipients [120].

Despite its great benefits (Table 2), the implementation of daily/nocturnal HD has not gained much attraction among patients, treating physicians and decision makers. Kjellstrand et al [34] contributed the slow and difficult introduction of daily dialysis to multiple factors including logistic problems, conservatism by physicians and nurses, patient worries and worries about expenses by governments and administrators, which is expected to be a major obstacle. However, the clinical and quality of life improvement brought by daily/nocturnal HD has been associated with dose reduction in different pharmaceutical medications (antihypertensive medications, phosphorus binders and erythropoetin dosage and iron supplements), extended use of dialyzers and tubing and decreased waste production and transportation upon implementation of home HD, and significant reduction in hospitalization and morbidity (and mortality) rates, all of which may result in reduction in management costs and total annual expenses [32, 119]. A recent economic assessment model for in-center, conventional home and more frequent home HD has shown that home-based conventional and more frequent HD are similar in cost to in-center HD in the first year but can be less costly than in-center HD from the second year onward [121]. The higher cost for more frequent home HD in first year is mainly due to higher consumables usage due to dialysis frequency. Frequent home HD (and conventional home HD), however, have been associated with much lower hospitalization costs than for in-center HD treated patients in first and subsequent years.

| | |
|---|---|
| 1 | Improved uremic toxins and fluid removal |
| 2 | Less cramping and no "washout" feeling |
| 3 | Less hypotension episodes, better blood pressure control, less antihypertensive drugs |
| 4 | Improvement in anemia, reduction in EPO dose and iron supplements |
| 5 | Reduction in left ventricular mass index |
| 6 | Improvement in mineral metabolism and reduction in phosphorus binders |
| 7 | Improvement in nutritional status |
| 8 | Enhanced quality of life |
| 9 | Reduction in hospitalization rates and costs |
| 10 | Increased cumulative survival rate |

**Table 2.** Benefits of Frequent (Daily/Nocturnal) Hemodialysis

## 10. Hemofiltration and hemodiafiltration

Attempts to increase the intensity or "dose" of HD with higher blood and dialysate flow rates, larger and adsorptive membranes and longer and more frequent dialysis sessions have improved the adequacy of HD, but failed to bring about the desired improvement in outcome [36, 37, 42, 83-85]. Recent innovations in the HD techniques have resulted in advancements in specifications of HD machines, HD medical devices, sterile ultrapure solutions and high quality water treatment plants [122]. These advancements have largely contributed to the ability to reconsider the implementation of the other physiologic principle of "convection" [123, 124]. This means that larger size uremic toxins can be dragged and removed from blood by filtering large volume of fluid pushed under high hydrostatic pressure through a larger pore size membrane (high cut-off membrane/high-flux dialyzer). This technique is known as "hemofiltration". Fluid balance is maintained by infusion of replacement solutions, which can be administered before the filter (pre-dilution) or after the filter (post-dilution). These solutions are infused directly into blood in order to replace the large volume of filtered fluids (convection volume). The replacement solutions, which also referred to as substitution fluid, are mixed with the blood and should, therefore, be sterile non-pyrogenic and endotoxin free buffered solutions with a composition similar to plasma water. Combination of the two physiologic principles of diffusion (hemodialysis) and convection (hemofiltration) in the management of patients with ESRD is known as "hemodiafiltration" [6]; a technique that has been described and implemented in 1974 [123] and a treatment modality that simulate to a large extent the natural function of a normal kidney.

## 11. Online hemodiafiltration

The implementation of hemofiltration (HF) or hemodialfiltration (HDF) as a renal replacement therapy in patients with ESRD requires the supply of large quantities of replacement solutions. These solutions are usually industrially prepared in autoclaved expensive plastic bags, which have been used in earlier studies, in order to fulfill the requirement of sterile non-pyrogenic and endotoxin free buffered solutions [125]. However, the need of large quantities of these bags makes the implementation of this technique rather costly and impractical. The recent advancement and improvement in the performance of water treatment plants that are capable of producing ultrapure water (almost nil bacterial growth and endotoxin free) have greatly contributed to the success of this technique [15, 126]. Such quality of water, which is available continuously and in unlimited amounts at the dialysis machine during each treatment, has been used directly from the water treatment plant to form the dialysate and the replacing solutions for the HDF [125], and hence this technique is known as "online hemodiafiltration" [127].

Online HDF offers the most physiologic clearance profile for a broad range of small, medium-sized and large toxic molecules (table 1). Like conventional HD, online HDF session is usually performed three times per week as an outpatient treatment that usually lasts for four hours. Prescription of effective online HDF should ensure higher blood and dialysate flow rates, ultrafiltration not less than 20% depending on the mode of HDF (it differs between post and pre-dilution HDF), and substitution/replacement fluids 5-25 liters/session. Earlier studies defined replacement fluids of 5–14.9 liters/session as low-efficiency HDF, and replacement fluids of 15–24.9 or more liters/session as high-efficiency HDF [15, 112]. However, the data from recent randomized controlled studies: CONTRAST [128, 129] and Turkish [130] studies suggested a convection volume higher than 15 liters in the post-dilution mode should be targeted in order to achieve successful HDF.

The implementation of both physiologic principles of diffusion and convection has enabled HDF, and in particular online HDF, over that of HD (low- and high-flux) in achieving better adequacy of dialysis and better clearance of small and middle-size uremic toxins [131]. In clinical practice, HDF (low- and high-efficiency) has been shown to be more effective than HD (low-flux and high-flux) in achieving significantly higher values of Kt/V (averages of 1.37 and 1.44 versus 1.35 and 1.33, respectively) [15].

Hyperphosphatemia, which has been associated with vascular calcification and considered as an independent predictor of mortality in dialysis patients [132], has been well controlled with efficient removal of phosphorus by online HDF [113, 129, 133] with marked reduction in phosphate binders [113]. Furthermore, the reduction ratio of $\beta_2$-M per session has been shown to be 20–30% higher with online HDF than with high-flux HD (72.7 versus 49.7%) [134]. Likewise, online high-efficiency HDF achieves higher serum free light chain removal than high-flux HD in multiple myeloma patients [135]. In addition, HDF is highly efficient in clearing other larger solutes such as myoglobin (16000 Dalton), retinol-binding protein (25000 Dalton) and the protein-bound p-cresol than high-flux HD [131, 136]. It has also been shown that online HDF efficiently reduces the circulating levels of advanced glycation-end products [74, 137]. The efficient removal of different types and sizes of uremic toxins by online HDF [138] has been associated with reduction of skin pigmentation [139], promotion of catch-up growth in children on chronic dialysis [140] and nutritional status improvement [141]. More recently, Maduell et al [113] have demonstrated a remarkable improvement in nutritional status with adequate social and occupational rehabilitation.

Online HDF is empowered with biocompatible high-cut-off membranes, ultrapure water and efficiency of removal of pro-inflammatory stimuli including oxidative stress molecules, advanced glycation end-products, homocysteine [142], p-cresol and pro-inflammatory cytokines, all of which would ensure abolishing virtually the possibility of stimulation of an inflammatory process in dialysis patients [124]. This effect of online HDF, at least in part, has been shown to improve the patients' responsiveness to erythropoetin and reduce the requirement of erythropoietin stimulating agents [143].

Hemodiafiltration, and in particular online HDF, had attracted much attention in recent years as a promising optimum modality of HD [144]. In addition to its efficient improvement in dialysis adequacy and clearing small and large-size uremic toxins [145], HDF significantly reduced inter-dialysis symptoms including less fatigue and cramps together with effective correction of intradialytic haemodynamic instability and blood pressure control [146, 147], especially for elderly, heart-compromised or patients prone to hypotension. A recent study by Maduell et al [113], where high volume (high efficiency) online HDF combined with more frequent (every-other-day nocturnal 7-8 hours) dialysis sessions, showed marked improvement in hypertension control with a substantial reduction in drug requirements and regression of left ventricular hypertrophy; an independent cardiovascular risk factor which has been associated with mortality in dialysis patients [148, 149].

Finally, observational studies have shown the benefit of online HDF in decreasing the mortality rate in patients on dialysis [150, 151]. Canaud et al [15] reported a significant 35% lower mortality risk with high-efficiency HDF compared to low-flux HD. Jirka et al [151] also observed a 35.3% reduction rate in mortality risk in online HDF-treated patients after adjustment for age, co-morbidities, and time on dialysis. More recently, in a randomized clinical trial the subgroup of HDF patients treated with a substitution volume over 17.4 liter per session (n=195), cardiovascular and overall survival were better than both the HDF subgroup with substitution volume ≤17.4 liter per session (n=196) (p=0.03) and the HD group (p=0.002). Primary outcome was similar in these 3 groups (85.2%, 83.8% and 81.2%, respectively, p=0.26). In adjusted Cox-regression analysis, HDF with substitution volume over 17.4 L was associated with a 46% risk reduction for overall mortality [RR=0.54 (95% CI 0.31-0.93), p=0.02] and a 71% risk reduction for cardiovascular mortality [RR=0.29 (95% CI 0.12-0.65), p=0.003] compared to HD [130].

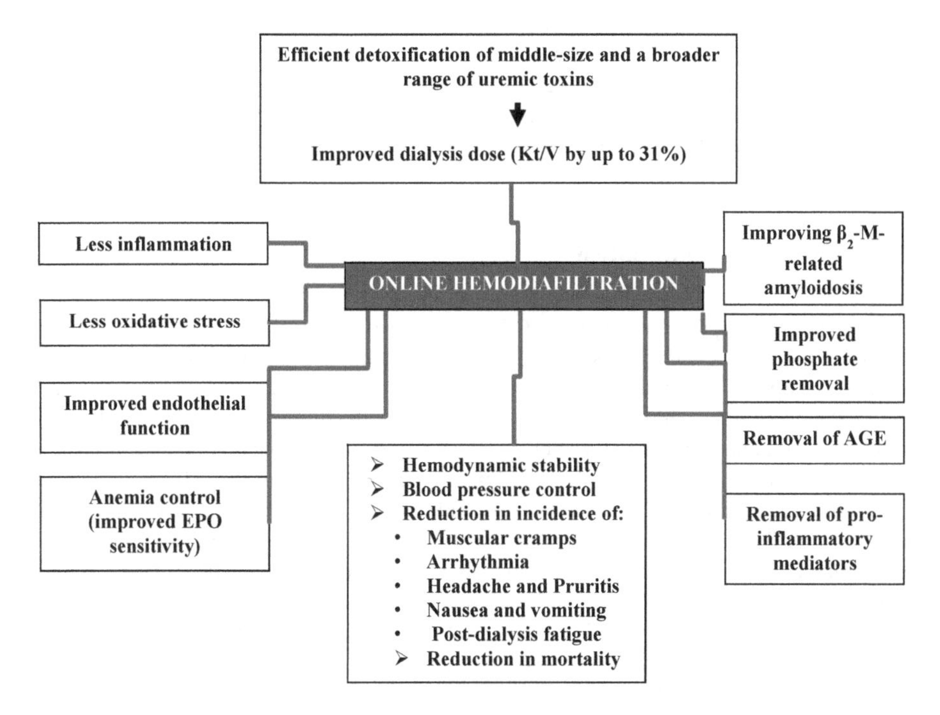


**Figure 2.** Benefits of online hemodiafiltration EPO: Erythropoetin, $\beta_2$-M: Beta 2-microglobulin, AGE: Advanced glycation end-product

The performance, success and benefits of online HDF (figure 2), however, depends on availability of special requirements. These include (1) experienced nephrologists and nursing staff, (2) high quality water treatment plant that can provide ultrapure water (bacterial growth < 0.1 colony factor unit/ml and endotoxin level < 0.03 endotoxin unit/ml) with frequent assessment of water quality [152-154], (3) dialysis machine specially designed and approved for online fluid preparation, (4) high-flux dialyzers and (5) good functioning vascular access with adequate blood flow. These essential requirements for ensuring successful online HDF therapy may incur extra costs and may limit its widespread implementation. However, training of medical and nursing staff is achievable, high flux dialyzers have already be recommended and in use in conventional HD with lower cost, different quality online HD machines are becoming cheaper and more affordable, and investing in quality ultrapure water treatment plant should not be a major barrier toward implementation of this premium modality of HD. In fact, investing in these requirements would not only improve the quality of life of dialysis patients but reduce the rates of morbidity and mortality. Furthermore, additional savings can be achieved by (1) reduction in the costs associated with hospitalization due to high morbidity rate of conventional HD [12, 155], (2) less requirements of phosphate binders due to better clearance of phosphorus [114], (3) better control of hypertension with less use of antihypertensive drugs [114], (4) less doses required of erythropoietin stimulating agents (ESA) and iron supplements, due to improved sensitivity to ESA as a result of abolishing or reducing the inflammatory response [125], and (5) improved hemodynamic stability, with no or less frequent hypotension episodes [114, 147], and consequently less consumption of normal saline and human serum albumin.

## 12. Continuous hemodialysis

Continuous renal replacement therapy (CRRT) is defined as "any extracorporeal blood purification therapy intended to substitute for impaired renal function over an extended period of time and applied for or aimed at being applied for 24hrs/day" [156]. CRRT modalities include slow continuous ultrafiltration (SCUF), continuous HD, continuous hemofiltration (HF), and continuous hemodiafiltration (HDF) [157]. SCUF technique is based on passing the blood through the dialyzer without dialysate or replacement fluids, and is basically used to remove excess body fluids as in patients with congestive heart failure and pulmonary edema [158]. The technique of continuous HD is similar in principle to that of intermittent/ conventional HD except that it is continuously applied for a longer period of time and at slower blood (100-200 ml/minute) and dialysate (40-70 ml/minute) flow rates. The techniques of hemofiltration (HF), which is based on the physiological principle of convection (dialysate is not used but replacement fluids) and hemodiafiltration (HDF), which based on the physiological principles of diffusion and convection (both dialysate and replacement fluids are used), are the same as those described earlier in this chapter, but are applied in continuous format and over a long period of time [159]. These techniques/modalities of CRRT are usually applied and used for critically ill patients with septic acute kidney injury and/or multi-organ failure in intensive care units. Other indications include cardiopulmonary bypass, fulminant hepatic failure, rhabdomyolysis, respiratory distress syndrome, severe burns, cerebral oedema, and tumor lysis syndrome [160]. The dialysis dose effect in these treatment modalities is assessed by adequacy and efficiency of fluid balance (and replacement/effluent fluids volume in HF/HDF), electrolyte balance, acid-base balance, and removal of small and middle-size uremic toxins [161]. Although expensive, these modalities provide smooth dialysis without fluctuation, hemodynamic/cardiovascular stability, improved fluid balance, removal of inflammatory mediators, allow supportive measures (nutrition), steady biochemical correction, and possibly improve survival rate [162, 163]. The disadvantages of these techniques include necessity for continuous anticoagulation, hypothermia, severe depletion of electrolytes (particularly potassium and phosphorus), where care is not taken, immobilization of the patient, possible side effects from lactate-containing replacement fluid or dialysate, 24 hour staffing (well trained and dedicated staff) and increased cost [160].

## 13. Slow low-efficiency hemodialysis

This slow low-efficiency dialysis (SLED) technique combines both intermittent and continuous modalities of HD [164]. It is based on providing intermittent/conventional HD but with low blood and dialysate flow rates (100-200 ml/minute) and for longer period of time usually 8-12 hours per session usually for 5 or 6 days per week [165]. SLED technique provides a gentle reduction of small solutes clearances over prolonged periods with an efficacy comparable to that of conventional intermittent HD and continuous hemofiltration [166, 167]. It has been considered an ideal technique of HD for critically ill patients with multi-organ failure and acute kidney injury in intensive care unit (ICU). SLED technique has several advantages which include easy-to-perform treatment, flexible timing of treatment (nocturnal SLED has the benefits of unrestricted physician access to the patient during the day and minimizing the interference of renal replacement therapy with other ICU activities), reduced costs [164], and hemodynamic/cardiovascular stability [168].

In conclusion, conventional or standard HD remains a valuable and basic life-supporting treatment for ESRD patients. This modality had over many years improved the survival rate of patients with end-stage renal disease. However, standard or conventional HD prescription is far from being optimal in replacing the function of normal kidneys. Its unphysiologic clearance pattern and inability to remove all types and sizes of uremic toxins results in inter and intra-dialysis complications and an unacceptable high rate of cardiovascular morbidity and mortality. The efficiency of HD can be improved by increasing blood and dialysate flow rates, the dialyzer size and surface area, and by increasing the duration and frequency of dialysis sessions. Home HD, where short daily or long slow nocturnal HD sessions can conveniently be performed, provides an excellent choice for quality of life improvement and reduction in morbidity and mortality. SLED technique is an ideal modality for critically ill patients in ICU with multiple organ failure and acute kidney injury. The recent innovations in the specifications of HD machines, HD medical devices and the improvement in dialysis membranes characteristics including the high-flux dialyzers, and water treatment technology paved the way for achieving quality HD. These advancements have resulted in efficient implementation of adsorption, diffusion and/or convection principles using adsorption HD, hemofiltration, hemodiafiltration and online hemodiafiltration modalities aiming at achieving optimum HD. High-flux dialyzer provides significantly less cardiac and cerebrovascular mortality rates, and has been associated with higher survival rate in dialysis patients with low serum albumin and diabetic patients. Therefore, since there have been no better results with low-flux dialyzers, high-flux dialysis should not be limited to high risk dialysis patients. Online HDF is an ideal HD technique with much less morbidity and mortality rates. In fact, online HDF is considered currently as the premium modality of HD that ensures optimum dialysis. Therefore, these HD modalities, and particularly online HDF, should be considered more seriously, if financial and human resources are available and/or affordable, to replace conventional HD should we aim at improving the quality of life and reducing the morbidity and mortality rates among HD patients, which are still unacceptably high, and reducing the costs associated with conventional HD.

## Author details

Ayman Karkar

Address all correspondence to: aymankarkar@yahoo.com

Kanoo Kidney Centre, Dammam Medical Complex, Dammam, Kingdom of Saudi Arabia

## References

[1] Himmelfarb J. Hemodialysis. N Engl J Med 2010;363:1833-1845.

[2] U.S. Renal Data System, the data supplied by the United States Renal Data System (USRDS): 2010 Annual Data Report: Atlas of End-Stage Renal Disease in the United States, National Institutes of Health, National Institute of Diabetes and Digestive and Kidney Diseases, Bethesda, MD, 2010 (http://www.usrds.org/faq.htm).

[3] European Renal Association-European Dialysis and Transplant Association. ERA-EDTA Registry 2004 Annual Report. Amsterdam, the Netherlands: Department of Medical Informatics, Academic Medical Center; 2006.

[4] Denhaerynck K, Manhaeve D, Dobbels F, Garzoni D, Nolte C, De Geest S. Prevalence and consequences of nonadherence to hemodialysis regimens. Am J Crit Care 2007;16:222-235.

[5] SCOT Data. Dialysis in the Kingdom of Saudi Arabia. Saudi J Kidney Dis Transplant 2010;21:789-797.

[6] Ledebo I, Blankestijn PJ. Haemofiltration-optimal efficiency and safety. Nephrol Dialysis Transplant Plus 2010;3:8-16.

[7] De Francisco ALM, Pinera C. Challenges and future of renal replacement therapy. Hemodialysis Int 2006;10:S19-S23.

[8] Dhondt A, Vanholder R, VanBiesen W, Lameire N. The removal of uremic toxins. Kidney Int 2000;58:S47-S59.

[9] Van Ypersele De Strihou C, Jadoul M, Malghem J, Maladague MB, Jamart and the working party on dialysis amyloidosis. Kidney Int1991;39:1012-1019.

[10] Kjellstrand CM, Evans RL, Petersen JR, von Hartitzsch B, Buselmeier TJ. The "unphysiology" of dialysis: A major cause of dialysis side effects? Hemodialysis Int 2004;8:24-29.

[11] Foley RN, Gilbertson DT, Murray T, Collins AJ. Long interdialytic interval and mortality among patients receiving hemodialysis. N Engl J Med 2011;365:1099-1107.

[12] Sehgal AR, Dor A, Tsai AC. Morbidity and cost implications of inadequate hemodialysis. Am J Kidney Dis 2001;37:1223-1231.

[13] Collins AJ, Kasiske B, Herzog C, Chen SC, et al. Excepts from the United States Renal Data System 2003 Annual Data Report: atlas of end-stage renal disease in the United States. Am J Kidney Dis. 2003;42:A5-A7.

[14] Rayner HC, Pisoni RL, Bommer J et al. Mortality and hospitalization in hemodialysis patients in five European countries: Results from the Dialysis Outcomes and Practice Patterns Study (DOPPS). Nephrol Dial Transplant 2004; 19: 108–120.

[15] Canaud B, Bragg-Gresham JL, Marshall MR, Desmeules S, et al. Mortality risk for patients receiving haemodiafiltration versus hemodialysis: European results from the DOPPS. Kidney Int 2006;69:2087-2093.

[16] Karkar A. The value of pre-dialysis care. Saudi J Kidney Dis Transplant 2011;22:419-427.

[17] Karkar A. Caring for patients with CRF: Rewards and benefits. Int J Nephrol 2011; Article ID 639840:1-6.

[18] Karkar A, Abdelrahman M, Ghacha R, Malik TQ. Prevention of viral transmission in HD units: The value of isolation. Saudi J Kidney Dis Transplant 2006;17:183-188.

[19] Karkar A. Hepatitis C in dialysis units: The Saudi experience. Hemodialysis Int 2007;11:354-367.

[20] Parker III T, Hakim R, Nissenson AR, Steinman T, Glassock RJ. Dialysis at a crossroads: 50 years later. Clin J Am Nephrolo 2011;6:457-461.

[21] Wizemann V, Wabel P, Chamney P, Zaluska W, et al. The mortality risk of overhydration in hemodialysis patients. Nephrol Dial Transplant 2009;24:1574-1579.

[22] Sutherland SM, Zappitelli M, Alexander SR, Chua AN, et al. Fluid overload and mortality in children receiving continuous renal replacement therapy: The prospective pediatric continuous renal replacement therapy Registry. Am J Kidney Dis 2010;55:316-325.

[23] Song MK, Gilet CA, Lin FC, MacHardy N, DeVito Dabbs AJ, et al. Characterizing daily life experience of patients on maintenance dialysis. Nephrol Dial Transplant 2011:26:3671–3677.

[24] Marshall MR, Byrne BG, Kerr PG et al. Associations of hemodialysis dose and session length with mortality risk in Australian and New Zealand patients. Kidney Int 2006;69:1229–1236.

[25] Brunelli SM, Chertow GM, Ankers ED, LowrieEG, Thadhani R. Shorter dialysis times are associated with higher mortality among incident hemodialysis patients. Kidney Int 2010;77:630-636.

[26] Block GA, Hulbert-Shearon TE, Levin NW, Port FK. Association of serum phosphorus and calcium x phosphate product with mortality risk in chronic hemodialysis patients: a national study. Am J Kidney Dis1988;31:607-617.

[27] Vanholder R, DeSmet R, Glorleux G, Argiles A, et al. Review on uremic toxins: Classification, concentration, and inter individual variability. Kidney Int 2003;63:1934-1943.

[28] Flythe JE, Kimmel SE, Brunelli SM. Rapid fluid removal during dialysis is associated with cardiovascular morbidity and mortality. Kidney Int 2011;79:250-257.

[29] Saran R, Bragg-Gresham JL, Levin NW, Twardowski ZJ, et al. Longer treatment time and slower ultrafiltration in hemodialysis: Associations with reduced mortality in the DOPPS. Kidney Int 2006;69:1222-1228.

[30] Woods JD, Port FK, Orzol S, Buonchristiani U, et al. Clinical and biochemical correlates of starting "daily" hemodialysis. Kidney Int 1999;55:2467-2476.

[31] Klarenbach S, Heidenheim AP, Leitch R, Lindsay RM, Daily/Nocturnal Dialysis Study Group. Reduced requirement for erythropoietin with quotidian hemodialysis therapy. ASAIOJ 2002;48:57–61.

[32] Agar JWM, Knight RJ, Simmonds RE, Boddington JM, et al. Nocturnal hemodialysis: An Australian cost comparison with conventional satellite hemodialysis. Nephrology 2005;10:557–570.

[33] Culleton BF, Walsh M, Klarenbach SW, Mortis G, et al. Effect of Frequent Nocturnal Hemodialysis vs Conventional Hemodialysis on Left Ventricular Mass and Quality of Life: A Randomized Controlled Trial. JAMA 2007;298:1291-1299.

[34] Kjellstrand CM, Buoncristiani U, Ting G, Traeger J, et al. Short daily hemodialysis: survival in 415 patients treated for 1006 patient-years. Nephrol Dial Transplant 2008;23:3283–3289.

[35] Peri J, Chan CT. Home hemodialysis, daily hemodialysis, and nocturnal hemodialysis: core curriculum. Am J Kidney Dis 2009;54:1171-1184.

[36] The FHN Trial Group. In-center hemodialysis six times per week versus three times per week. N Engl J Med 2010;363:2287-2300.

[37] Rocco MV, Lockridge RS, Beck GJ, Eggers PW, et al. The effects of frequent nocturnal home hemodialysis: the Frequent Hemodialysis Network Nocturnal Trial. Kidney Int 2011;80:1080-1091.

[38] Hemodialysis Adequacy 2006 Work Group. Clinical practice guidelines for hemodialysis adequacy, update 2006. Am J Kidney Dis 2006;48:S2–S90.

[39] Collins AJ, Ma JZ, Umen A, Keshaviah P: Urea index and other predictors of hemodialysis patient survival. Am J Kidney Dis 1994;23:272-282.

[40] Held PJ, Port FK,Wolfe RA, Stannard DC, et al. The dose of hemodialysis and patient mortality. Kidney Int 1996;50:550-556.

[41] Moret KE, Grootendorst DC, Dekker FW, Boeschoten EW, et al. Agreement between different parameters of dialysis dose in achieving treatment targets: results from the NECOSAD study. Nephrol Dial Transplant 2011;26:1-8.

[42] Eknoyan G, Beck G, Cheung AK, Daugirdas JT, et al. Effect of dialysis dose and membrane flux in maintenance hemodialysis. N Engl J Med 2002;347:2010-2019.

[43] Mendoza JM, Bayes LY, Sun S, Doss S, Schiller B. Effect of lowering dialysate sodium concentration on interdialytic weight gain and blood pressure in patients undergoing thrice-weekly in-center nocturnal hemodialysis: A quality improvement study. Am J Kidney Dis 2011;58(6):956-963.

[44] Ward RA: Blood flow rate: An important determinant of urea clearance and delivered Kt/V. AdvRen Replace Ther 1999;6:75-79.

[45] Kim YO, Song WJ, Yoon SA, Shin MJ, et al. The Effect of increasing blood flow rate on dialysis adequacy in hemodialysis patients with low Kt/V. Hemodialysis Int 2004;8:85.

[46] Borzou SR, Gholyaf M, Zandiha M, Amini R, et al. The effect of increasing blood flow rate on dialysis adequacy in hemodialysis patients. Saudi J Kidney Dis Transpl 2009;20:639-642.

[47] Hassell DRM, van der Sande FM, Kooman JP, Tordoir JP, Leunissen KML. Optimizing dialysis dose by increasing blood flow rate in patients with reduced vascular-access flow rate. Am J Kidney Dis 2001;38(5):948-955.

[48] Hauk M, MD, Kuhlmann MK, Riegel W, Köhler H. In vivo effects of dialysate flow rate on Kt/V in maintenance hemodialysis patients. Am J Kidney Dis 2000;35:105-111.

[49] Azar AT. Increasing dialysate flow rate increases dialyzer urea clearance and dialysis efficiency: an in vivo study. Saudi J Kidney Dis Transpl 2009;20:1023-1029.

[50] Alp Ikizler T, Schulman G. Hemodialysis: techniques and prescription. Am J Kidney Dis 2005;46:976-981.

[51] Kerr PG. International differences in hemodialysis delivery and their influence on outcomes. Am J Kidney Dis 2011;58:461-470.

[52] Ronco C, Brendolan A, Crepaldi C, Rodighiero M, Scabardi M. Blood and dialysate flow distributions in hollow-fiberhemodialyzers analysed by computerized helical scanning technique. J Am SocNephrol 2002;13[Suppl 1]:S53-S61.

[53] Ward RA, Idoux JW, Hamdan H, Ouseph R, et al. Dialysate flow rate and delivered Kt/V urea for dialyzers with enhanced dialysate flow distribution. Clin J Am Soc-Nephrol 2011;6:2235-2239.

[54] Lafrance JP, Rahme E, Lelorier J, Iqbal S. Vascular access–related infections: definitions, Incidence rates, and risk factors. Am J Kidney Dis 2008;52(5):982-993.

[55] Pisoni RL, Arrington CJ, Albert JM, Ethier J, Kimata N, Krishnan M, Rayner HC, et al. Facility hemodialysis vascular access use and mortality in countries participating in DOPPS: an instrumental variable analysis. Am J Kidney Dis 2009;53(3):475-491.

[56] Lacson E, Wang W, Lazarus JM, Hakim RM. Change in vascular access and mortality in maintenance hemodialysis patients. Am J Kidney Dis 2009;54(5):912-921.

[57] Becker BN, Breiterman-White R, Nylander W, Van Buren D. Care pathway reduces hospitalizations and cost for hemodialysis vascular access surgery. Am J Kidney Dis 1997;30(4):525-531.

[58] Polkinghorne KR. Vascular Access Practice in Hemodialysis: Instrumental in Determining Patient Mortality. Am J Kidney Dis 2009;53(3):359-362.

[59] Lee H, Manns B, Taub K, Ghali WA. Cost analysis of ongoing care of patients with end-stage renal disease: The impact of dialysis modality and dialysis access. Am J Kidney Dis 2002;40(3):611-622.

[60] Ng LJ, Chen F, Pisoni RL, Krishnan M, Mapes D, Keen M, Bradbury BD. Hospitalization risks related to vascular access type among incident US hemodialysis patients. Nephrol Dial Transplant 2011;26: 3659–3666.

[61] Ocak G, Halbesma N, le Cessie S, Hoogeveen EK, van Dijk S, et al. Hemodialysis catheters increase mortality as compared to arteriovenous accesses especially in elderly patients. Nephrol Dial Transplant 2011;26: 2611–2617.

[62] National Kidney Foundation. K/DOQI Clinical Practice Guidelines for Vascular Access, 2000. Am J Kidney Dis 2001;37:S137-S181 (suppl 1).

[63] Lynch JR, Wasse H, Armistead NC, McClellan WM. Achieving the goal of the fistula first breakthrough initiative for prevalent maintenance hemodialysis patients (www.fistulafirst.org). Am J Kidney Dis 2011;57(1):78-89.

[64] Pisoni RL, Young EW, Dykstra DM, Greenwood RN, Hecking E, Gillespie B, Wolfe RA, Goodkin DA, Held PJ. Vascular access use in Europe and the United States: Results from the DOPPS. Kidney Int2002;61:305–316.

[65] 2010 Annual Report of the Dialysis Outcomes and Practice Patterns Study: Hemodialysis Data 1999-2010. Arbor Research Collaborative for Health, Ann Arbor, MI. http://www.dopps.org.

[66] Vanholder R, Glorieux G, Van Biesen W. Advantages of new hemodialysis membranes and equipment. Nephron ClinPrac 2010;114:c165-c172.

[67] Humes HD, Fissell WH, Tiranathanagul K. The future of hemodialysis membranes. Kidney Int 2006;69:1115-1119.

[68] Fischer KG. Essentials of anticoagulation in hemodialysis. Hemodialysis Int 2007; 11:178–189.

[69] Ikizler TA, Schulman G. Hemodialysis: techniques and prescription. Am J Kidney Dis 2005;46(5):976-981.

[70] Davenport A. What are the anticoagulation options in intermittent hemodialysis? Nat Rev Nephrol 2011;7:499-508.

[71] Chanard J, Levaud S, Maheut H, Kazes I, Vitry F, Rieu P. The clinical evaluation of low-dose heparin in hemodialysis: a prospective study using the heparin-coated AN69ST membrane. Nephrol Dial Transplant 2008;23:2003-2009.

[72] Henderson L, Ward RA, Mion CA, et al. Should hemodialysis fluid be sterile? Semin Dial 1993;6:26-36.

[73] Meijers BKI, Bammens B, De Moor B, Verbeke K, Vanrenterghem Y, Evenepoel P. Free p-cresol is associated with cardiovascular disease in hemodialysis patients. Kidney Int 2008;73:1174-1180.

[74] Lin CL, Huang CC, Yu CC, et al. Reduction of advanced glycation end product levels by on-line haemodiafiltration in long-term hemodialysis patients. Am J Kidney Dis 2003;42:524-531.

[75] Calo LA, Naso A, Carraro G, Wratten ML, et al. Effect of haemodiafiltration with on-line regeneration of ultrafiltrate on oxidative stress in dialysis patients. Nephrol Dial Transplant 2007;22:1413-1419.

[76] Weber KT. Oxidative stressand cardiovascular injury: A symposium presented at the Southern Society for Clinical Investigation. Am J Clin Sciences 2011;342:111-113.

[77] Wizemann V, Külz M, Techert F, Nederlof B. Efficacy of haemodiafiltration. Nephrol Dial Transplant 2001;16:S27-S30.

[78] Evenepoel P, Bammens B, Verbeke K, Vanrenterghem Y. Superior dialytic clearance of b2-microglobuli and p-cresol by high-flux hemodialysis as compared to peritoneal dialysis. Kidney Int 2006;70:794-799.

[79] Hornberger JC, Chernew M, Petersen J, Garber AM.A multivariate analysis of mortality and hospital admissions with high- flux dialysis. J Am SocNephrol 1992;3:1227–1237.

[80] Koda Y, Nishi SI, Miyazaki S, Haginoshita S, et al. Switch from conventional to high-flux membrane reduces the risk of carpal tunnel syndrome and mortality of hemodialysis patients. Kidney Int 1997;52:1096-1101.

[81] Woods HF, Nandakumar M. Improved outcomes for hemodialysis patients treated with high-flux membranes. Nephrol Dial Transplant 2000;15:S36-S42.

[82] Port FK, Wolfe RA, Hulbert-Shearon TE, Daugirdas JT, et al. Mortality risk by hemodialyzer reuse practice and dialyzer membrane characteristics: Results from the USRDS dialysis morbidity and mortality study. Am J Kidney Dis 2001;37:276–286.

[83] Cheung AK, Levin NW, Greene T, Agodoa L, et al. Effect of high-flux hemodialysis on clinical outcome: Results of the HEMO study. J Am Society of Nephrol 2003;14:3251-3263.

[84] Delmez JA, Yan G, Bailey J, Beck GJ, et al. Cerebrovascular disease in maintenance hemodialysis patients: Results of the HEMO study. Am J Kidney Dis 2006;47:131-138.

[85] Locatelli F, Martin-Malo A, Hannedouche T, Loureiro A, et al. Effect of membrane permeability on survival of hemodialysis patients. J Am SocNephrol 2009;20:645-654.

[86] Tattersall J, Canaud B, Heimburger O, Pedrini L, et al. High-flux or low-flux dialysis: a position statement following publication of the membrane permeability outcome study. Nephrol Dial Transplant 2010;25:1230-1232.

[87] Blankestijn PJ, Ledebo I, Canaud B. Hemodiafiltration: clinical evidence and remaining questions. KidenyInt 2010;77:581-587.

[88] Premru V, Kovač J, J Buturović-Ponikvar, Ponikvar R. High Cut-Off Membrane Hemodiafiltration in Myoglobinuric Acute Renal Failure: A Case Series. Therapeutic Apheresis and Dialysis 2011;15(3):287-291.

[89] Heyne N, Weisel KC, Hutchison CA, Friedrich B, Goehl H, et al. Characterization of extra corporal serum free light chain elimination kinetics via high cut-off protein permeable membrane in light chain multiple myeloma. Nephrol Dial Transplant 2007;22Suppl 6:123.

[90] Gondouin B, Hutchison CA. High cut-off dialysis membranes: current uses and future potential. Adv Chronic Kidney Dis 2011;18(3):180-187.

[91] Naka T, Haase M, Bellomo R. 'Super high-flux' or 'high cut-off' hemofiltration and hemodialysis. ContribNephrol 2010;166:181-189.

[92] Contin C, Pitard V, Itai T, Nagata S, et al. Membrane-anchored CD40 is processed by the tumor necrosis factor-a-converting enzyme. J BiolChem 2003;278:32801–32809.

[93] Tessitore N, Lapolla A, Aric NC, Poli A, et al. Effect of protein leaking BK-F PMMA-based hemodialysis on plasma pentosidine levels. J Nephrol 2004;17:707–714.

[94] Contin-Bordes C, Lacraz A, de Précigout V. Potential role of the soluble form of CD40 in deficient immunological function of dialysis patients: new findings of its amelioration using polymethylmethacrylate (PMMA) membrane. Nephrol Dial Transplant Plus 2010;3:i20-i27.

[95] Aucella F, Vigilante M, Gesuete A. Review: the effect of polymethylmethacrylate dialysis membranes on uraemicpruritis. NDT Plus 2010;3:S8-S11.

[96] Santoro A, Guadagni G. Dialysis membrane: from convection to adsorption. Nephrol Dial Transplant Plus 2010;3:i36–i39.

[97] Hayama M, Miyasaka T, Mochizuki S, Asahara H, Tsujioka K, Kohori K, Sakai K, Jinbo Y, Yoshida M. Visualization of distribution of endotoxin trapped in an endotoxin-blocking filtration membrane. J Membrane Sci 2002;210(1):45-53.

[98] Wernert V, Schäf O, Faure V, Brunet P, et al. Adsorption of the uremic toxin p-cresol onto hemodialysis membranes and microporous adsorbent zeolite silicalite. J Biotechnol 2006;123:164-173.

[99] Aoike I. Clinical significance of protein adsorbable membranes-long-term clinical effects and analysis using a proteomic technique. Nephrol Dial Transplant 2007;22:13–19.

[100] Dimkovic N, Djukanovic L, Radmilovic A, Bojic P, Juloski T. Uremic pruritus and skin mast cells. Nephron 1992;61:5–9.

[101] Yamada S, Kataoka H, Kobayashi H, et al. Identification of an erythropoetic inhibitor from the dialysate collected in the hemodialysis with PMMA membrane (BK-F). ContribNephrol 1999;125:159–172.

[102] Hutchison CA, Harding S, Hewins P, et al. Quantitative assessment of serum and urinary polyclonal free light chains in patients with chronic kidney disease. Clin J Am SocNephrol2008;3:1684–1690.

[103] Cohen G, Rudnicki M, Schmaldienst S, Hörl WH. Effect of dialysis on serum/plasma levels of free immunoglobulin light chains in end stage renal disease patients. Nephrol Dial Transplant 2002;17:879–888.

[104] Hata H, Nishi K, Oshihara W, et al. Adsorption of Bence–Jones protein to polymethylmethacrylate membrane in primary amyloidosis. Amyloid 2009;16:108–110.

[105] Oshihara W, Nagao H, Megano H, Arai J, et al. Trial use of a polymethylmethacrylate membrane for the removal of free immunoglobulin light chains in dialysis patients. Nephrol Dial Transplant Plus 2010;3 [Suppl 1]:i3–i7.

[106] Contin C, Pitard V, Delmas Y, et al. Potential role of soluble CD40 in the humoral immune response impairment of uraemic patients. Immunology 2003;110:131–140.

[107] Van Kooten C, Gaillard C, Galizzi JP, et al. B cells regulate expression of CD40 ligand on activated T cells by lowering the mRNA level and through the release of soluble CD40. Eur J Immunol 1994;24:787–792.

[108] Sykora R, Chvojka J, Krouzecky, Rade J, et al. Coupled Plasma Filtration Adsorption in Experimental Peritonitis-Induced Septic Shock. Shock 2009;31:473-480.

[109] Lucisano G, Capria M, Matera G, Presta P, et al. Coupled plasma filtration adsorption for the treatment of a patient with acute respiratory distress syndrome and acute kidney injury: a case report. Nephrol Dial Transplant Plus 2011;4:285-288.

[110] Locatelli F, Buoncristiani U, Canaud B, KöhlerH,PetitclercT,Zucchelli P. Dialysis dose and frequency. Nephrol Dial Transplant 2005;20:285-296.

[111] Achinger SG, Ayus JC. The role of daily dialysis in the control of hyperphosphatemia. Kidney Int 2005;67:S28-S32.

[112] Basile C, Liputti P, Di Turo AL, Casino FG, et al. Removal of uraemic retention solutes in standard bicarbonate hemodialysis and long-hour slow-flow bicarbonate hemodialysis. Nephrol Dial Transplant 2011;26:1296-1303.

[113] Maduell F, Arias M, Dura′n CE, Vera M, et al. Nocturnal, every-other-day, online haemodiafiltration: an effective therapeutic alternative. Nephrol Dial Transplant 2011; 0: 1–13, doi:10.1093/ndt/gfr491.

[114] Ayus JC, Achinger SG, Mizani MR, Chertow GM, et al. Phosphorus balance and mineral metabolism with 3 h daily hemodialysis. Kidney Int 2007;71:336-342.

[115] David S, K°umpers P, Eisenbach GM, Haller H, Kielstein JT. Prospective evaluation of an in-centre conversion from conventional hemodialysis to an intensified nocturnal strategy. Nephrol Dial Transplant 2009;24:2232–2240.

[116] Rao M, Muirhead N, Klarenbach S, et al. Management of anaemia with quotidian hemodialysis. Am J Kidney Dis 2003;42:S18–S23.

[117] Fagugli RM, Reboldi G, Quintaliani G, Pasini P. Short daily hemodialysis: Blood pressure control and left ventricular mass reduction in hypertensive hemodialysis patients. Am J Kidney Dis 2001;38:371-376.

[118] Galland R, Traeger J, Arkouche W, Cleaud C, DelawariE,Fouque D. Short daily hemodialysis rapidly improves nutritionalstatus in hemodialysis patients. Kidney Int 2001;60:1555–1560.

[119] Mowatt G, Vale L, MacLeod A. Systematic review of the effectiveness of home versus hospital or satellite unit hemodialysis for people with end-stage renal failure. IJTAHC 2004;20:258-268.

[120] Pauly RP, Gill JS, Rose CL, Asad RA, et al. Survival among nocturnal home hemodialysis patients compared to kidney transplant recipients. Nephrol Dial Transplant 2009;24:2915–2919.

[121] Komenda P, Gavaghan MB, Garfield SS, Poret AW, Sood MM. An economic model for in-center, conventional home, and more frequent home hemodialysis. Kidney Int. advanced online publication 12 October 2011;1-7.

[122] Lameire N, Van Biesen W, Vanholder R. Did 20 years of technological innovations in hemodialysis contribute to better outcomes? Clin J Am Nephrol 2009;4:S30-S40.

[123] Henderson LW, Colton CK, Ford CA, Bosch JP. The Kinetics of hemodiafiltration. II. Clinical characterization of a new blood cleansing modality. 1975 classical article. J Am SocNephrol 1997;8:494-508.

[124] Bolasco P, Altieri P, Andrulli S, Basile C, et al. Convection versus diffusion in dialysis: an Italian prospective multicenter study. Nephrol Dialysis Transplant 2003;18:vii50-vii54.

[125] Vaslaki L, Karatson A, Voros P, Major L, et al. Can sterile and pyrogen-free on-line substitution fluid be routinely delivered? A multicentric study on the microbiological safety of on-line haemodiafiltration. Nephrol Dial Transplant 2000;15:74-78.

[126] Ramirez R, Carracedo J, Merino A, Nogueras S, et al. Microinflammation induces endothelial damage in hemodialysis patients: the role of convective transport. Kidney Int 2007;72:108-113.

[127] Van Laecke S, De Wild K, Vanholder R. Online haemodiafiltration. Artif Organs 2006;30:579-585.

[128] Penne EL, Blankestijn PJ, Bots ML, et al. Effect of increased convective clearance by on- line hemodiafiltration on all cause and cardiovascular mortality in chronic hemodialysis patients—the Dutch CONvectiveTRAnsport Study (CONTRAST): rationale and design of a randomised controlled trial [ISRCTN38365125]. Curr Control Trials Cardiovasc Med. 2005;6(1):8.

[129] Penne EL, Van der Weerd NC, Van den Dopel MA, et al. Short-term effects of on-line hemodiafiltration on phosphate control: a result from the randomized controlled convective transport study (CONTRAST). Am J Kidney Dis 2009;55:77-87.

[130] Ok E, Asci G, Ok ES, et al. Comparison of post-dilution on-line hemodiafiltration and hemodialysis (Turkish HDF Study). Nephrol Dial Transplant Plus 2011;4:Suppl 2 (Abstracts from the 48th ERA-EDTA Congress, June 23-26 2011, Prague, Czech Republic).

[131] Meert N, Eloot S, Waterloos MA, Van Landschoot M, et al. Effective removal of protein-bound uremic solutes by different convective strategies: a prospective trial. Nephrol Dialysis Transplant 2009;24:562-570.

[132] Block GA, Hullbert-Shearon TE, Levin NW, et al. Association of serum phosphorus and calcium x phosphate product with mortality risk in chronic hemodialysis patients: a national study. Am J Kidney Dis 1998;31:607-617.

[133] Davenport A, Gardner C, Delaney M. The effect of dialysis modality on phosphate control: hemodialysis compared to haemodiafiltration. The Pan Thames Renal Audit. Nephrol Dialysis Transplant 2010;25:897-901.

[134] Wizemann V, Lotz C, Techert F, Uthoff S. On-line haemodiafiltration versus low flux hemodialysis. A prospective randomized study. Nephrol Dial Transplant 2000;15:43–48.

[135] Valle'e AG, Chenine L, Leray-Moragues H, Patrier L, et al. Online high-efficiency haemodiafiltration achieves higher serum free light chain removal than high-flux hemodialysis in multiple myeloma patients: Preliminary Quantitative Study. Nephrol Dial Transplant 2011;0:1–7.

[136] Bammens B, Evenepoel P, Verbeke K, Vanrenterghem Y. Removal of the protein-bound solute p-cresol by convective transport: a randomized crossover study. Am J Kidney Dis 2004;44:278–285.

[137] Gerdemann A, Wagner Z, Solf A, et al. Plasma levels of advanced glycation end products during hemodialysis, haemodiafiltration and haemofiltration: potential importance of dialysate quality. Nephrol Dial Transplant 2002;17:1045–1049.

[138] Vanholder R, Van Laecke S, Glorieux G. The middle-molecule hypothesis 30 years after: lost and rediscovered in the universe of uremic toxicity. J Nephrol 2008;21:146-160.

[139] Shibata M, Nagai K, Usami K, Tawada, H, Taniguchi S. The quantitative evaluation of online haemodiafiltration effect on skin hyperpigmentation. Nephrol Dial Transplant 2011;26:988–992.

[140] Fischbach M, Terzic J, Menouer S, Dheu C, et al. Daily online haemodiafiltration promotes catch-up growth in children on chronic dialysis. Nephrol Dial Transplant 2010;25:867–873.

[141] Basile C. The effect of convection on the nutritional status of hemodialysis patients. Nephrol Dialysis Transplant 2003;18:vii46-vii49.

[142] Badiou S, Morena M, Bargnoux AS, Jaussent I, et al. Does hemodiafiltration improve the removal of homocysteine? Hemodialysis Int 2011;15:515-521.

[143] Maduell F, Del Pozo C, Garcia H, Sanchez L, et al. Change from conventional haemodiafiltration to on-line haemodiafiltration. Nephrol Dial Transplant 1999;14:1202-1207.

[144] Van der Weerd NC, Penne EL, Van den Dorpel MA, Grooteman MPC, et al. Haemodiafiltration: promise for the future? Nephrol Dial Transplant 2008;23:438-443.

[145] Pedrini LA, De Cristofaro V, Comelli M, Casino FG, et al. Long-term effects of high-efficiency on-line haemodiafiltration on uraemic toxicity. A multicentre prospective randomized study.Nephrol Dial Transplant 2011; 26:2617–2624.

[146] Altieri P, Sorba G, Bolasco P, Ledebo I, et al. On-line hemofiltration in chronic renal failure: Advantages and limits. Saudi J Kidney Dis Transplant 2001;12:387-397.

[147] Locatelli F, Altieri P, Andrulli S, Bolasco P, et al. Hemofiltration and hemodiafiltration reduce intradialytic hypotension in ESRD. J Am SocNephrol 2010;21:1798-1807.

[148] Silberberg JS, Barre PE, Prichard SS, et al. Impact of left ventricular hypertrophy on survival in end-stage renal disease. Kidney Int 1989;36:286-290.

[149] Foley RN, Parfrey PS, Harnett JD, et al. Clinical and echocardiographic disease in patients starting end-stage renal disease therapy. Kidney Int 1995;47:186-192.

[150] Vilar E, Fry AC, Wellsted D, Tattersall JE et al. Long-term outcomes in online haemodiafiltration and high-flux hemodialysis: A comparative analysis. Clin J Am Soc-Nephrol 2009;4:1944-1953.

[151] Jirka T, Cesare S, Di Benedetto A, et al. Mortality risk for patients receiving hemodiafiltration versus hemodialysis. Kidney Int 2006;70:1524-1525.

[152] Canaud B, Bosc JY, Leray H, Stec F. Microbiological purity of dialysate for on-line substitution fluid preparation. Nephrol Dial Transplant 2000;15:S21-S30.

[153] Canaud B. Rapid assessment of microbiological purity of dialysis water: the promise of solid-phase cytometry assessment and the epifluorescence microscopy method. Nephrol Dial Transplant 2011:26:3426–3428.

[154] Penne EL, Visser L, Van den Dorpel MA, Van der Weerd NC, et al. Microbiological quality and quality control of purified water and ultrapure dialysis fluids for online haemodiafiltration in routine clinical practice. Kidney Int 2009;76:665-67.

[155] Locatelli F, Del Vecchio L, Manzoni C, et al. Morbidity and mortality on maintenance hemodialysis. Nephron 1998;80:380-400.

[156] Bellomo, R, Ronco C, Mehta, RL. Nomenclature for Continuous Renal Replacement Therapies. Am J Kidney Dis 1996;28(5):S2-S7.

[157] Bellomo R, Ronco C. Continuous haemofiltration in the intensive care unit. Crit Care 2000;4(6):339–345.

[158] Geronemus, R, Schneider, N. Continuous arteriovenous hemodialysis: A new modality for treatment of acute renal failure. Trans Am SocArtif Intern Organs 1984;30:610–612.

[159] Dirkes S, Hodge K. Continuous renal replacement therapy in the adult intensive care unit: History and current trends. Crit Care Nurse 2007;27:61-80.

[160] Vanholder R, Biesen WV, Lameire N. What is the renal replacement method of first choice for intensive care patients? Am SocNephrol 2001;12:S40–S43.

[161] Bouchard J, Macedo E, Mehta RL. Dosing of renal replacement therapy in acute kidney injury: lessons leaened from clinical trials. Am J Kidney Dis 2010;55(3):570-579.

[162] Davenport A, Will EJ, Davidson AM. Improved cardiovascular stability during continuous modes of renal replacement therapy in critically ill patients with acute hepatic and renal failure. Crit Care Med 1993;21:328-338.

[163] Ronco C, Bellomo R, Homel P, et al. Effects of different doses in continuous venovenous haemofiltration on outcomes of acute renal failure: a prospective randomised trial. Lancet 2000;356:26-30.

[164] Marshall MR, Golper TA, Shaver MJ, Alam MG, Chatoth DK. Urea kinetics during sustained low-efficiency dialysis in critically ill patients requiring renal replacement therapy. Am J Kidney Dis 2002;39(3):556-570.

[165] Salahudeen AK, Kumar V, Madan N, Xiao L, Lahoti A, et al. Sustained low efficiency dialysis in the continuous mode (C-SLED): dialysis efficacy, clinical outcomes, and survival predictors in critically ill cancer patients. Clin J SocNephrol 2009;4:1338-1346.

[166] Marshall MR, Ma T, Galler D, Rankin APN, Williams AB. Sustained low-efficiency daily diafiltration (SLEDD-f) for critically ill patients requiring renal replacement therapy: towards an adequate therapy. Nephrol Dial Transpl 2004;19(4):877-884.

[167] Berbece AN, Richardson RMA. Sustained low-efficiency dialysis in the ICU: cost, anticoagulation, and solute removal. Kidney Int 2006;70:963-968.

[168] Fliser D, Kielstein JT. Technology Insight: treatment of renal failure in the intensive care unit with extended dialysis. Nature Clin Practice Nephrol 2006;2:32-39.

Chapter 5

# Implementation and Management of Strategies to Set and to Achieve Clinical Targets

Bernard Canaud, Ciro Tetta, Daniele Marcelli, Guido Giordana, Stefano Stuard, Katrin Koehler, Flavio Mari, Carlo Barbieri, Miryana Dobreva, Andrea Stopper and Emanuele Gatti

Additional information is available at the end of the chapter

## 1. Introduction

Today health care and care provider organizations are facing new challenges. They must continually improve their services to provide the highest quality at the lowest cost. Pressures to increase the quality and lower the costs are coming from accreditation and certification boards, public health authorities and the media that publish comparisons and rank facilities by performance. In addition, new demands on health care systems require action accountability with hard outcome data based on morbidity and mortality. Quality control, quality assurance and continuous quality improvement (CQI) processes derived from the manufacturing and industrial world have been progressively applied with success to medicine and in particular to the treatment of end stage renal disease.

[1,2]. It is generally accepted that quality control describes the process for reviewing and checking that targets according to whether a defined set of criteria has been achieved, while quality assurance is the process in which systematic monitoring, collecting and evaluating the performance of a facility or a care network are assessed to ensure that standards of care are met [3]. CQI describes the action that takes place after analyzing outcomes with the intent of improving the results and reducing variation from the target. In this respect, renal replacement therapy by dialysis represents a particular field of application where quality control and quality assurance processes have been shown to be very efficient tools for optimizing treatment adequacy and improving patient outcomes.

Over the last ten years, it has been well documented that survival and outcomes of stage 5 chronic kidney disease patients on dialysis are depending on age, comorbid status at the start of treatment, but also on quality care and practice patterns [4,5,6]. Renal replacement therapy by dialysis is a clear paradigm where results are quite closely tied to quality assurance and CQI processes. Dialysis adequacy is a multi-target concept developed to face complexity of uraemia disorders and to provide physicians with an easy tool based on a 'checklist' to address the patients' vital metabolic needs. Dialysis prescription and adjunctive medical treatment are intended to provide over time (from years to decades) an adequate and regular correction of metabolic disorders to each patient, to prevent side-effects and 'un-physiology' of intermittent dialysis and to preserve quality of life at an affordable cost. Treatment adequacy is then closely tied to the quality assurance process that links prescription and treatment delivery [7]. On one hand, prescription of the haemodialysis treatment relies mainly on the patient's metabolic needs, cardiovascular and general tolerance of sessions, dietary compliance, residual renal function [8] and local health care and economic offer. It is not our intent to revisit here the principle of prescribing dialysis but just to remind that it relies on five primary elements: dialysis modality (haemodialysis, haemodiafiltration, ect), dialyzer type, total weekly treatment duration (number of sessions per week and duration of session), blood flow and 'dry weight' achievement. Additional components need to be considered as secondary part of the prescription being part of the prescription such as dialysate flow, substitution flow in convective therapies, dialysate electrolytic composition, antithrombotic drugs, specific medications (iron, erythropoiesis-stimulating agents, vitamins ect) [9]. On the other hand, adequate delivery of haemodialysis relies on the continuous achievement of pre-specified targets using quality control markers intended to monitor major metabolic disorders of the uraemic syndrome. The markers clearly identified and recommended by international best practice guidelines (formerly the European Best Practice Guidelines, EBPG, now the European Renal Best Practice, ERBP, KDOKI at http://www.european-renal-best-practice.org/, the National Kidney Foundation Kidney Disease Outcomes Quality Initiative, NKF KDOQI, Kidney Disease: Improving Global Outcomes, KDIGO) are summarized in clinical performance measures (CPM) covering 10 main domains: 1.[7]; 1. Lack of clinical uraemic symptoms; 2. Fluid volume control; 3. Blood pressure control; 4. Adequate dialysis dose delivery (small and middle molecules); 5. Acidosis correction; 6. HyperkalemiaHyperkalemia control; 7. Divalent ion metabolism (phosphatemia, calcaemia and magnesaemia); 8. Iron repletion and anaemia correction; 9. Prevention of malnutrition; 10. Prevention of inflammation and oxidative stress. As shown by the international Dialysis Outcome Practice Patterns (DOPPS) study, clinical practices should be now considered as a major component of quality of care having a direct impact on dialysis patient outcomes. By linking country and unit, specific practices to patient outcomes, the DOPPS study introduced a new dimension in the control of the overall quality of care of haemodialysis patients. Among the main findings of DOPPS it must be stressed that less use of central venous catheter [10,11], longer duration of dialysis with reduced ultrafiltration rate [12], adequate dialysis schedule [13], higher dialysis dose delivered [14], better control of fluid overload and blood pressure control [15], prevention of metabolic bone disease [16,17], better control of anaemia with lower erythropoiesis-stimulating agent dose requirement [18,19], enhanced convective dose [20] are all beneficial to patient outcomes. In addition, DOPPS has also shown that overall clinical practices at the facility level were essential for improving patient outcomes [21]. In other words, dialysis facilities achieving optimal targets for a core of selected quality control items in the majority of patients were extending life expectancy to each patient individually [[21]]). In this new perspective, it is then necessary to implement complementary items of quality control probing the degree of compliance of dialysis facilities with best clinical practices [22,23]. A quality control tool in this case may be simply expressed as the percentage of patients within the predefined target range per unit. Combining clinical performance measures and percentage of patients complying with targeted objectives, a new key performance indicators (KPI) may be elaborated for a group of patients treated either within a dialysis unit and/or within a network. In addition to directly addressing clinical practices and patient outcomes, DOPPS has been used as a platform for economic and policy analyses [24]. Fresenius Medical Care as the world's largest integrated provider of products and services for individuals undergoing dialysis because of chronic kidney failure was historically involved in the development of continuous quality improvement processes of dialysis care. We take this opportunity to present additional results collected within the Fresenius Medical Care network system (EuCliD, European Clinical Database). In this article, we discuss some practical ways of implementing the CQI process based on real time collection of clinical performance measures and KPI. Using selected indicators we explore the beneficial effects over time of achieving targeted criteria of good medical practice in terms of patient outcome and cost saving effect. In developed countries, health care costs are currently progressively increasing and in case of U.S. exceeds 17% of the Gross Domestic Product (GDP). Other countries spend less of their GDP on health care but demonstrate the same increasing trend.

Today, national health care systems worldwide are expected to deliver more and better services to a greater number of patients, while dealing with ever more reduced economical resources on the one hand and increased costs on the other hand. Major challenges posed to healthcare systems include global ageing and increase in so-called civilization diseases, growing budget deficits and slowing economic growth, worldwide health care workers shortage and commodity shortage. The need to provide innovative and high-quality, innovative products and treatments should able to contribute to improving outcomes and to be in balance with new perspectives addressing the health care change. Innovation has to contribute to solving the challenge of the economic pressure, though innovation will need standardization according to the rules of good clinical practice and proved by evidence-based medicine. Perverted incentives may also contribute to rising costs as well as reimbursement as providers are reimbursed for performed procedures rather than achieved ones. Moreover, a common weakness of health care systems is linked to the low level of responsibility for the costs generated by the patients at the time they require the medical service. The costs for renal replacement therapy is exceedingly high and are consuming a significant proportion of health care budgets. The global prevalence of kidney failure continues to rise, and treatment is costly; thus, the burden of illness is growing and the resources allocated to treatment are increasing. According to the U.S. Renal Data System (USRDS) Annual Report 2011, total Medicare costs in 2009 rose 8%, to $491 billion; costs for ESRD rose

3%, to $29 billion, accounting for 6% of the total Medicare budget. ESRD data for 2009, however, do not include Part D (costs of drugs), which amounted to $2 billion in 2008 (Best Dialysis Centres at [25]. In European health care systems, the costs of treatment for the growing population of chronically ill patients (including those requiring renal replacement therapy) are considered an emerging public health problem. Indeed, renal failure persists as a chronic worldwide epidemic with an exponential growth trend on a global scale. Over the last decade, the prevalence of ESRD in Europe grew by an annual average rate of 5%. By the end of 2011, the number of ESRD patients in Europe was estimated to be 657,000 and, of these, approximately 433,000 (around 66%) received dialysis treatment [26]. Currently, many healthcare systems in Europe try to address the growing budget pressures by savings. Savings alone can provide relief to the challenged financial situation only to a very limited extent. Providers and payors turn to simplistic actions such as across-the-board cuts in expensive services, staff compensation, and head count. Imposing arbitrary spending limits on discrete components of care, or on specific line-item expense categories, achieves only marginal savings that often lead to higher total systems costs and poorer outcomes. The inability to properly measure cost and compare cost with outcomes is at the root of the incentive problem in health care and has severely retarded the shift to more effective reimbursement approaches. Moreover, poor measurement of cost and outcomes also means that effective and efficient providers go unrewarded preventing them from making systemic and sustainable cost reductions. A broad consensus exists regarding targets for best medical practice in renal care [27]. Concepts regarding how to achieve these targets in the most efficient way, however, vary significantly. The variety of solutions, reflected by different national models of renal care as well as ongoing reforms and recent reform proposals, suggest that the search for an optimum is still ongoing.

Achieving the right balance between high-quality service for chronically ill patients and its cost is now one major challenge for the health care industry. It is crucial to recognize the benefit of collecting and analyzing large amounts of data, comparing treatment modalities and opting for the highest quality. The wide use of evidence-based medicine and the implementation of national and international guidelines for optimal care play a very important role in this process of improvement of care, drawing a clear line of effective treatment. A recent study by the DOPPs emphasizes how quality of treatment may diverge among centers [28]. In the present context of an ever-growing number of patients requiring treatment in a system of scarce available resources, the optimization of care protocols in terms of "improved care for less money" has become a very complicated challenge. Standardized guidelines coupled with innovative models for process improvement have made it possible to accomplish this otherwise herculean task.

Fresenius Medical Care, has included QPI in an elaborate system called Balanced Scorecard, aimed at evaluating and comparing clinics, countries and regions, providing the stakeholders with an important tool allowing an insight into what is the actual level of care provided in the clinics, besides from the usual financial data [29]. Fresenius Medical Care's approach to 'optimal care' is being applied in more than 3,000 dialysis clinics in North America, Europe, Latin America, Asia-Pacific and Africa. NephroCare, the service provider for Fresenius

Medical Care in Europe, coordinates the clinics in Europe, Middle East, Africa and Latin America, that use state-of-the-art dialysis products, renal pharmaceuticals and therapies (all of which are constantly being improved), as well as care from qualified, motivated clinic personnel who regularly participate in training programs. In every country of its European network, NephroCare adapts its care model to reflect the national health care architecture and to further develop concepts within the predefined regulatory frame [[29]]. To impact the quality and efficacy of a health care service, patient and cost related information must be captured, updated, and shared with all stakeholders in a timely and effective manner to not only ensure universal access to quality data, but also to extend essential information to key clinical decision makers [30]. The Balanced Scorecard tool has allowed NephroCare to promote the collaboration between public institutions and the private provider in more than 20 European countries, giving in the hands of the public a way to control the quality outcomes achieved in the clinics [31,[29]]. This has been an important achievement for quality in the European healthcare context where dialysis is still mainly provided by public hospitals. It has to be noted that all this would not be possible without the implementation of the electronic medical record EMR). Like in the rest of the health care context, the use of a specialized software to keep track of the patients' medical history has made it possible for the nephrologist to have immediate access to an enormous amount of patient information. In the last few years, a large number of software platforms have been proposed and some of them offer personalized versions, which could be customised to the needs of the nephrologist (The DoctorsPartner Nephrology EMR, by DoctorPartner LLC ectectect).

## 2. The Electronic Medical Record (EMR): Benefits of the worldwide web, quick and simple data collection and analysis, statistics as a tool to predict outcomes

Paper-based records are still by far the most common method of recording patient information for most hospitals and practices in the world. A critical aspect of paper-based records is legibility. Handwritten paper medical records can be associated with poor legibility, which can contribute to medical errors [32]. Pre-printed forms, the standardization of abbreviations, and standards for penmanship were encouraged to improve reliability of paper medical records. The majority of physicians still find it easier to handle paper-based records and consider entry of data into an EMR tedious. However, paper-based data require a significant amount of storage space and to retrieve information is quite difficult and time-consuming [[2]]. This is particularly true in the case of person-centred records, which are impractical to maintain if not electronic. For this reason, retrospective analysis based on large historical case series and programs based on data, as Continuous Quality Improvement, are only recently becoming popular with the deployment of EMR. Because of these many "after entry" benefits, governments, insurance companies and large medical institutions are heavily promoting the adoption of EMR. The benefits can be especially high considering the different uses of the same information, i.e. for monitoring a patient, CQI requirements, for reporting purposes or for billing a service. A critical aspect of EMR is the codification of information.

In human communication, free text is the natural approach used not only for oral communication but also for written medical records. Free text offers the option to maximize the benefit of a given language to describe situations well, but it may be difficult to maintain the same content once translated into another language. Additionally, it cannot be used for statistical purposes. Codification is somehow universal, and a code is a kind of ideogramme readable by people of different languages. To get more out of an EMR, information has to be codified as much as possible, allowing an easier use. In general electronic records help with the standardization of forms, terminology and abbreviations, and data input. However, the increased portability and accessibility of electronic medical records may also increase the risk of unauthorized access and theft by as acknowledged by increased security requirements. The ability to exchange records between different EMR systems ("interoperability") facilitates the co-ordination of health care delivery in non-affiliated health care practices. Nowadays it is very common to see primary physicians working with computerized systems in their practice. However, very often they use systems which could be described as minimally functional since they include only orders for prescriptions, orders for tests, viewing laboratory or imaging results, and clinical notes. A more sophisticated use, including further analytical elaboration of the data as required by the CQI approach, is normally not part of the routine. To ensure the quality of care delivered to patients treated in its dialysis units, Fresenius Medical Care continuously monitors its dialysis services. The overall quality management system of the company, which is based on CQI, provides the necessary framework. CQI programs, incorporating the implementation of clinical practice guidelines and CPM by dialysis providers, demand the development of computerized monitoring systems in order to collect and supply information on the dialysis treatment. Therefore, Fresenius Medical Care developed a specific clinical database as a tool to monitor critical aspects of dialysis care and improve the quality of care.. This central database is called EuCliD, the acronym for European Clinical Database as the database was first developed in Europe. EuCliD collects the most-important medical information on the treatment of dialysis patients. The data provide a basis for clinical trials and help improve the treatment of dialysis patients by comparing the different treatments. The description of the first version of the database has already been published [33]. Right from the outset, EuCliD was structured to follow a logical information flow. During the last years the software has been updated and a new project based on an enlarged scope has been initiated. EuCliD 5 now includes daily treatments performed throughout European, Latin American and African Countries. The new project was aimed not only at supporting quality assurance, but also to facilitate the day-to-day work of the clinical staff. As a result, EuCliD 5, is a multilingual and fully codified software using, as much as possible, international standard coding tables (ICD10, WHO: International Statistical Classification of Diseases and Related Health Problems 1992; ISCED, UNESCO, 1997;ISCO-88, International Standard Classification of Occupations 1988 etc.). EuCliD 5 collects and handles sensitive medical patient data, and ensures the confidentiality of these data [34]. EuCliD 5 has been approved by the respective national or regional authorities prior to data entry and the initiation of data transfer. Of course, the transfer of private patient data out of the dialysis center is not permitted. The availability of EuCliD 5 data, as well as the increasing interoperability of data present in other systems has allowed the practical implementation in a clinical environment of tools like the Balanced Scorecard, a tool developed in the scientific domain of complex system management. Key characteristic of Balanced Scorecard is the aim of maximizing concurrent interests of different stakeholders in a balanced form, concentrating on KPIs able to describe variables whose improvement can improve the overall system behavior [29,30]. Each KPI is not a reported value only, but much more the headline of a project or program to improve performance in a strategic relevant, target oriented way. KPIs are dynamic and when they approach saturation need to be substituted by new ones in a continuous development process of quality improvement and know-how and operational excellence Related to the use of a Balanced Scorecard, there are certain *caveat* to consider: since the Balanced Scorecard is nothing else than a model of stege 5 chronic kidney disease management, Wrong or inadequate model design and definition and wrong or inadequate implementation (or execution) can lead to erroneous conclusions. In this sense the right selection of KPI and the appropriateness of the derived actions are of crucial importance as well as the validation of data and their causal relationships with outcomes. It is fundamental to understand how to manage and not just measure performance and this will not happen without regular review sessions at all levels

## 3. Self-organizing maps for continuous quality improvement

In order to derive improvements from the clinical data Self-Organizing Maps (SOMs), an innovative approach recently introduced by Fresenius Medical Care, could complement standard statistical methods used to extrapolate information. A brief description of SOMs follows: As an example, let us consider a dataset containing the values of four variables (Weight, Height, Body Mass Index – BMI –, and Fat) for 251 patients, for which we built a SOM with 84 neurons (Fig. 1). In this case, each neuron is characterized by a vector of four elements, one for each variable: each neuron can be seen as an "average patient", whose height is the average height of all patients associated with that neuron, and the same goes for the other three variables. Neurons that are close in the SOM represent patients that are similar from the point of view of the considered variables. Once the SOM has been configured, different effective views of the distribution of the data can be obtained. In particular, one can focus on a specific variable of the input data by color-coding each neuron of the SOM based on the value of that variable. This kind of plot is called component plane of the SOM (see, for instance, Fig. 1). By comparing different planes (i.e., different variables) it is possible to identify relations existing among the variables. Notice that each given neuron (depicted in Fig. 1 as a hexagon) always represents the same subset of data, over all the different component planes. For example, in Fig. 1 it can be noticed that the same units in the top left of the four component planes represent patients with large weight, medium to small height, large BMI, and large percentage of fat. The units in the bottom right of the graph represent patients with small weight, medium to small height, small BMI, and small percentage of fat. It should be noted that, although the SOM algorithm is not aware of how the BMI is computed, the relation between height and weight that determines the BMI clearly emerges from the component planes. This example shows how the SOM can be effectively used to extract the relations among the variables of interest.

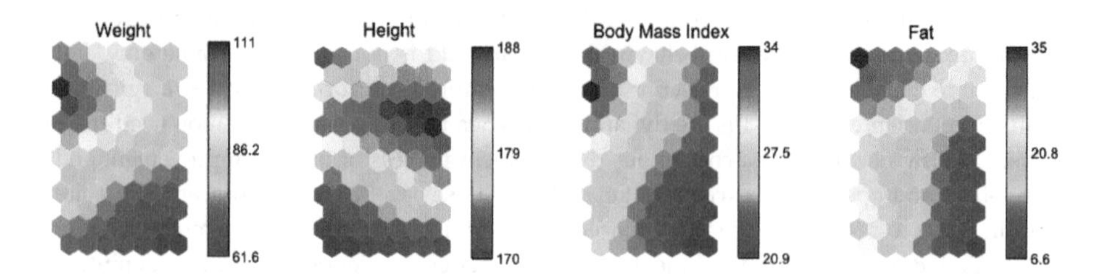


**Figure 1.** Example of SOMs of different variables (Weight, Height, Body Mass Index – BMI –, and Fat) for 251 patients.

To ensure the implementation of CQI policies, extensive data collection from the care units, and their reassembly into meaningful performance indexes need to be put in place. Such processes generate massive amounts of data, which carry information that is not always easily extracted by means of standard statistical approaches. On the other hand, the wealth of the available data allows the application of machine learning approaches, which are able to find structure in complex datasets, even in the absence of an a priori hypothesis about what should be looked for. In other words, the data-driven approach of such techniques *lets the data speak for themselves,* allowing interesting, possibly unanticipated information to emerge. In turn, such information can be used by the management to discover areas of excellence, or clinics where a margin for improvement exists, as well as strategies for achieving such improvement. In the context of the Balanced Scorecard, the available data are organized as vectors of KPI scores, one per clinic-month. Given these data, it is of particular interest to extract the relations existing among different KPIs for particular groups of clinics, in order to identify clusters that share a similar performance pattern, as characterized by correlated scores on specific KPIs.

For this reason, we have recently introduced the use of SOMs to analyze BSC data [34]. SOMs have already been validated as reliable tools in health care, for instance for population studies [35](Basara H, Yuan M, 2008) and for organization [36] or economic evaluations [37]. A Self-Organizing Map is a machine learning paradigm mainly used for clustering and visualization of data in high dimensional spaces (ie, data with a large number of variables) [38]. The SOM model is composed of units, often referred to as *neurons,* organized in a low dimensional reticular structure (generally in bi-dimensional or tri-dimensional space), which act as prototypes of the input data in such lower-dimensional space. The SOM learns in an *unsupervised* way to assign each input data point to the neuron that is most similar to it, by means of a training procedure that aims at preserving the topological characteristics of the input space – that is, similar input vectors are mapped to close regions in the SOM. Once the SOM has been configured, different effective views of the distribution of the data can be obtained. In particular, one can focus on a specific dimension of the input vectors (in our case, one specific KPI) by colour-coding each neuron of the SOM based on the value that the

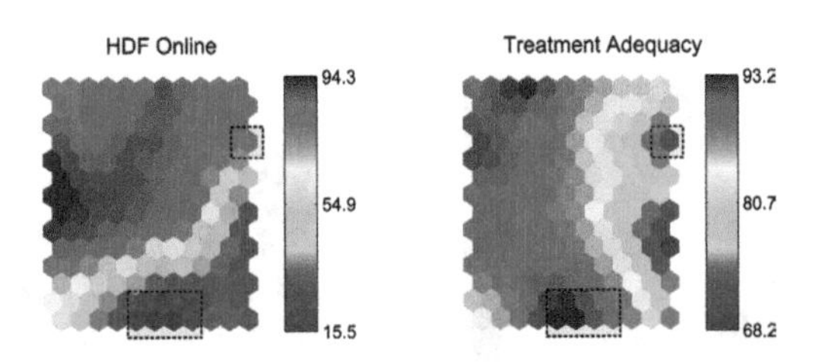


**Figure 2.** Two component planes (relative to the HDF online KPI and to the Treatment Adequacy KPI, respectively) of an SOM trained on BSC data from Portuguese clinics of the NC network. The dashed rectangles superimposed on the planes indicate regions of the SOM where interesting groups of clinics can be found (see discussion in the text). SOM training and visualization were performed in MATLAB using the SOM toolbox [39]. The SOM is shown as a collection of neurons (hexagons) placed in a two-dimensional grid, where the focus is on the relative, rather than the absolute, position of each neuron: that is, the main information content lies in the neighborhood relationships among neurons, as adjacent neurons contain similar KPI records. We can therefore compute the average score for a given KPI in each neuron: this is represented by a color code (colorbar shown on the right) in the component plane relative to that KPI

prototype takes on that particular dimension. This kind of plot is called *component plane* of the SOM (Fig. 2).

Many interesting insights can be achieved when running an SOM-based analysis on BSC data. For instance, Fig. 2 shows two component planes obtained from an SOM trained on the BSC data of Portuguese clinics (33 clinics, monitored for 28 months, from January 2008 to March 2010). By comparing different planes (*i.e,* different KPIs), it is possible to identify groups of data (in our case, clinic-month KPI vectors) that share a similar pattern of performance (as they are located in the same region of the map) and characterize such patterns in terms of specific KPI relations. Thus, for instance in Fig. 2, all KPI vectors that are assigned to the upper left corner of the SOM share a similar structure, which is characterized, among other things, by a high score both on the HDF Online and the Treatment Adequacy KPIs (positive correlation). From these planes one can notice that, while these two KPIs are positively correlated for most clinics in the dataset, there are also cases where treatment adequacy is low (see marked unit on the right side of the map), and cases where a good treatment adequacy is achieved (bottom part of the map). These groups of clinics thus show an interesting performance pattern that might prompt further investigations, and possibly corrective measures. To this end, one can easily trace back the clinics falling into these regions of the map to retrieve all relevant information about them. Similarly, in Fig. 3, two different component planes from the same SOM as above are shown: as expected, the patient growth and new patient inflow KPIs are, in general, directly correlated. However, it is also possible to identify groups of clinics that show a moderately high new patient Iinflow while maintaining a low patient growth score (upper left corner).

This observation can allow to quickly identifying those clinics where, presumably, there is a relevant outflow of patients and, therefore, there might be the need for corrective measures. As a final example, consider Fig. 4 where two component planes of a different SOM, trained on data from Turkey (46 clinics monitored during the same period as those in Portugal), are shown.

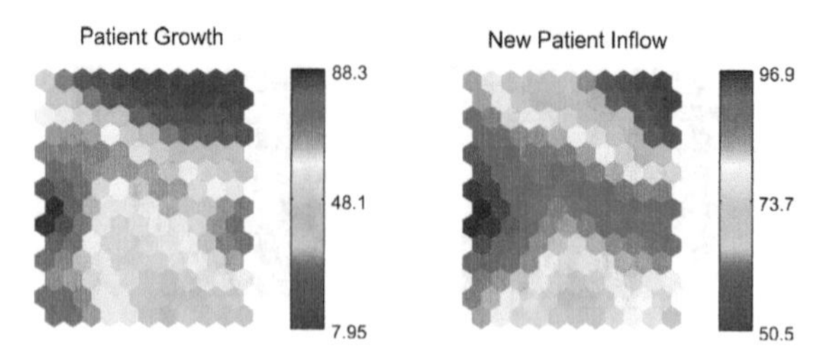


**Figure 3.** Two component planes from the SOM for the Portuguese clinics of the NC network. The shown planes refer to the Patient Growth and New Patient Inflow KPIs, respectively.

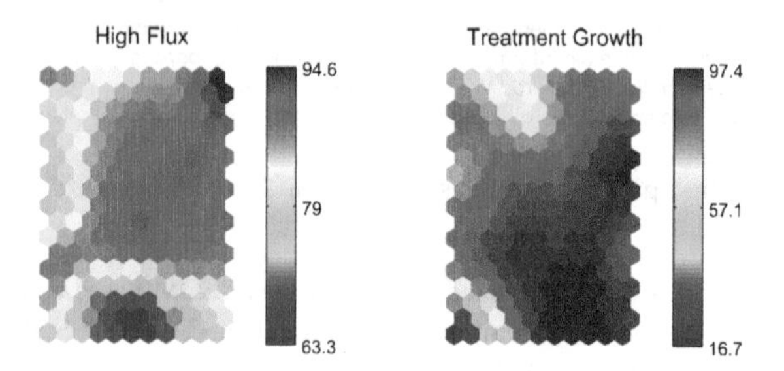


**Figure 4.** The High Flux and Treatment Growth component planes of an SOM trained on data from Turkish clinics of the NC network.

Here, it can be noticed, in particular, that an interesting group of clinics exists (bottom part of the map) where high Treatment growth is observed but the use of High Flux dialysis is low. This means that patients may be referred to this group of clinics for reasons different than quality of treatment (*i.e.* proximity) as expressed by this KPI. These were just a few examples of benefits from an SOM-based analysis on performance data; other results are extensively described [35]. Together, these results show how SOMs have the potential to unveil significant relationships among KPIs and to identify groups of clinics with different performance patterns, which in turn may require different corrective actions. Thus, SOMs offer valuable hints on the potential areas of intervention in the context for CQI. Information about correlated features emerges directly from the data, without the need for the management to specify a working hypothesis in advance; in this way, also relationships that were not previously advanced can be unveiled, which underlines the greater power of the SOM approach with respect to more traditional statistical analyses. Moreover, it should be remarked that another attractive feature of SOMs is that they can be visualized in an intuitive way so as to immediately convey the correlation structure of the data: this is an extra value of the approach that makes it particularly suited for prompt communication at the management level. This innovative approach to intelligent analysis of clinical data could be a contributing factor to more effective guidance of disease management.

## 4. Conclusions

Every care process and particularly chronic care has to be centered on patients; therapeutic performance should therefore be measured on outcomes and not on inputs and/or procedures. This holistic approach of organizational models shall encompass all therapeutic aspects. Full availability of data and transparency are fundamental to make this patient orientation possible and long term sustainable for all involved stakeholders. Furthermore data will allow the extensive use of tools like the Balanced Scorecard and CQI. Tools of the domain of Computational Intelligence will help to develop unconsidered working hypothesis that could open to physicians new horizons of clinical research and improve understanding of functional processes in an "in vivo" environment at affordable costs. Collecting comparable and meaningful data requires the adoption of therapeutic protocols and the extensive use of guidelines. This will not lead to mere standardization and flattening of clinical activity but to a conscious personalization of clinical path. In complex models, with multiple correlated variables, consistent implementation of standards is fundamental to isolate the therapeutic change doctors want to initiate. In an environment of limited resources. their correct utilization could reduce the number of therapeutic errors with consequent reduction of waste of chances for the patient, doctor time, pharmaceutical and biomedical therapies. This would be reached through induction of error-free behaviours, increase of doctor time dedicated to real relevant things (*e.g.* using proven algorithms instead of calculating every time therapetic effort) and a patient orientation focused on relevant issues. A strong distinction has to be made between formal and substantial adoption and application of guidelines: it is not about formally adopting a given guideline, it is much more about their correct and consistent implementation and maintenance along the years. In this sense, it has to be highlighted role and relevance of training and continuous education. Finally, the complex nature of systems like the ones dealing with chronic illness care has to be considered. Complex systems tend to adapt to changes and to adsorb variations; the focus on execution and the application of guidelines tend to decrease and/or reduce their marginal benefit. To achieve the step from performance measurement to performance management, it is necessary to understand the real nature of KPIs as projects, with a start, an execution and an end according to a certain plan and with given resources. And to be ready to exchange new *vs.* old KPIs as soon as the project target has been achieved (e.g. when the KPI tends to saturation).

## Acknowledgement

The authors are grateful to Ms Gerdi Klinkner for the revision of the text.

## Disclosure

All the authors are full-time employees of Fresenius Medical Care.

## Author details

Bernard Canaud[1], Ciro Tetta[1*], Daniele Marcelli[1], Guido Giordana[2], Stefano Stuard[2], Katrin Koehler[1], Flavio Mari[3], Carlo Barbieri[3], Miryana Dobreva[2], Andrea Stopper[2] and Emanuele Gatti[4]

*Address all correspondence to: ciro.tetta@fmc-ag.com

1 Medical Board EMEALA, Fresenius Medical Care Deutschland GmbH, Bad Homburg, Germany

2 Nephrocare Coordination EMEALA, Fresenius Medical Care Deutschland GmbH, Bad Homburg, Germany

3 Healthcare and Business Advanced Modeling Fresenius Medical Care Deutschland GmbH, Palazzo Pignano, Italy

4 CEO EMEALA, Global Chief Strategist, Fresenius Medical Care, Bad Homburg, Germany and Center for Biomedical Technology, Danube University, Krems, Austria

## References

[1] Mendelssohn, D. C., & Benaroia, M. (2008). The modern haemodialysis factory: must quality improvement trump personalized care? Nephrol Dial Transplant X: , 1-3.

[2] Hegbrant, J., Gentile, G., & Strippoli, G. F. (2011). The quest to standardize hemodialysis care. Contrib Nephrol , 171, 39-49.

[3] Marcelli, D., Moscardó, V., Steil, H., Day, M., Kirchgessner, J., Mitteregger, A., Orlandini, G. C., & Gatti, E. Data Management and Quality Assurance for Dialysis Network ((2002). Ronco C, La Greca G (eds): Hemodialysis Technology. Contrib Nephrol., Karger (Basel) , 137

[4] Canaud, B., Tong, L., Tentori, F., Akiba, T., Karaboyas, A., Gillespie, B., Akizawa, T., Pisoni, R. L., Bommer, J., & Port, F. K. (2011). Clinical practices and outcomes in elderly hemodialysis patients: results from the Dialysis Outcomes and Practice Patterns Study (DOPPS). Clin J Am Soc NephrolJul;, 6(7), 1651-62.

[5] Robinson BM, Joffe MM, Pisoni RL, Port FK, Feldman HI(2006). Revisiting survival differences by race and ethnicity among hemodialysis patients: the Dialysis Outcomes and Practice Patterns Study. J Am Soc Nephrol. , 17(10), 2910-8.

[6] Port, F. K., Pisoni, R. L., Bommer, J., Locatelli, F., Jadoul, M., Eknoyan, G., Kurokawa, K., Canaud, B. J., Finley, M. P., & Young, E. W. (2006). Improving Outcomes for Dialysis Patients in the International Dialysis Outcomes and Practice Patterns Study. Clin J Am Soc Nephrol , 1(2), 246-255.

[7] Canaud, B., Wabel, P., & Tetta, C. (2010). Dialysis prescription: A modifiable risk factor for chronic kidney disease patients. Blood Purif., 29(4), 366-74.

[8] Canaud, B., Chenine, L., Leray-Moragués, H., Wiesen, H., & Tetta, C. (2006). Residual renal function and dialysis modality: is it really beneficial to preserve residual renal function in dialysis patients? Nephrology (Carlton) , 11(4), 292-6.

[9] Di Benedetto, A., Richards, N., Marcelli, D., Basci, A., Cesare, S., Ponce, P., Scatizzi, L., & Marotta, P. (2008). Is it necessary to check outcomes to improvequality of care? The example of anemia management. J Nephrol 21 (suppl 13): SS152, 146.

[10] Ng, L. J., Chen, F., Pisoni, R. L., Krishnan, M., Mapes, D., Keen, M., & Bradbury, . (2011). Hospitalization risks related to vascular access type among incident US hemodialysis patients. Nephrol Dial Transplant , 26(11), 3659-66.

[11] Rayner HC, Pisoni RL(2010). The increasing use of hemodialysis catheters: evidence from the DOPPS on its significance and ways to reverse it. Semin Dial , 23(1), 6-10.

[12] Tentori, F., Zhang, J., Li, Y., Karaboyas, A., Kerr, P., Saran, R., Bommer, J., Port, F., Akiba, T., Pisoni, R., & Robinson, B. (2012). Longer dialysis session length is associated with better intermediate outcomes and survival among patients on in-center three times per week hemodialysis: results from the Dialysis Outcomes and Practice Patterns Study (DOPPS). Nephrol Dial Transplant Mar 19. [Epub ahead of print]

[13] Zhang, H., Schaubel, D. E., Kalbfleisch-Gresham, Bragg., Robinson, J. L., Pisoni, R. L., Canaud, B., Jadoul, M., Akiba, T., Saito, A., Port, F. K., & Saran, R. (2012). Dialysis outcomes and analysis of practice patterns suggests the dialysis schedule affects day-of-week mortality. Kidney Int , 81(11), 1108-15.

[14] Robinson BM, Port FK(2009). International Hemodialysis Patient Outcomes Revisited: The Role of Practice Patterns and Other Factors. Clin J Am Soc Nephrol. 4 Suppl 1:S, 12-17.

[15] Lopes-Gresham, Bragg., Ramirez, J. L., Andreucci, S. P. B., Akiba, V. E., Saito, T., Jacobson, A., Robinson, S. H., Port, F. K., Mason, N. A., & Young, E. W. (2009). Prescription of antihypertensive agents to hemodialysis patients: Time trends and associations with patient characteristics, country, and survival in the DOPPS. Nephrol Dial Transplant , 24, 2809 2816.

[16] Tentori, F. (2010). Mineral and bone disorder and outcomes in hemodialysis patients: Results from the DOPPS. Semin Dial 10; , 23(1), 10-14.

[17] Blayney, Tentori. F. (2009). Trends and Consequences of Mineral Bone Disorder in Hemodialysis Patients: Lessons from the Dialysis Outcomes and Practice Patterns Study (DOPPS). Invited paper for Supplement to the Journal of Renal Care. J Ren Care 35: (Suppl 1) 7-13

[18] Hasegawa, T., Bragg-Gresham, J. L., Pisoni, R. L., Robinson, Fukuhara. S., Akiba, T., Saito, A., Kurokawa, K., & Akizawa, T. (2011). Changes in anemia management and

hemoglobin levels following revision of a bundling policy to incorporate recombinant human erythropoietin. Kidney Int , 79, 340-346.

[19] Mc Farlane, P. A., Pisoni, R. L., Eichleay, Wald. R., Port, F. K., & Mendelssohn, D. International trends in erythropoietin use and hemoglobin levels in hemodialysis patients. Kidney Int (2010). , 78(2), 215-223.

[20] Canaud, B., Bragg-Gresham, J. L., Marshall, M. R., Desmeules, S., Gillespie, B. W., Depner, T., Klassen, P., & Port, F. K. (2006). Mortality risk for patients receiving hemodiafiltration versus hemodialysis: European results from the DOPPS. Kidney Int , 69, 2087-2093.

[21] Canaud, B., Bragg-Gresham, J. L., Marshall, M. R., Desmeules, S., Gillespie, B. W., Depner, T., Klassen, P., & Port, F. K. (2006). Mortality risk for patients receiving hemodiafiltration versus hemodialysis: European results from the DOPPS. Kidney Int , 69, 2087-2093.

[22] Hornberger, J., & Hirth, R. A. (2012). Financial implications of choice of dialysis type of the revised medicare payment system: an economic analysis. Am J Kidney Dis , 60(2), 280-7.

[23] Richards, N., Ayala, J. A., Cesare, S., Chazot, C., Di Benedetto, A., Gassia, J. P., Merello, J., Rentero, R., Scatizzi, L., & Marcelli, D. (2007). Assessment of Quality Guidelines Implementation Using a Continuous Quality Improvement Programme. Blood Purif , 25, 221-228.

[24] Hirth RA(2010). International economics of dialysis: Lessons from the DOPPS. Semin Dial 20; , 23(1), 16-18.

[25] http://dialysis-centers.findthebest.com/, 2012

[26] Fresenius Medical Care Market & Competitor Survey, 2011

[27] Directive 95/46 of the European Parliament and of the Council, 1995

[28] Pisoni, R. L., Bragg-Gresham, J. L., Fuller, Morgenstern. H., Canaud, B., Locatelli, F., Li, Y., Gillespie, B., Wolfe, R. A., Port, F. K., & Robinson, . (2011). Facility-level interpatient hemoglobin variability in hemodialysis centers participating in the Dialysis Outcomes and Practice Patterns Study (DOPPS): Associations With mortality, patient characteristics, and facility practices. Am J Kidney Dis , 57(2), 266-275.

[29] Stopper, S., Amato, C., Gioberge, S., Giordana, G., Marcelli, D., & Gatti, E. (2007). Managing Complexity at Dialysis Service Centers across Europe. Blood Purif , 25, 77-89.

[30] Stopper, A., Raddatz, A., Grassmann, A., Stuard, S., Menzer, M., Possnien, G., Scatizzi, L., Marcelli, D., & (2011, . (2011). Delivering Quality of Care while Managing the Interests of All Stakeholders. Blood Purif , 32(4), 323-30.

[31] de Francisco, A. L. M., & Piñera, C. (2011). Nephrology around Europe: organization models and management strategies: Spain. J. Nephrol. , 24(4), 438-45.

[32] Institute of Medicine(1999). To Err Is Human: Building a Safer Health System (1999)". The National Academies Press. http://fermat.nap.edu/catalog/9728.html#toc.

[33] Marcelli, D., Kirchgessner, J., Amato, C., Steil, H., Mitteregger, A., Moscardo, V., Carioni, C., Orlandini, G., & Gatti, E. (2001). EuCliD (European Clinical Database): a database comparing different realities. J Nephrol 14 (Suppl 4): SS101., 94.

[34] Cattinelli, I., Bolzoni, E., Barbieri, C., Mari, F., Martin-Guerrero-Olivas, Soria., Martinez-Martinez, E., Gomez-Sanchis, J. M., Amato, J., Stopper, C., Gatti, A., & , E. (2012). Use of Self-Organizing Maps for Balanced Scorecard analysis to monitor the performance of dialysis clinic chains, Health Care Manag Sci , 15, 79-90.

[35] Basara, H., & Yuan, M. (2008). Community health assessment using self-organizing maps and geographic information systems. Int J Health Geogr 7:67

[36] Lloyd-Williams, M., & Williams, T. (1996). A neural network approach to analyzing health care information. Top Health Inf Manage , 17(2), 26-33.

[37] Montefiori, M., & Resta, M. (2008). A computational approach for the health care market. Health Care Manag Sci , 12(4), 344-350.

[38] Kohonen, T. (2001). Self-organizing maps, Springer, 3rd edition.

[39] Vesanto, J., Himberg, J., Alhoniemi, E., & Parhankangas, J. (2000). SOM Toolbox for MATLAB 5, Technical Report, Helsinki University of Technology.

Chapter 6

# Analysis of the Dialysis Dose in Different Clinical Situations: A Simulation-Based Approach

Rodolfo Valtuille, Manuel Sztejnberg and
Elmer. A. Fernandez

Additional information is available at the end of the chapter

## 1. Introduction

End Stage Renal Disease (ESRD) is an important public health concern around the globe. It is associated with high morbidity and mortality being Hemodialysis (HD) the main applied therapy. [1]

A recent study (HEMO study) could not show any decrease in the morbidity and/or mortality associated with increases in the dose -expressed as equilibrated Kt/V (eqKt/V)- and/or the flow (comparing high versus low flux, where high flux is defined as a Kt/V of Beta 2 microglobulin (B2M) ≥ 20 ml/min) when utilizing the three-times-a-week (3-times/wk HD) schedule therapy. [2]

This led to development of several HD schedules proposals based on the variation of the session time duration (TD) as well as on its weekly frequency (Fr). However, more frequent HD schedules require new indexes to measure the delivered dose. In this context, the Equivalent Renal Clearence (EKR) [Casino y López] [3] and Standard Kt/V (stdKt/V) [Gotch] [4] indexes have been proposed to quantify the dialysis dose for different HD frequency schedules.

The EKR concept equalizes the time-averaged concentration (TAC) of Urea (U) for different therapies which is then normalized by U distribution Volume. Gotch has proposed that the weekly dialysis dose (WDD) is better expressed as standardized kt-V (stdKt/V) when dialysis is more frequent than 3-times/wk. Standard Kt/V combines treatment dose and frequency allowing comparison of intermittent (HD, High flux HD, Hemofiltration, etc) and continuous (Continuous Ambulatory Peritoneal Dialysis) therapies; the formula is expressed as U generation rate (G) rate divided by the average peak concentration. [4]

EqKt/V is the true dialysis dose per session occurring when U rebound (R), which is related to compartments and flow disequilibrium produced during HD treatment, is completed 30-60 minutes after the end of the HD session.

The determination of eqKt/V requires the measurement or the "prediction" of the true Eq U because the value of sp (single pool)Kt/V - a dimensionless ratio which includes Clearence of dialyzer (K), duration of treatment (TD) and volume of total water of the patient (V) - is greater than the Kt/V achieved in the patient which is calculated using the immediate postHD blood U concentration.

In the last decade, several formulas were developed to predict eq Kt/V trying to avoid the extraction of an additional blood sample. The Daugirdas and Schneditz "rate formula" is the most popular and validated equation and it is based in the prediction of eqKt/V as a linear function of spKt/V and the rate of dialysis (K/V). [5]

An alternative and robust formula, based in the double pool analysis by Smye, [6] is the equation of Tattersall where he described a soluble time constant: the patient equilibration time (tp). [7]

The majority of these formulas of prediction have been validated in the 3-times/wk HD schedules.

New formulas to predict eq Kt/V have been recently published. Examples include the eqKt/V formula based on observations of the HEMO [8] study and two others developed by Leypoldt (based on blood sample analysis during hemofiltration and short and daily HD) [9].

The high accuracy of the extracellular U concentration evolution during and after (UR) an HD session by double pool U kinetic model has been verified in several studies. [10]

Access and cardio-pulmonary recirculation can both influence the UR, but the effect occurs in the first minutes after the end of HD and is considered to be mild. [10]

Several factors other than clearance of U might play a role in morbidity and mortality of hemodialyzed patients.

One of them, recently revised, is the role of the "denominator" to normalize the Kt. The results derived from the HEMO study showed that Kt/V failed to explain the paradoxical outcomes related to size (underweight versus obese patients) and gender. This factor was considered in the Frequent Hemodialysis Network (FHN) study which is currently underway. The investigators included the body surface area (BSA) as a potential tool for a better normalization of Kt and to allow more appropriate comparison among different HD populations. [11]

Since 1980 the idea of emulating reality in a computer environment by simulation rapidly spread among biomedical researchers, being accepted as one of the most powerful tools both for understanding phenomenological aspects of a chosen physics or physiological complex and for predicting functional or operative conditions of technological systems. The main concept of this approach relies in numerically solving a mathematical model that governs a chosen physical system, whose the analytical solution is not known or potentially dangerous to reach for a specific application. In spite of many efforts spent in the past for formulating accurate and robust algorithms for solving mathematical models, the effectiveness of that approach heavily dependent on computational resources. This led to only recent widespread use of simulation strategy both scientific and medical problems [12].

A variable volume double-compartment (VVDC) kinetic model can reflect the behavior of different molecules and can be used as a mirror to analyze the profile in vivo by taking blood samples during the HD procedure. [13]

In this scenario, the computational simulation including all the variables which affect the dialysis procedure can be a safe and useful tool to mimic many treatment schemes to help improve our knowledge of the dialysis therapy. [14]

The aim of this study is to utilize a variable volume double-compartment (VVDC) kinetic model to simulate:

1. Several clinical situations that allow comparison between the true eqKt/V and all the developed predictors, including the effect of increasing the TD and Fr.
2. Changes in Kt/V, EKR and stdKt/V related to changes in TD and Fr.
3. Comparison between using V with BSA to normalize K.

## 2. Materials and methods

### 2.1. Simulation and analysis

A variable volume double-compartment (VVDC) kinetic model has been implemented based on the existing models of the U concentration behaviour. The model is described in Figure 1 and the equations are as follows:

$$\frac{d(V_eC_e)}{dt}(t) = G - K_c(C_e(t) - C_i(t)) - C_e(t)(K_e(t) + K_r + K_d) \tag{1}$$

$$\frac{d(V_iC_i)}{dt}(t) = K_c(C_e(t) - C_i(t)) \tag{2}$$

$$\frac{dV}{dt}(t) = \alpha(t) \tag{3}$$

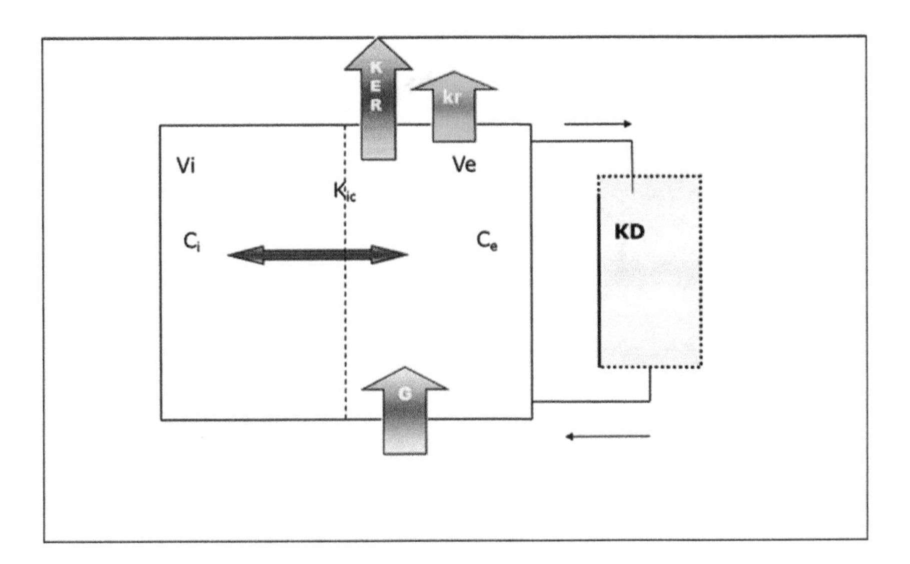


**Figure 1.** Scheme of Variable-Volume Double Compartment dialysis kinetic model

Whereas "V" is: solute distribution volume, "C": solute concentration, "K": clearance constant, "G": solute generation, "c": cellular, "e": extracellular, "i": intracellular, "r": renal, "d": dialyser, a: volume change velocity (this constant is positive between dialysis sessions and negative during them), "t": time. Equations 1, 2 and 3 make a dependent differential equation system that can be numerically solved. Through these simulations, it is possible to obtain the time profile of intra and extracellular volumes and concentrations of the studied solutes (figure 2).

By defining a behaviour determined for several time intervals on certain variables, such as $\alpha$ and Kd, it is possible to simulate different dialysis schedules, regarding session duration times (TD) and time between dialysis sessions or dialysis frequency (Fr).

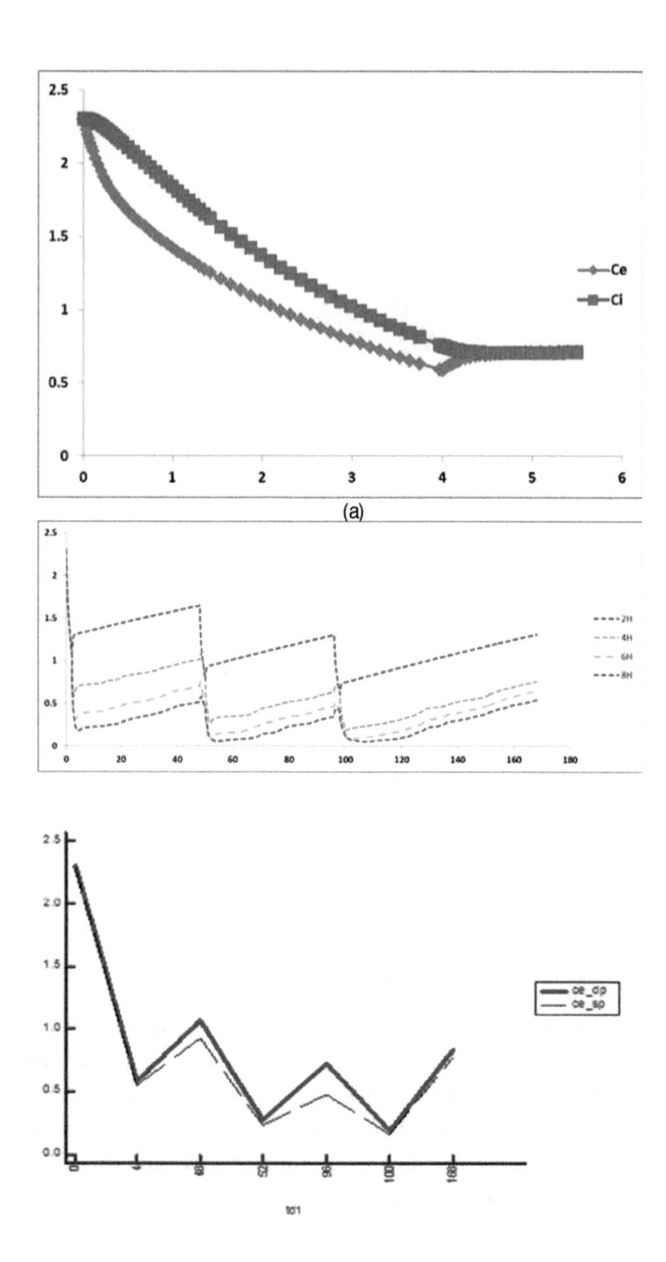


**Figure 2.** (a) Simulation of a profile during HD and the rebound of the solute immediately after the end. (b) Simulation of the weekly HD profile showing the effect of increasing the TD with fixed Kd and Kc. (c) Urea dinamycs simulated with double or single pool.

### 2.2. Simulated systems

*2.2.1. Comparison between the true eq Kt/V and all the developed predictors*

The simulations assumed that the subjects had a solute distribution volume of 580 ml/Kg and the intra and extracellular distribution relation is 2/3 and 1/3 of the total V. The extra-renal clearance constant (Ker) was considered invalid for the U.

Residual renal clearance (Kr) was 0. 1ml/min in all the cases.

Dialysis schedules with a duration between 2 and 8 hours at 2-hour-intervals of 2 hour were simulated and the weekly frequency of treatment were 3 and 7 days/wk.

The simulations resulted in a time-dependent evolution of the molecule concentration under study (U) in each of the compartments, that is, the intracellular (Ci) and extracellular (Ce) compartments.

We analysed 1005 determinations of U pre HD, U posHD and eqU (60 minutes after the end of the simulated session). This determinations were obtained in the midweek of the 4th and 10th week of simulation

These determinations were product of the manipulation of six (6) variables-Table 1-

| Weight | Kc(ml/min) | Kd(ml/min) | $U_{onset(mg\%)}$ | UF(ml/session) | UR% |
|---|---|---|---|---|---|
| 60-120 | 400-1000 | 100-250 | 160 -240 | 500-4000 | 3.65-17.8 |

**Table 1.** Range of values of the different simulated variables.

U G was 6. 25mg/min in all the simulations.

*2.2.2. Formulas*

Simulated eqKt/V was compared with the previously described predictors with the next formulas :

$$Kt/V = Ln\left(\frac{U_{poo}}{U_{pre}}\right) \tag{4}$$

$$Kt/V = Ln\left(\frac{U_{eq}}{U_{pre}}\right) \tag{5}$$

$$Kt/V_{TATTERSALL} = Kt/V * \left[\frac{t}{t+35}\right] \tag{6}$$

$$Kt / V_{DAUGIRDAS} = Kt / V - 0.6 * \frac{Kt / V}{t} + 0.03 \quad (7)$$

$$Kt / V_{HEMO} = Kt / V - 0.39 * \frac{Kt / V}{t} \quad (8)$$

$$Kt / V_{LEYPOLDT1} = 0.924 * Kt / V - 0.395 * \frac{Kt / V}{t} + 0.056 \quad (9)$$

$$Kt / V_{LEYPOLDT2} = 0.915 * Kt / V - 0.485 * \frac{Kt / V}{t} + 0.106 \quad (10)$$

### 2.3. Changes in Kt/V, EKR and stdKt/V related to changes in TD and Fr

Typical 80-kg-patient with a residual renal clearance (Kr) of 0. 1ml/min and a weight gain a (interdialysis) and ultrafiltration (intradialysis) of 0. 65 ml/min was chosen to simulate the different therapeutic dialysis schedules.

The assumption was that this typical patient would have a solute distribution volume of 580 ml/Kg (46. 4 litres) and when the solute is U, the intra and extracellular distribution relation is 2/3 and 1/3 of the total V. The extrarenal clearance constant (Ker) was considered invalid for the U.

Dialysis schedules with a duration between 1 and 8 hours at intervals of 1 hour were simulated and the weekly frequency of treatment was changed from 3 to 7 days a week on each of them thus obtaining 28 different schemes.

The Fr applied to the simulations does not represent sessions uniformly distributed through the week; it was implemented according to the time tables used in the usual HD practice. For the 3-times/wk Fr, three sessions with an interval between the beginning of sessions of 48, 48 and 72 hours (that is, Monday, Wednesday and Friday) were performed. For the 4-times/wk sessions, the intervals are 24, 48, 24 and 72 hours. For the 5-and 6 -times/wk sessions, 4 and 5 intervals of 24 hours and the last one of 72 and 48 hours, respectively, are established. When the Fr is of 7-times/wk, the distribution is uniform.

The simulations resulted in a time-dependent evolution of the molecule concentration under study (Urea) in the intracellular (Ci) and extracellular (Ce) compartments.

Over the U time profiles, the real Time Average Concentration (TAC) is calculated. Since the main objective was to evaluate which of the proposed indexes more accurately showed the dose changes caused by the scheme changes, the behaviour of the weekly Kt/V, EKR (Casino), std Kt/V (Gotch) and the rebound percentage (% rebound), were compared according the following formulas:

$$\frac{Kt}{V} = \sum_{j=1}^{N} \ln\left(\frac{C_{ePre}}{C_{ePost}}\right)_j \tag{11}$$

$$TAC = \frac{1}{2N}\sum_{j=1}^{N}\left(C_{ePre} + C_{ePost}\right)_j \tag{12}$$

$$EKR = \frac{G}{TAC} \tag{13}$$

$$std\frac{Kt}{V} = \frac{G}{\frac{1}{N}\sum_{j=1}^{N}\left(C_{ePre}\right)_j} \tag{14}$$

$$\%R = \frac{100}{N}\sum_{j=1}^{N}\left(\frac{C_{eq} - C_{ePost}}{C_{eq}}\right)_j \tag{15}$$

## 2.4. Hemodialysis simulation tool: HD-SIM

The simulations of hemodyalisis kinetics were performed through the utilization of a software specially developed for hemodyalisis simulation: HD-SIM. [15] This software was developed on MATLAB (c) platform and consists of a calculation core and a graphical user interface (GUI).

HD-SIM calculation core utilizes MATLAB ® (version 6. 5) simulation package SIMULINK® to support the VVDC kinetics model. Given the set of required parameters through the GUI, solute compartmental concentrations (Ce and Ci) and volumes (Ve and Vi) are calculated as functions of time. Concentration-time profiles are used for the calculation of different hemodyalisis quantity-quality estimators such as: TAC, EKR, Kt/V, and stdKt/V. The calculation core solver is used with: ode113 algorithm (Adams – variable step) that is recommended by MathWorks for narrow tolerances, automatic integration step, maximum step of 1 (1 hr), duration of 1680 (10 weeks), absolute tolerance of $10^{-7}$ ($10^{-7}$ mg/ml) and relative tolerance of $10^{-7}$.

HD-SIM GUI provides a friendly set of windows that allows inserting patient and dialyzer specific data into the simulation system that is required to feed the VVDC model, defining sets of TDs and Frs to evaluate a wide range of treatment schedules, and managing the outcome of the simulations from visualizing estimator values and concentration profiles to file-saving selected results. (figures 3, 4 and 5)

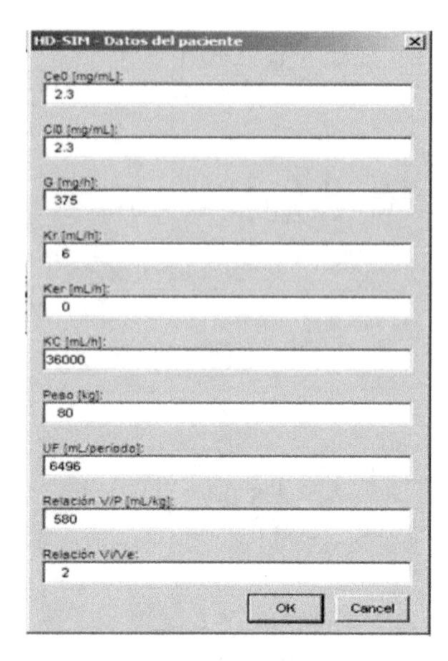


**Figure 3.** Patient and simulation data displayed by HD-SIM

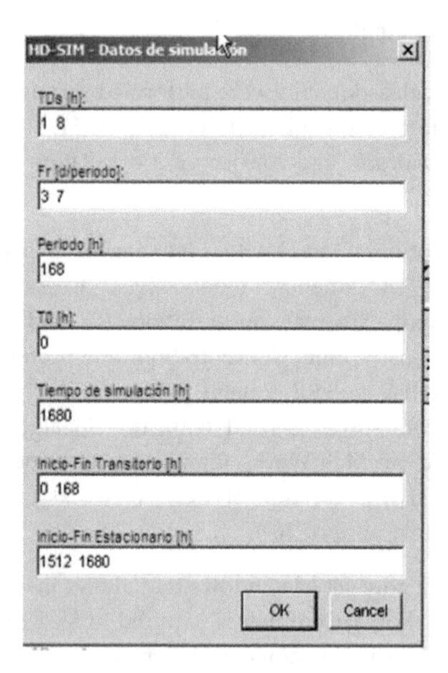


**Figure 4.** Patient and simulation data displayed by HD-SIM

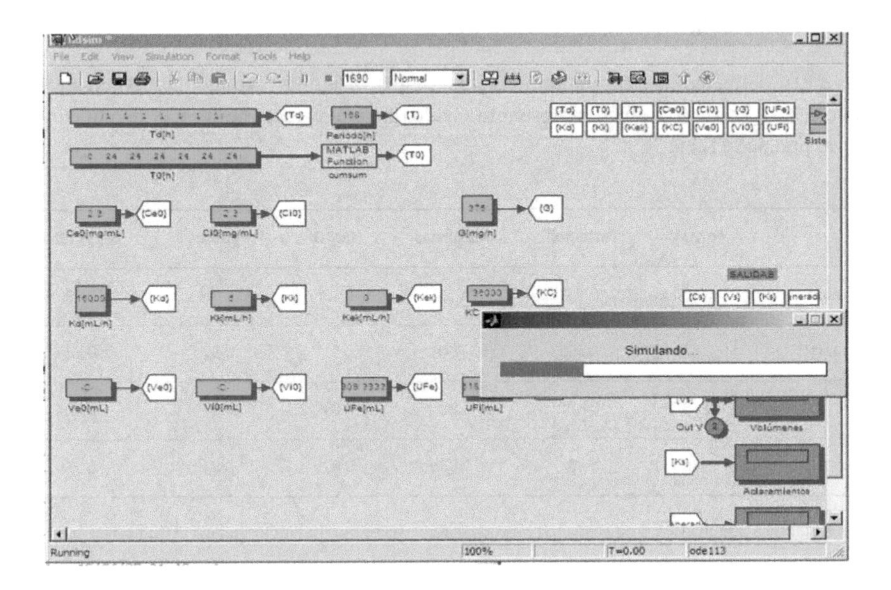


**Figure 5.** HDSIM running the simulations.

Table 2 shows the values at the the beginning of the simulation.

| Solute | Ce onset (mg %) | G (mg/min) | Kc(ml/min) | Kd(ml/min) |
|---|---|---|---|---|
| Urea | 230 | 6.25 | 600 | 250 |

**Table 2.** Values at the beginning of the simulation

## 3. Statistical analysis

All values are expressed as mean±standard deviation (sd) or median (range) as appropriate. Correlation coefficients were determined using the Pearson method. For analysis of agreement between methods (for example simulated (sim) eqKtV versus EqKtV predictors) we used Bland Altman analysis. To compare sim eqKtV with predictors we also used analysis of error: mean error (sim eqKtV-predictor) and % mean error ( (sim eqKtV-predictor)/ sim eqKtV) x 100). We used MedCalc version 12. 3. 0(MedCalc Software,Mariakerke,Belgium) for the statistical analysis.

# 4. Results

## 4.1. Prediction of the eqKt/V

The eq KtV delivered in 1005 simulations was 0. 84±0. 47 with a median of 0. 78 and a range between 0. 10 and 2. 54, which represent the wide range of values commonly seen in current clinical practice. (Table 3)

| | eqKt/V | Tattersall | Daugirdas | HEMO | Leypoldt 1 | Leypoldt 2 |
|---|---|---|---|---|---|---|
| **Minimum** | 0.10 | 0.13 | 0.14 | 0.13 | 0.18 | 0.13 |
| **1st Quart** | 0.47 | 0.50 | 0.50 | 0.51 | 0.52 | 0.46 |
| **Mean** | 0.85 | 0.87 | 0.88 | 0.89 | 0.87 | 0.80 |
| **Median** | 0.78 | 0.80 | 0.82 | 0.82 | 0.81 | 0.75 |

**Table 3.** Statistical summary of Simulated and predicted eqKt/V values by different formulas. (1st Quart=first quartile)

## 4.2. Behaviour of predictors

All predictors showed a high Pearson correlation coefficient (≥ 0. 99) with sim eqKt/V and among themselves.

Daurgidas, Tattersall, HEMO and Leypoldt1 underestimated sim eqKt/V. Leypoldt2 was the only one to overestimate the sim eqKtV. (Tables 4 and 5)

| | Daugirdas | Tattersall | HEMO | Leypoldt1 | Leypoldt2 |
|---|---|---|---|---|---|
| **Mean** | -0.0302 | -0.0199 | -0.0435 | -0.0244 | 0.0428 |
| **SD** | 0.03680 | 0.03255 | 0.02959 | 0.05039 | 0.05670 |
| **Median** | -0.0350 | -0.0241 | -0.0459 | -0.0300 | 0.0304 |
| **Minimum** | -0.101 | -0.0836 | -0.110 | -0.110 | -0.0454 |
| **Maximum** | 0.0783 | 0.0827 | 0.0721 | 0.170 | 0.259 |

**Table 4.** Mean Error (ME) between sim eqKt/V and predictors

| | Daugirdas | Tattersall | HEMO | Leypoldt1 | Leypoldt2 |
|---|---|---|---|---|---|
| **Mean** | 5.63 | 4.32 | 7.47 | 7.63 | -3.18 |
| **SD** | 7.7 | 6.9 | 7.42 | 11.83 | 6.67 |
| **Median** | 4.65 | 3.23 | 5.89 | 4.60 | -3.9 |
| **Minimum** | -2.14 | -2.26 | -1.95 | -1.14 | -2.82 |
| **Maximum** | 5.37 | 3.54 | 4.08 | 8.55 | 3.43 |

**Table 5.** % Error (% ME) between sim eqKt/V and predictors

The lower error of prediction expressed as ME or % ME was obtained with the Tattersall and the Daurgidas formula. Leypoldt1 and 2 showed the worst predictive performance.

One interesting point was the effect of increase TD of Fr it was used in unconventional schedules (different from 3-times/wk). Error was higher in schemes shorter than 4 hours and the increasing of Fr did not affect the prediction (Figures 6 and 7)

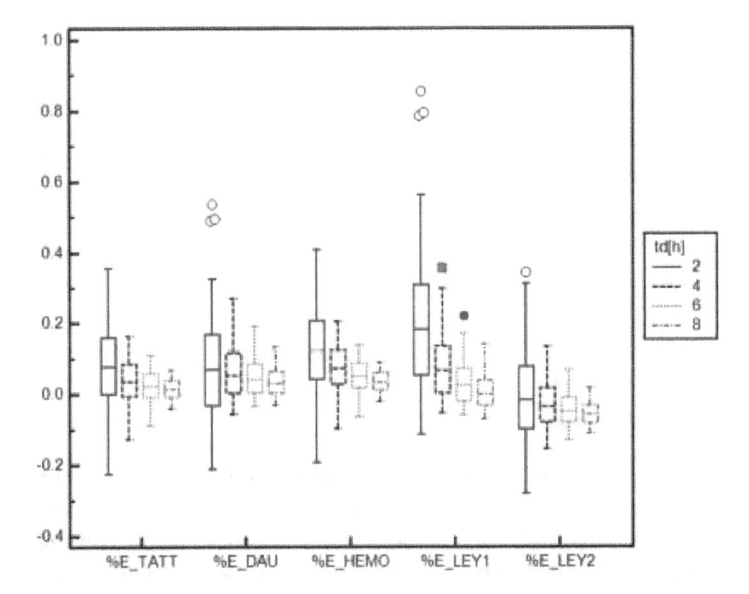


**Figure 6.** Effect of the TD and increased Fr in the % error prediction of eqKt/V

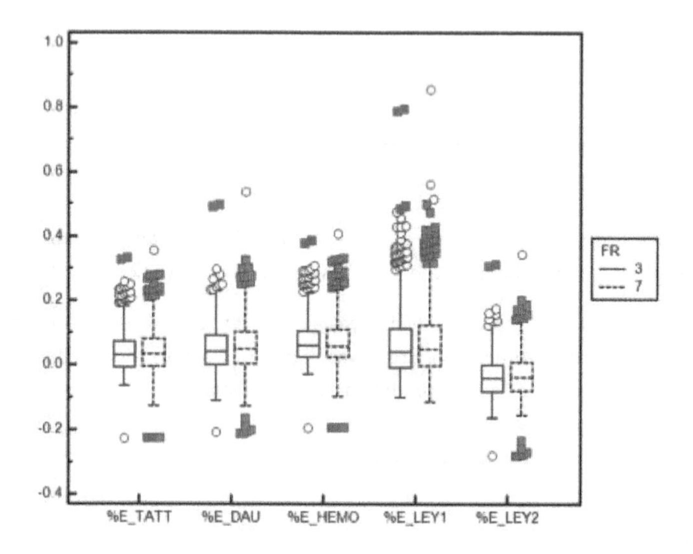


**Figure 7.** Effect of the TD and increased Fr in the % error prediction of eqKt/V

### 4.3. Bland-Altman analysis

A Bland-Altman analysis of agreement between gold standard (sim KtV) and eqKt/V predictors was performed. Tattersall and Daugirdas formulas showed the lower mean difference (±2sd): -0. 02 (+0. 04 -0. 08) and -0. 03 (+0. 04 -0. 1) respectively with a Gaussian distribution of error. Both Leypoldt formulas showed higher error with the increasing of the magnitude of eqKtV. HEMO study formula showed a higher mean difference than Tattersall and Daugirdas formulas with a lower 95% agreement interval (+0. 01-0. 1) (figure 8)

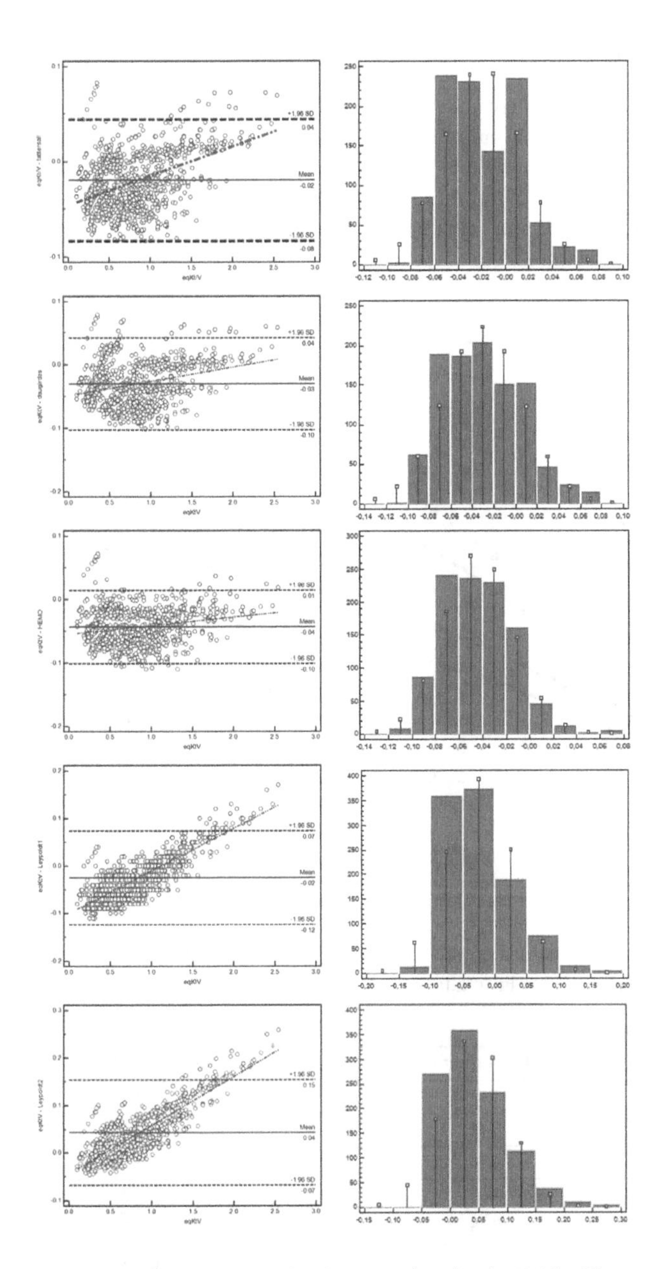

**Figure 8.** Left side: Bland Altman plot comparing simulated eq Kt/V and predicted eq Kt/V by different predictors formulaes. Right side: Histogram of Error between simulated eq Kt/V and predicted eq Kt/V by different predictors formulas.

### 4.4. Quantification of the Weekly Dialysis Dose (WDD)

The minimal dialysis dose recommended by the DOQI standards (Kt/V U/session = 1. 2) corresponded to EKR U =3. 17 ml/min and stdKt/V U = 2. 07 ml/min in a usual scheme of 3 days/4 hours (3d4hs) and the high dose equivalent similar to HEMO study (EqKt/V=1. 4) was 4. 28 ml/min and 2. 57 ml/min for stdKt/V in a schedule of 3 days 6 hours. Figure 9 shows the stdKt/V behaviour related to increase of TD and Fr as well as the equivalent values of minimal and high Kt/V.

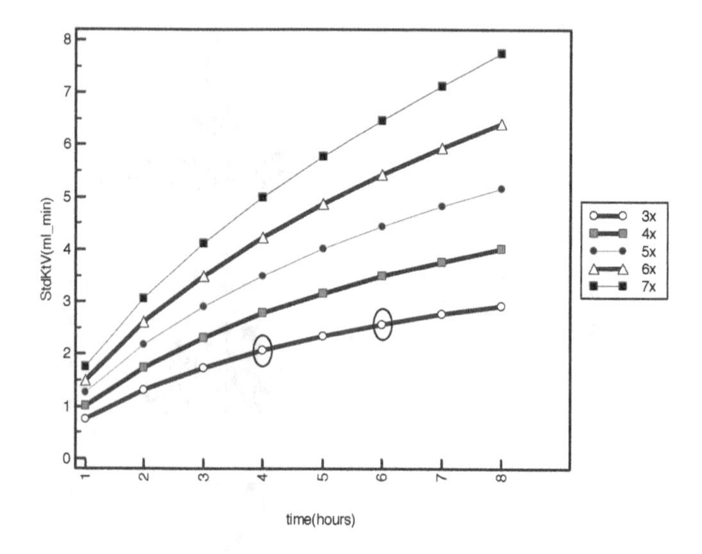


**Figure 9.** stdKt/V behaviour related to increase of TD and Fr as well as the equivalent values of minimal and high Kt/V.

Table 6 shows tipical values of EKR, stdKt/V, wk Kt/V (weekly Kt/V) and Kt/V by session according changes in TD y Fr in a typical 80-kg-patient.

| Frequency | time[h] | EKR (ml/min) | stdKt/V(ml/min) | wk Kt/V(ml/min) | KTV/Session |
|---|---|---|---|---|---|
| 3 | 4 | 3.17 | 2.07 | 3.55 | 1.18 |
| 3 | 8 | 5.11 | 2.92 | 5.82 | 1.94 |
| 4 | 4 | 4.23 | 2.78 | 4.61 | 1.15 |
| 7 | 2 | 4.06 | 3.05 | 4.78 | 0.68 |
| 7 | 4 | 7.45 | 5 | 7.52 | 1.07 |
| 7 | 8 | 12.69 | 7.75 | 10.54 | 1.51 |

**Table 6.** EKR, stdKt/V, wkKt/V and Kt/V by session according changes in TD and Fr in a typical 80-kg-patient. (Ce onset=230;KD=250 ml/min;Kc=600ml/min.

The weekly Kt/V, EKR and std Kt/V showed a high correlation to express increasing of TD and Fr (weekly Kt/v-std Kt/V r= 0. 987 EKR-stdKt/V r=0. 9937) showing the weekly Kt/V (5. 68±2. 46) and the EKR (5. 55±3. 02) values to be higher than std Kt/V (3. 56±1. 76)

The behaviour proved different when the three indexes were separately analysed. When they are compared to quantify 3-times/wk and weekly schedules, the ekr and std Kt/V have a similar behaviour, the EKR tending to overestimate the WDD as the TD increases. (Figure 11) When the difference EKR-std Kt/V is showed in a graph (Figure 10) a high correlation of it (R2=0. 99) is verified, with a logarithmic increase of the Kt/V/session and is lower with the increase of Fr in a fixed TD. The weekly Kt/V has a behaviour similar to that of the EKR in the 3-times/wk schedules but clearly fails in the daily schedules, especially in the TD schedules >4 hours.

When the Kt/V-session is analysed, the results match. The Kt/V/session increases as the TD increases when a certain number of sessions are fixed (Fr). When it is analysed for different Frs, the Kt/V/session only shows differences when duration is > 4 hours; however, if the Fr varies and the TD is fixed, instead we can observe that the Kt/V/session is not able to respond to the dose increases and tends to decrease as the WDD increases due to an increment of the Fr. (Figure 11)

The U rebound is complete one hour after the end of the HD session in all the simulations, decreasing as the TD increases.

Figure 11 showed the effect of TD and Fr on different predictors of the WDD (wkKt/V, EKR and stdKt/V) as well the changes Kt/V-session.

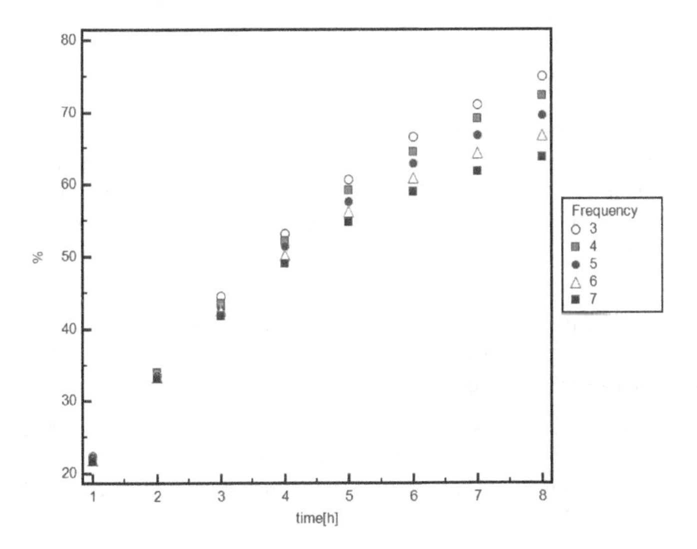


**Figure 10.** Difference (%) EKR-stdKtV related to Kt/V by session

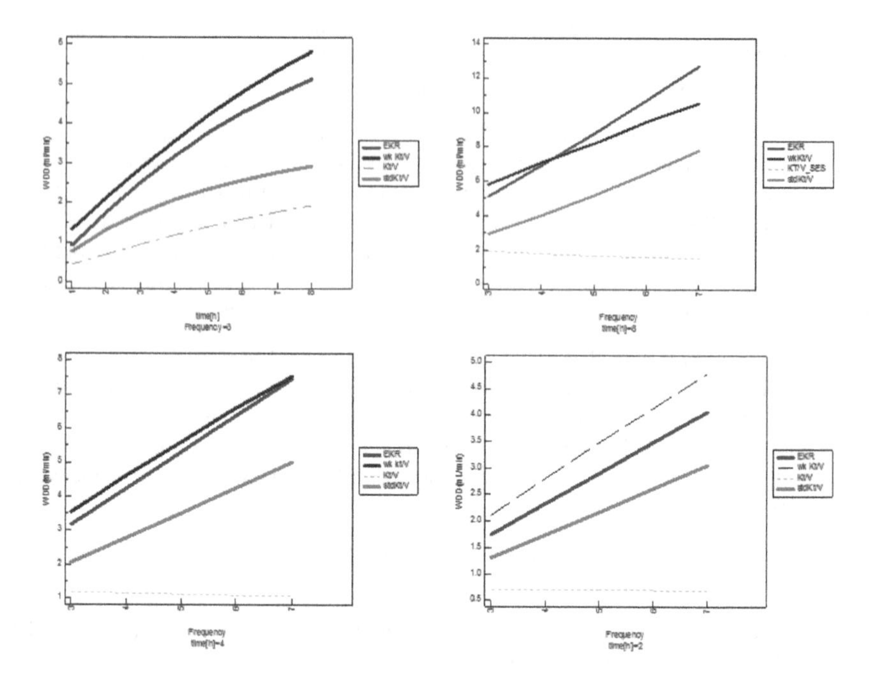

**Figure 11.** Effect of changes in increasing of TD and Fr on the behavior of WDD predictors (wkKt/V, stdKt/V, EKR) and Kt/V by session. (WDD=Weekly Dialysis Dose (ml/min)

## 4.5. Comparison of V with BSA to normalize Kt/V

In the last four decades dialysis dose expressed as KtV has been widely used due to its low complexity and ability to predict to be a strong predictor or mortality in HD population. However, recent studies showed paradoxical outcomes related to sex and higher mortality in patients with high Kt/V and low Volume, leading to the proposal of a normalized volume using and the correction by a Volumen normalized by Body Surface Area (BSA). has been proposed. [16]

We randomly simulated 1031 K*t with a range of between 14400 ml/min and 57600 ml/min and then Kt/V (using Watson formula for Volume) and Kt/V corrected by BSA (Dubois formula) were calculated and analysed

KtV values delivered by simulation showed a mean of 1. 01, a median of 0. 99, a range between 0. 29-2. 44 and a standard deviation of 0. 40 The results of the allometrical correction of Volume Watson formula by BSA were 0. 084*V 0. 86 (female) r=0. 98 and 0. 1229*V 0. 73 (male) r=0. 99. (Figure 12)

The results after V normalized by BSA clearly changed between men and women and the overestimation in patients with lower volumes was corrected (Table 7 and figures 13 and 14)

| | Sex | | | |
|---|---|---|---|---|
| | f | | m | |
| | Mean | SD | Mean | SD |
| Kt/V | 1.158 | 0.4354 | 0.921 | 0.3415 |
| Kt/Vcorr | 1.862 | 0.6891 | 2.489 | 0.8909 |

**Table 7.** Kt/V and Kt/V corrected by BSA (Dubois) according to sex.

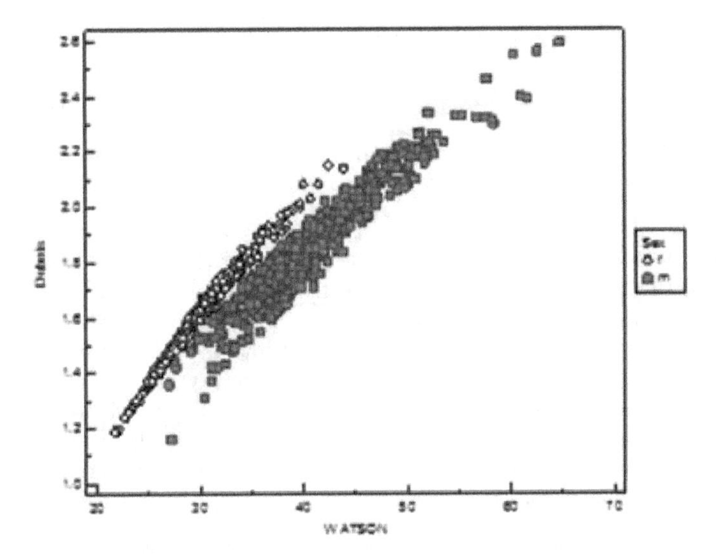


**Figure 12.** Allometric regression between Body Surface Area (Dubois) and Volume (Watson)

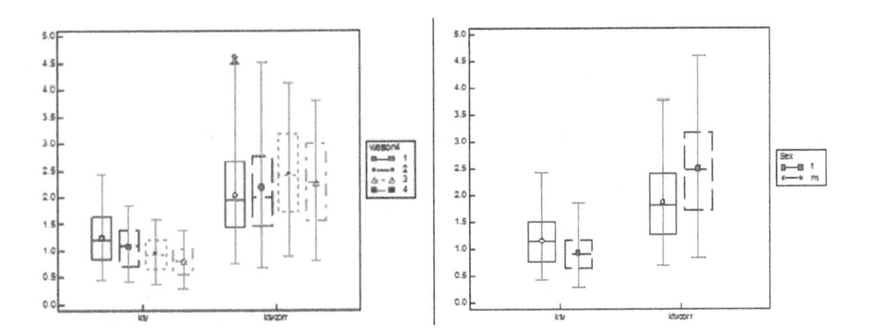


**Figure 13.** Effect of changes in Volume and Sex on BSA-normalized Kt/V and Watson Kt/V

## 5. Discussion

In this work we propose the simulation with a VVDC kinetic model as a useful and safe tool to investigate, learn and find out the numerous aspects of the HD treatment related to dialysis dose. Single pool models used by Gotch [10] to developed the pharmaco- kinetic concept of Kt/V are simpler and also useful but it frequently leads to errors in showing the true behaviour of little known molecules or not yet validated treatments. VVDC kinetic model is used in current studies that analyze the influence of increasing TD and Fr in HD outcomes after the failure of HEMO study to demonstrate better results with high dose expressed as eqKtV. [2]

Exponencial decay curves defined by WWDC to fit dialysis dose by session are actually used in several medical devices based on ionic dialysance or urea sensors. [17] [18]

We used WWDC based curve fitting and neural networks to predict dialysis dose from samples provided by an on-line urea monitor. [17]

The main interpretation of the double compartment [19] represent intra and extracellular fluid spaces, with diffusion of molecules between the spaces characterised by a mass transfer coefficient, Kc. This interpretation is based on the observation that Kc correlated with patient size. This model had been deeply developed by Smye and it had been the basis of the Tattersall formula. However, Scheneditz et al suggests that the two compartment based in different regional tissue flows (high and low blood flow) may describe urea distribution, and transport during dialysis, more accurately. This theorical approach also permited the development of a formula for dialysis dose that accounts for molecular rebound but only is based only on measurements of urea made during HD procedure. This formula has proved higher clinical usefulness: the Daurgirdas formula.

In this study we confirmed the robustness of the two widespread eqKtV predictors developed under the two different ways: Tattersall [7] and Daugirdas formulas. They showed a high accuracy in the numerous simulated schedules. The lower error of Tattersall formula has been validated in clinical situations and could be explained in our study because it was developed under a theorical approach using a diffusion –based VVDC.

Formula emerged from the blood U samples analysis of 1131 patients in the HEMO study [8] showed as an interesting approach. It behaved with a higher error than Tattersall and Daurgirdas formulas but showing a very low bias in all the simulations.

Eq KtV was confirmed as the metric of dialysis session in the thrice a week schedule. Equivalent dose of stdKt/V for eqKt/V in schedules>3-times/wk may be easily calculated in a graphical fashion (Figure 9)

The main issue which justifies the fact that Kt/V U is considered the key of the adequacy of dialysis is that it is related to mortality. However, many studies have questioned the utility of Kt/V: mainly, scaling for the volume is a confounding factor since gender and body mass index directly affect morbidity and mortality in HD patients. [20]

In our study the influence of the denominator to achieve a real dose independent of sex and volume showed similar results with others studies.

VVDC proved particularly useful when we analysed the new proposed predictors of the WDD: EKR and standard Kt/V.

Std KtV was confirmed as the best project to explain the different schedules. EKR was showed closely related with Kt/V and sensitive to changes in TD, overestimating the dose in daily HD schedules. VVDC allowed to graph different weight, dialyzer and patient clearences, etc.

Other molecules such as B2M [21] and phosphorus related to mortality and different behaviour with urea have not been simulated in this work but VVDC have been successfully used for both. B2M is a molecule of high molecular weight, with typical lower levels in plasma and lower distribution Volume fully explained by VVDC when we know completely their characteristics. On the contrary, Phosphorus [22] shows a heterogeneous and complex behaviour that cannot be completely validated with a VVDC kinetic model.

In addition to U kinetics, clinicians must consider clinical indicators (in example extracellular volume control, blood pressure, anemia and cardiovascular status) and comorbidities (diabetes, ageing, undernutrition) when using frequent or prolonged dialysis no forgetting to provide the best possible clinical results and quality of life.

## 6. Conclusions

In our experience, a VVDC kinetic model proved to be showed as a useful and safe tool to analyse different HD schedules and novels techniques before the clinical validation. The use of graphical interfaces to extrapolate the numerical results enhanced the VVDC simulation. Clinical practice and simulation interact in a permanent feedback. Std KtV was confirmed as the best project to explain the different schedules. Tattersall and Daugirdas showed highly accurate in the numerous simulated schedules.

## Author details

Rodolfo Valtuille[1], Manuel Sztejnberg[2] and Elmer. A. Fernandez[3]

1 Centro Hemodialisis Burzaco, Buenos Aires, Argentina

2 Instrumentation and Dosimetry Division, National Atomic Energy Commission, Argentina

3 Catholic University of Cordoba, Cordoba, Argentina

## References

[1] Hecking E, Bragg-Gresham JL, Rayner HC, Pisoni RL, Andreucci VE, Combe C, Greenwood R, McCullough K, Feldman HI, Young EW, Held PJ, Port FK. Haemodialysis prescription, adherence and nutritional indicators in five European countries: results from the Dialysis Outcomes and Practice Patterns Study (DOPPS). Nephrol Dial Transplant. 2004 Jan;19 (1): 100-7.

[2] Eknoyan G, Beck GJ, Cheung AK, Daugirdas JT, Greene T, Kusek JW, Allon M, Bailey J, Delmez JA, Depner TA, Dwyer JT, Levey AS, Levin NW, Milford E, Ornt DB, Rocco MV, Schulman G, Schwab SJ, Teehan BP, Toto R; Hemodialysis (HEMO) Study Group. Effect of dialysis dose and membrane flux in maintenance hemodialysis. N Engl J Med. 2002 Dec 19;347 (25): 2010-9

[3] Casino FG, López T. The equivalent renal urea clearance: a new parameter to assess dialysis dose. Nephrol Dial Transplant 1996 Aug;11 (8): 1574-81.

[4] Gotch FA. The current place of urea kinetic modelling with respect to different dialysis modalities. Nephrol Dial Transplant 1998;13 Suppl 6: 10-4.

[5] Daugirdas JT. Second generation logarithmic estimates of single-pool variable volume Kt/V: an analysis of error. J Am Soc Nephrol. 1993 Nov;4 (5): 1205-13.

[6] Smye SW, Will EJ. A mathematical analysis of a two-compartment model of urea kinetics. Phys Med Biol. 1995 Dec;40 (12): 2005-14.

[7] Tattersall JE, DeTakats D, Chamney P, Greenwood RN, Farrington K. The post-hemodialysis rebound: predicting and quantifying its effect on Kt/V. Kidney Int. 1996 Dec;50 (6): 2094-102.

[8] Daugirdas JT, Depner TA, Gotch FA, Greene T, Keshaviah P, Levin NW, Schulman G. Comparison of methods to predict equilibrated Kt/V in the HEMO Pilot Study. Kidney Int. 1997 Nov;52 (5): 1395-405.

[9] Leypoldt JK, Cheung AK, Deeter RB, Goldfarb-Rumyantzev A, Greene T, Depner TA, Kusek J. Kinetics of urea and beta-microglobulin during and after short hemodialysis treatments. Kidney Int. 2004 Oct;66 (4): 1669-76.

[10] Gotch, F ;Keen, Marcia. kinetic modeling in hemodialysis. In: Clinical Dialysis>Nissenson, Fine (eds). Mc Graw-Hill, 2005. p 153-203.

[11] Suri RS, Garg AX, Chertow GM, Levin NW, Rocco MV, Greene T, Beck GJ, Gassman JJ, Eggers PW, Star RA, Ornt DB, Kliger AS; Frequent Hemodialysis Network Trial. Frequent Hemodialysis Network (FHN) randomized trials: study design. Kidney Int. 2007 Feb;71 (4): 349-59.

[12] Petrone, G;Camaratta, G. Recent Advances in Modeling and Simulation. I-Tech. Vienna. 2008.

[13] Canaud B, Bosc JY, Cabrol L, Leray-Moragues H, Navino C, Verzetti G, Thomaseth K. Urea as a marker of adequacy in hemodialysis: lesson from in vivo urea dynamics monitoring. Kidney Int Suppl. 2000 Aug;76: S28-40.

[14] Clark WR, Leypoldt JK, Henderson LW, Mueller BA, Scott MK, Vonesh EF. Quantifying the effect of changes in the hemodialysis prescription on effective solute removal with a mathematical model. J Am Soc Nephrol 1999 Mar;10 (3): 601-9.

[15] Sztejnberg ML, Valtuille R, Fernández EA, Willshaw P, Efecto del Aumento de la Frecuencia y el Tiempo sobre la Dosis Semanal de Dialisis: Comportamiento Cinetico de la Urea, in: Memorias del XIV Congreso Argentino de Bioingeniería, III Jornadas de Ingeniería Clínica. SABI 2003. Ciudad de Córdoba, Córdoba, Argentina. October 2003.

[16] Daugirdas JT, Depner TA, Greene T, Kuhlmann MK, Levin NW, Chertow GM, Rocco MV. Surface-area-normalized Kt/V: a method of rescaling dialysis dose to body surface area-implications for different-size patients by gender. Semin Dial. 2008 Sep-Oct; 21 (5): 415-21.

[17] Fernández EA, Perazzo CA, Valtuille R, Willshaw P, Balzarini M. Molecular kinetics modeling in hemodialysis: on-line molecular monitoring and spectral analysis. ASAIO J. 2007 Sep-Oct;53 (5): 582-6.

[18] Uhlin F, Fridolin I, Magnusson M, Lindberg LG Dialysis dose (Kt/V) and clearance variation sensitivity using measurement of ultraviolet-absorbance (on-line), blood urea, dialysate urea and ionic dialysance. Nephrol Dial Transplant. 2006 Aug;21 (8): 2225-31.

[19] Smye SW, Clayton RH. Mathematical modelling for the new millenium: medicine by numbers. Med Eng Phys. 2002 Nov;24 (9): 565-74.

[20] Daugirdas JT, Greene T, Chertow GM, Depner TA. Can rescaling dose of dialysis to body surface area in the HEMO study explain the different responses to dose in women versus men? Clin J Am Soc Nephrol. 2010 Sep;5 (9): 1628-36.

[21] David S, Bottalico D, Tagliavini D, Mandolfo S, Scanziani R, Cambi V. Behaviour of beta2-microglobulin removal with different dialysis schedules. . Nephrol Dial Transplant 1998;13 Suppl 6: 49-54.

[22] Spalding EM, Chamney PW, Farrington K. Phosphate kinetics during hemodialysis: Evidence for biphasic regulation. Kidney Int. 2002 Feb;61 (2): 655-67.

Chapter 7

# Adsorption in Extracorporeal Blood Purification: How to Enhance Solutes Removal Beyond Diffusion and Convection

Fabio Grandi, Piergiorgio Bolasco,
Giuseppe Palladino, Luisa Sereni,
Marialuisa Caiazzo, Mauro Atti and
Paolo Maria Ghezzi

Additional information is available at the end of the chapter

## 1. Introduction

Uremic syndrome is linked to a plethora of uremic toxins circulating in the body in ESRD patients. Their overall spectrum is partly or entirely unexplored despite the need to urgently define the specimens and the patho-physiology beyond their high blood levels to address new or more selective removal strategies.

It is generally accepted that convective hemodialysis is the best choice to remove large part of the molecular spectrum, even though it is not fully demonstrated its superiority in terms of clinical outcomes. Then, transport mechanisms can benefit from maximizing all the physico-chemical principles including diffusion for small solutes, convection for middle molecules and adsorption for large molecular size uremic toxins. The latter has not been fully adopted in hemodialysis and this transport mechanisms is limited to the intrinsic capability of dialysis membrane to adsorb macromolecules while transporting solutes by diffusion and/or convection. However, poorly has been explored about the use of sorbents to enhance the solute removal in hemodialysis.

The purpose of this chapter is to summarize the main contributions of so far published clinical and technical experiences.

The chapter will be structured as follow: first we introduced a summary of the basic principles of solutes transport and relative contribution of the different mechanisms to the overall solutes removal; then, we described the extracorporeal techniques using adsorption as further transport mechanism; third we introduced the filtration adsorption architecture and we described the proteomic profile in extracorporeal adsorption hemodialysis; finally we reviewed the main clinical experiences with two techniques, the hemofiltration reinfusion (HFR) and coupled plasma-filtration adsorption (CPFA).

## 2. Some basic principle of solutes transport through a semipermeable membrane and relative contribution of the different mechanisms to the overall clearance

Main purposes of extracorporeal blood purification treatments are the elimination of toxins from the body and in the presence of renal failure (acute or chronic), the recover of the hydro-electrolytic and acid-base homeostasis. Beyond this direct aims, the extracorporeal treatments can also help, particularly in chronic diseases, to recover the anaemic, the nutritional status and to control the inflammatory body response. Extracorporeal blood purification treatments refer usually to three major techniques: hemodialysis (HD), hemofiltration (HF) and hemodiafiltration (HDF) which can be delivered as intermittent therapiesor continuous ones.

Mass transfer through a semipermeable membrane are governed by three major mechanisms: diffusion (described by Fick's law); convection (described by the Staverman law, solvent drag principle driven by the hydrostatic pressure drop); adsorption (which refers to the separation of a solute from a mixture by binding the specimen to a sorbent surface).

Usually, all the three mechanisms occur simultaneously through a semipermeable membrane but the relative contribution of each transport mechanism is given by the chemical-physical properties of the media respect to the specific solute (diffusivity, hydraulic permeability and solute affinity), and the driving forces (concentration gradient, hydrostatic pressure gradient). Then, depending on the specific membrane characteristics and operating conditions we can have only diffusive transport (HD) with negligible effect form convection and adsorption, only convection (HF, without any contribution from diffusion and negligible from adsorption), only adsorption (hemoperfusion - HP) or a combination of those.

In HD, a hydrosoluble solute movement through two phases is driven by its concentration gradient, but it is partially limited by the diffusive permeability, sieving coefficient and membrane cut-off in relation to its molecular weight and geometry. Then, the mass flow is usually high for low molecular weight, like urea and poor for middle-high molecular weight solutes, like β2-microglobulin.

In HF, a hydrosoluble solute movement is driven by the hydrostatic pressure gradient but it is limited by the hydraulic permeability of the membrane, the sieving coefficient and the membrane cut-off. The clearance and mass transfer are equal to ultrafiltration (*uf*) flow which is limited by the blood flow rate, hematocrit (Hct), total protein content. As a consequence middle-high molecular weight toxin are easier removed than in the only diffusive case, while small molecular weight toxins do not take so much benefit from the convective transport.

Adsorption, especially of proteins, always occur onto the inner surface of the membrane and inside the porous frame along the membrane wall. This phenomenon has two major implications during extracorporeal treatment: 1) it allows for mediating the hemocompatibility of the artificial surface and its thrombogenicity; 2) the adsorbed protein layer can significantly interfere with both diffusion and convection. Adsorption can be advocated as further removal mechanisms especially for low molecular weight protein, like β2-microglobulin, inflammatory mediators, like endotoxin fragment, IL-1 and IL-6, and in some extent also large molecular weight protein like immunoglobulin G [1].

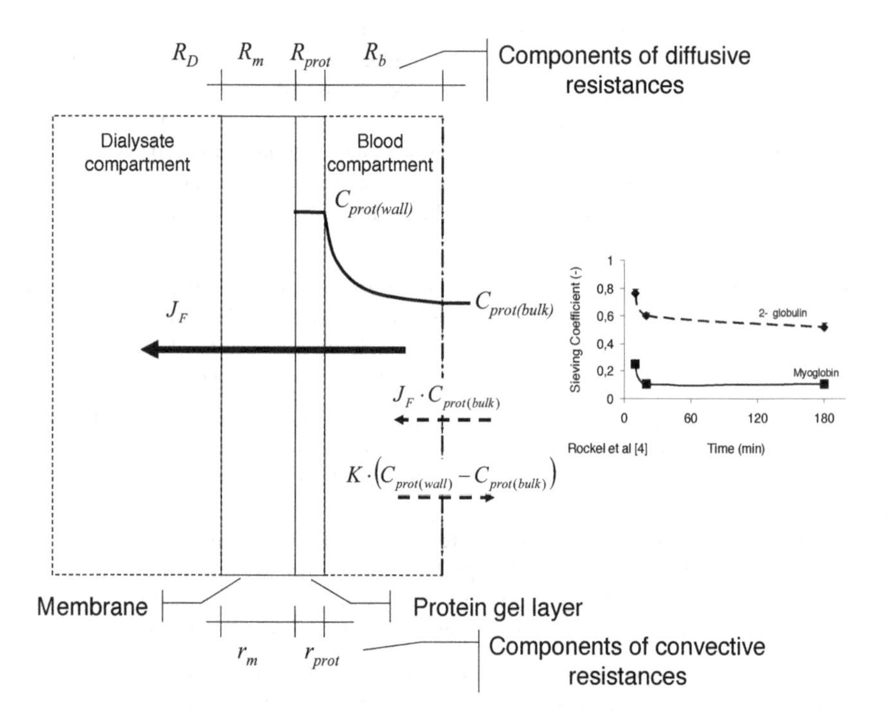


**Figure 1.** Major determinants of diffusive an convective transport behaviour through a semi permeable membrane. Legend of the figure: $J_F$=water flow rate, $K$=free diffusion coefficient, $C$ protein concentration at wall or at the centre of the fiber.

In normal operating conditions it exists an interference among these three transport mechanisms. Indeed, convective solute removal can be heavily influenced by the membrane fouling or gelling and concentration polarization. Fouling refers to the formation of a protein layer onto the inner surface of the membrane which has been shown to significantly decrease the sieving coefficient of the membrane [2]. Concentration polarization indeed consists of a second protein layer which is a function of theamount of protein delivered to the inner membrane surface by convective flow, and the amount of protein back diffusing from this high protein concentration boundary layer to the inner bulk phase of plasma at the center of the fiber (Figure 1). Again, the concentration polarization constitutes a barrier to solute movement toward the membrane surface decreasing both resistances to solute transport through the media and the overall sieving coefficient. In fact, the sieving membrane coefficient can be thought composed as: 1) intrinsic sieving coefficient ($s_i = C_d / C_{wall}$), (where $C_d$ is the solute concentration in the dialysate and $C_{wall}$ is the solute concentration at the membrane wall) which is inherent to the membrane characteristic and solute and 2) the observed sieving coefficient ($S = C_d / C_{bulk}$), (where $C_{bulk}$ is the solute concentration at the center of fiber) which is also influenced by fouling and polarization [3].

In vitro data indicate that both hydraulic permeability and middle-high molecular weight solute sieving coefficient fall down during convection with high permeable membranes. Rockel et al [4] showed that middle-high molecular weight molecules decrease the sieving coefficient during the first minutes of dialysis with synthetic Polysulfone membranes. The extent of reduction was by 21% after 20 min and 32% after 180 min from the peak value of the sieving coefficient of 0.76 at 10 min for β2-microglobulin. Even more was the reduction of $S$ for myoglobin which achieved -56% just after the firs 20 min of treatment.

Finally, fouling and concentration polarization also influences diffusion and convection by changing or introducing some further flow resistance components to the intrinsic characteristic membrane resistances (Figure 1).

Hemodiafiltration was initially proposed as a mixed technique that offered the advantages of two systems of transmembrane transport: diffusion and convection. This combination allowed better removal both middle molecules, particularly with respect to HD, and small uremic toxins when compared to HF [5, 6].

Although HDF is characterized by processes that can negatively interfere between diffusion and convection, leading to academic and clinical arguments over the choice between pre-, post- or pre/post dilution, overall the development of HDF offers, without doubt, an important positive evolution in dialytic strategy. Beyond the convection diffusion interference HDF is objectively associated with further two issues: a) quantity and quality of the reinfusion fluid; b) loss of important physiologic components in the *uf*. In fact, the choice of the $Q_{uf}$ rate depends on several factors; first, from a practical point of view, the $Q_{uf}$ must always be considered within the limits permitted by the blood flow ($Q_b$), Hct, total protein determining factors of fractional filtration. Elevated $Q_{uf}$ improves the depurative efficiency of the treatment, but it also necessitates large quantities of reinfusion solution that must absolutely have a guarantee of safety for the patient. The utilization of *ready-to-use* reinfusion bags produced by the pharmaceutical industry are associated with notable problems including handling (repeated connections to the hematic lines, storage) and cost. This has led to interest in on-line production of reinfusion fluids that can guarantee sterility and allow elevated $Q_{uf}$, thus leading to economic and practical handling issues to give a good cost/benefit ratio. Furthermore, high $Q_{uf}$ can often lead to severe depletion of substances such as vitamins, essential and branch chain amino acids (aa), as far as the albumin. Chronic renal failure patients often have high nutritional losses during both convective and diffusive dialytic treatments that may be closely linked to other patient comorbidities or that may aggravate patient health and well being. HDF, in particular, is associated with remarkable losses of amino acids and it is not surprising that higher losses are found with higher hydraulic permeability membranes [7].

As far the interference between convection and diffusion is of concerned, convective clearance (and therefore mass transfer) of a diffusible solute in HDF can not be fully represented by the *uf* flow ($Q_{uf}$), in that the simultaneous process of both convection and diffusion diminish the solute's concentration.

The overall interferences can be simply accounted knowing the overall dialyzer clearance as a function of operating condition ($Q_b$,$Q_{uf}$, ) and overall mass transfer coefficient-area (*KoA*). Assuming the same approach described by Sargent and Gotch [8] the overall dialyzer clearance, $K_T$, is:

$$K_T = K_d\left(1 - \frac{S \cdot Q_{uf}}{Q_b}\right) + S \cdot Q_{uf} \tag{1}$$

Where $K_d$, $S$, $Q_{uf}$ and $Q_b$ represent respectively the diffusive clearance, the sieving coefficient, the ultrafiltration rate and blood flow rate.

In turn, $K_d$, can be expressed as a function of the membrane characteristics, and operative condition of the dialyzer, as follow [9]:

$$Kd = Q_b \cdot \frac{e^{\left[\frac{KoA}{Qb}\cdot\left(1-Q_b/Q_b\right)\right]}}{e^{\left[\frac{KoA}{Q_b}\cdot\left(1-Q_b/Q_d\right)\right]} - \frac{Q_b}{Q_d}} \tag{2}$$

Where *KoA* is the overall mass transfer coefficient per surface area ($KoA=1/\sum_i R_i$) and $Q_d$ the dialysate flow rate. The mass transfer coefficient is a function of the transmittance (inverse of the overall resistance *R*). From the equations above it can been simply accounted what is the $K_T$ change for variations of *KoA* up to -50% and of $Q_{uf}$ in the allowed range for a given $Q_b$ (maximum 30%).

The overall clearance is plotted in Figure 2 as a function of $Q_{uf}$ and *KoA* for two solutes like urea and vitamin B12 (molecular weight of 60 and 1355 Da, respectively), often used as markers to characterize the dialyzer performances. Values are shown as percentage respect to the nominal value of $K_d$. It is worth to note that $K_T$ does not change linearly with $Q_{uf}$ but it is proportional to its change with a slope <1. Moreover the change is much more marked for middle-high molecular weight solutes. In fact, in absence of *KoA* variations the urea $K_T$ increases up to +3% with $Q_{uf}$, while in presence of high *KoA* impairment when no convection is applied ($Q_{uf}$=0) the $K_T$ decreases to -15%. The Vitamin B12 $K_T$ increases linearly with $Q_{uf}$ up to +16% in absence of *KoA* variations but decreases by -30% in case of *KoA* impairment in absence of convection. Nonetheless, when convection and fouling occur simultaneously, the positive contribution from convection itself, can be even knock down by *KoA* impairment and at higher $Q_{uf}$ one should expect higher *KoA* changes especially for high molecular weight solutes. This observation is in line with the results by Rockel [4] who found that protein adsorption has a negligible impact on membrane characteristic of polysulphone membrane for low molecular weight solutes while it significantly alters the sieving coefficient of molecular weight substances above 11'000 Da.

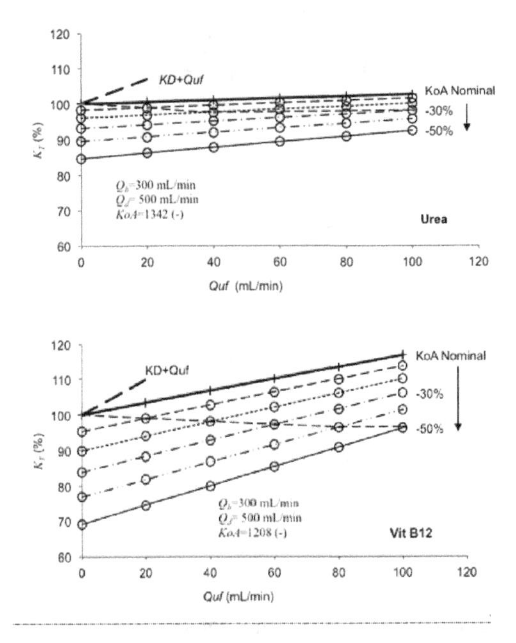


**Figure 2.** Relationship between $K_T$ and changes of $Q_{uf}$ and *KoA*.

Then according to these results, it is almost evident that less interference among the transport mechanisms should lead to better $K_T$. Maximum transport mechanisms can be achieved when they take place separately even though not all the interference like fouling and concentration polarization can be avoided at all but only minimized.

To solve this problem, Ghezzi et al [10] proposed a novel form of HDF that used a twin stage filter, in series, to separate diffusion from convection. The two stages permitted simultaneous convection and diffusion but also offered several benefits over traditional HDF combined in one filter unit. The first stage of the filter used a membrane with high hydraulic permeability for convective solute removal, while the second stage used a membrane with low hydraulic permeability for diffusive solute removal and to control the patient weight. Reinfusion of substitution fluids prepared on-line or in bags occurred between the two filter stages.This fluid was equal to the $Q_{uf}$, in order to maintain the effective $Q_b$. Therefore, this technique physically separates convection from diffusion, thus leading to two main results: a) the continuous availability of pure *uf* during the whole duration of the session; b) the absence of dialysate backfiltration. The method was called Paired Filtration Dialysis (PFD) [figure 3], and his efficiency and tolerance have been proven [11].

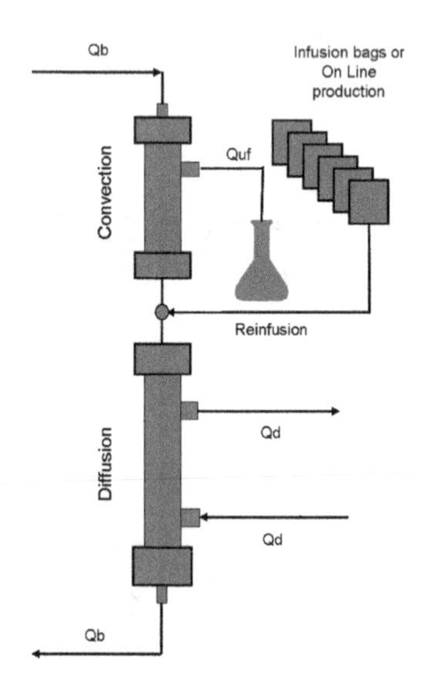


**Figure 3.** Paired Filtration Dialysis (PFD).

## 3. Extracorporeal techniques using adsorption

According to the "Consensus Conference on Biocompatibility," [12] adsorption is a method for removal of molecules from blood or plasma by molecules attachment to a surface incorporated in a device within an extracorporeal circuit. Sorbents are substances that, because of their physical and chemical characteristics, adsorb on their surface other elements in solution. In medicine, sorbents have been used to rapidly eliminate both industrial and pharmacological toxins, as well as some endogenous toxins such as bilirubin or porphyrines. They can be divided in two large categories: (1) those that have hydrophobic properties and therefore adsorb the molecules present in the solution in contact with the sorbent, and (2) those that eliminate solutes by chemical affinity [13]. Within the first category, hydrophobic sorbents, there are two subgroups: charcoal and non-ionic macroporous resin.

Charcoal is produced both from biological substances, such as coconut shells or peach pits and from non-biological substances, such as petroleum. The charcoal is activated by controlled oxidation in air (carbon dioxide) or steam. Adsorption into charcoal occurs through its pores, and therefore, its efficiency depends on the total number of pores and their radius. The charcoal may be coated or uncoated. Coating charcoal reduces some of its adverse effects, such as platelets entrapment, but it also reduces its efficiency, since the diffusion of the toxin from the blood to the charcoal is limited by the thickness of the polymer membrane, which covers it. The non-ionic macroporous resins are very similar to charcoal and are micro-sphere agglomerates, which adsorb the toxins they eliminate in their surface. Styrene-divinylbenzene polymers are generally used in clinical practice. The sorbents, which eliminate substances by chemical affinity, are fundamentally ion exchange resins, which exchange one ion for another of the same electrical charge. Some substances, which act by chemical links between the sorbent and the solute, are also considered "chemi-sorbents."

The use of sorbents in clinic can be divided in two big categories: hemoperfusion (HP) and plasma or *uf* perfusion.

Hemoperfusion is the passage of blood across material that adsorbs various solutes or substances [12]. In nephrology, sorbents were first used by Muirhead and Reid in 1948 [14] and later by Yatzidis in 1964 [15] in HP to eliminate uremic toxins. However, the adverse effects, principally platelets depletion, hemolysis, hemorrhage, and hypotension, outweighed the advantages. Although the majority of these adverse effects were solved thanks to the introduction of coated charcoal by Chang in 1966 [16, 17], the isolated use of HP for the treatment of uremia has been discontinued. At present, the use of HP is an accepted treatment for certain exogenous intoxication (pharmacological or suicidal).

After the abandonment of HP alone in the treatment of chronic renal failure, sorbents were used in combination and simultaneously with other dialysis methods. Gordon et al in 1969 [18] first described a HD technique in which the blood system, including the dialyser, was the usual one, but only six litres of dialysis fluid were used in the entire session, as the dialysate was regenerated by sorbents. The cartridge containing the sorbents consisted of four compartments: the first with urease, which transformed urea into ammonia; the second with zirconium phosphate, which eliminated ammonia, potassium, calcium, and magnesium; the third compartment, containing hydrated zirconium oxide, which eliminated phosphates; and the final compartment using charcoal, which eliminated a large number of both small and middle molecules. The system, called "Redy®," had the advantage of not needing running water nor any type of special installation and, therefore, could be quickly operated anywhere, for example, intensive care units and catastrophe sites, such as earthquakes. It also had various disadvantages, like unbalance of the sodium and acid-base equilibrium, but the most important was the release of aluminium to the dialysis fluid [19].

Another possibility of combining sorbents with HD was the inclusion of these substances in the dialyser membrane [20]. In this way, the patients blood was purified by diffusion as well as by adsorption on passing through the dialyser. The disadvantage to this method was its short efficiency period, as the sorbent became saturated in the first hour of dialysis and then stopped eliminating the uremic toxins. The Redy® sorbent cartridge was used by Shaldon et al [21] to regenerate the ultrafiltrate for reinfusion. This study was discontinued because of the appearance of osteomalacia in the patients [22].

## 4. Filtration adsorption architecture

The easy availability of isolated continuous *uf* during PFD led to the hypothesis that it could be "regenerated" and used as an endogenous reinfusion fluid. In 1992 [23] the first attempt to regenerate the *uf* was done with 130 mL of non-coated mineral carbon sorbent along the *uf* stream. The method was called Hemo Filtrate Reinfusion (HFR) and it is illustrated in Figure 4. HFR is a renal replacement therapy that utilizes convection, diffusion and adsorption. It uses a double stage filter that consists of a high permeability filter in the first convective stage and a low flux filter in the second diffusive stage.

The stages of the filter allow complete separation of convection from diffusion. The convective part of the first stage allows pure *uf* to flow through a sorbent resin cartridge. The potential of non-coated carbon sorbent to activate the contact phase [24,25], lead to switch the carbon cartridge to a hydrophobic styrenicdivinylbenzene resin (40mL). This has the potential advantage of a high affinity for several uremic toxins and middle molecules such as β2-microglobulin, homocystein, angiogenin, PTH, and several chemokines and cytokines [26, 27].

The resin structure allows molecules to flow through many pores and channels enlarging the sorbent surface area up to approximately 700 $m^2$/ gram. Despite its high affinity for many different uremic toxins, the resin has been proven not to [28] retain albumin and essential physiological molecules. Toxins are adsorbed to the resin beds and the purified *uf* is then reinfused between the first and second stage of the filter. The first convective/adsorption stage has no net fluid removal. The blood and reinfused regenerated *uf* then undergo traditional dialysis. The second stage works as conventional HD which also includes the patient net fluid loss.

Reasons to clear plasma water instead of whole blood are: a) a lower plasma water flow rate than the blood flow and consequently longer contact time with the resin and higher toxin adsorption; b) low sequestration of coagulative factors improving the hemocompatibility; c) absence of any depletion of inflammatory cells and platelets. The technique proved easy to use and offered high treatment tolerance, an optimal balance of bicarbonate (since it is not adsorbed and therefore it is reinfused) and was also associated with diminished inflammatory response often related to the exogenous reinfusion. Urea, creatinine, uric acid, $Na^+$, $K^+$, phosphates and bicarbonates are not adsorbed and remain unchanged after flowing through the cartridge. These can be managed during the second stage of the diffusive stage of the circuit. Thus the regenerated *uf* in the closed circuit is an endogenous reinfusion of patient plasmatic water. In particular, HFR has been associated with an aa loss similar to that observed with low flux HD, and surely much lower than other high flux HD or HDF on average as high as 33% [29]. The amino acids loss during HFR and low flux HD is approximately 10-11%.

The *uf* is much more than merely plasma water containing a few uremic toxins. Studies using proteomics and other chromatographic analyses have shown that *uf* contains between over 18,000 proteins and peptides [30-32]. Richter et al [30] found that *uf*, analyzed by MALDI-TOF mass spectrometry, consisted of approximately: 95% masses that were smaller than 15 kDa; 55% of the masses were found to be fragments from plasma protein (fibrinogen, albumin, β2-microglobulin, cystatin); 7% were hormones, growth factors and cytokines; 33% consisted of complement, enzymes, enzyme-inhibitors and transport proteins. Weissinger et al. [32] also found a wide polypeptide's spectrum in a recent study that analyzed *uf* from uremic patients using either high or low flux hemodialyzer. In this study they found a higher number of polypetides in samples obtained from uremic patients with high flux dialyzers compared to low flux dialyzers (1394 polypeptides with high flux ones vs. 1046 with low flux dialyzers), as well as a significant differences when they used healthy donors *uf* by filtering plasma with a 5 kDa or 50 kDa cut-off membranes (590 polypeptides for the high cut off, 490 polypeptides for the low cut off).

Although the study focused on characterization of uremic toxins, there are certainly a lot of beneficial substances that are also lost during HDF with high convection. In conclusion, peculiar characteristic of HFR over classical HDF, is that the technique allows a better removal of high molecular weight toxins, and the reinfusion of vitamins, hormones and other physiologic compounds.

The cartridge adsorption was optimized progressively as investigated by different studies, to determine the maximal adsorption at different *uf* flow rates for different cartridge diameters and quantities of resin. The treatment is performed on the Formula Plus™ dialysis machine (Bellco, Mirandola, Italy) which is equipped with a dedicated algorithm which automatically determines the best *Quf* based initially on the maximal linear velocity (the flow rate that gives the best adsorption). The machine also determines the patient's Hct and transmembrane pressure to adjust the *Quf* based on these parameters.Thus the *Quf* is usually higher at the start of the treatment and then adjusts if necessary to reduce the flow rate based on changes in hemoconcentration [33]. For the handling point of view, this therapy does not add much more respect to an on-line hemodiafiltration, since it adds an external cartridge to be connected along the reinfusion pathway. The remaining extracorporeal circuit is fully preassembled and do not introduce any extra work for the nurses. On the contrary, the advantage of endogenous reinfusion relies in the reduction of extra costs and extra work associated to the analysis of the on-line substitution fluids and to the need of devices and preventive maintenance to guarantee the fluid purity. Finally, the complexity of intra-session management is located inside the dialysis machine being the $Q_{uf}$ automatically adjusted according to the operative conditions in terms of pressures and flow. This tool, again, reduces the complexity of manual adjustment of ultrafiltration rate which must cope with the intra-session changing trans-membrane pressure developed in the hemodialyzer in conventional on-line hemodiafiltration. Very often, this aspect represents one of the major limitations to achieve high exchange volumes OL-HDF.

The HFR architecture has been next extended in terms of plasma water solutes selectivity and sorbent capacity. In fact, the use of more permeable membranes, in the convective chamber, with higher cut-off allows for high molecular weight solute to flow through the sorbent.

In chronic dialyzed patients in order to reduce the effect of high molecular weight toxins retention, the micro-inflammation and the malnutrition status it is necessary remove molecule with high molecular weight over the albumin limit. For this purpose, the evolution of the HFR technique in SUPRA HFR (by the use of new super high cut-off membrane in the convective chamber: Synclear 0,2 with albumin sieving in water of 0.2), has allowed to achieve this purpose without loss of albumin. This is possible because the resin contained in the cartridge doesn't adsorb the albumin and therefore re-infuse that to the patient [28].

End stage renal disease patient is not the only one that could take advantage of the filtration and adsorption mechanism. Septic shock patients with or without Acute Kidney Injury (AKI) require the removal of high molecular weight inflammation mediators (like, IL-1β, IL-6, IL-8, IL-10, Macrophage Inflammatory Protein-α and β, TNF-α) which cannot be achieved with only ultrafiltrate flowing through the sorbent resin [34,35, 66, 67].

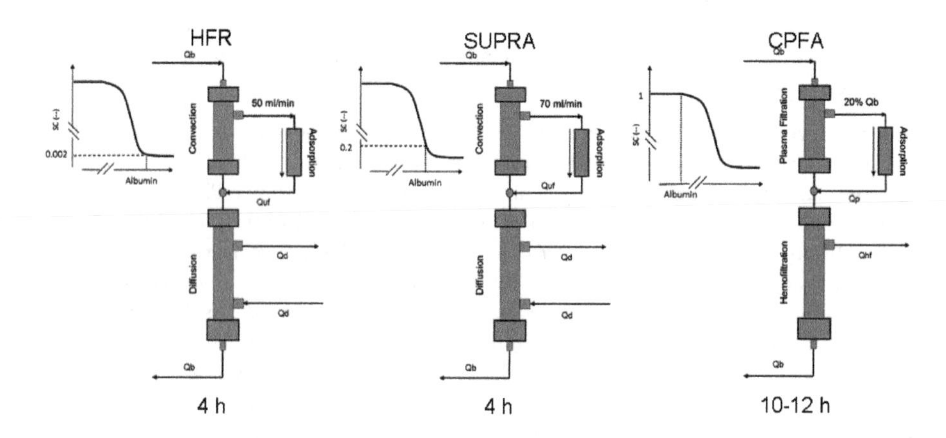


**Figure 4.** The Filtration Adsorption architecture, form left to right: standard HFR, super high-flux HFR (SUPRA) and CPFA. Figure shows also the albumin sieving coefficient o each convective chamber, the typical *uf* or plasma flow rate and the length of each session.

For this purpose a special technique, dedicate to this kind of patients, that couple plasma filtration with adsorption have been parallelly developed. The name of this technique is Coupled Plasma Filtration Adsorption (CPFA) [36].

The first stage is now a plasma filter (MICROPES 0.45 $m^2$ polyethersulfone which separates the corpuscular part of the blood from plasma) replacing the convective membrane. Obviously, the fluids treated are very different from those in HFR and then they required to develop a new cartridges with high sorbent properties and performances. Then, a nonselective hydrophobic styrene resin cartridge with macroporous structure 50'000 $m^2$/cartridge is used. Finally, a synthetic, high-permeability, 1.4 $m^2$ polyethersulfone hemofilter clears the reconstituted blood in a post-dilution mode to restore the hydro-electrolytic and acid-base balance and the removal of small molecular weight toxins. The outline of the development of this architecture is shown in Figure 4.

The post-dilution re-infusion rate can be set for up to a maximum of 4 liters/h. The blood flow is usually 150-180 ml/min while the plasma filtration rate is maintained at a fractional filtration of the blood flow (approximately 15-20%).

The treatment is performed for a 10 h period, after which haemofiltration in postdilution mode can continue according to the clinical conditions if needed for renal support.

## 5. Proteic profiles in extracorporeal filtration adsorption systems

The high-throughput technique Surface Enhanced Laser Desorption/Ionization Time-of-Flight Mass Spectrometry (SELDI-ToFMS) is powerfully used to analyze the protein content of various biological samples [37]. In particular it helps to identifies the types of molecules that could cross the convective membranes and to quantify their relative adsorption onto the resin bed.

The extraction capability could be evaluated as regard to specific pro-inflammatory proteins such as Tumor Necrosis Factor-$\alpha$ (TNF–$\alpha$), Interleukin 6 (IL-6), $\alpha$-1-acid glycoprotein [AAG] and Albumin,.

Three different permeability membrane, Polyphenylene High Flux (pHF), polyphenylene Super High-Flux (pSHF) and Synclear 0.2 (Synclear 0.2), whose sieving coefficient are shown in Figure 5, have been investigated and analyzed for their permeability [38].

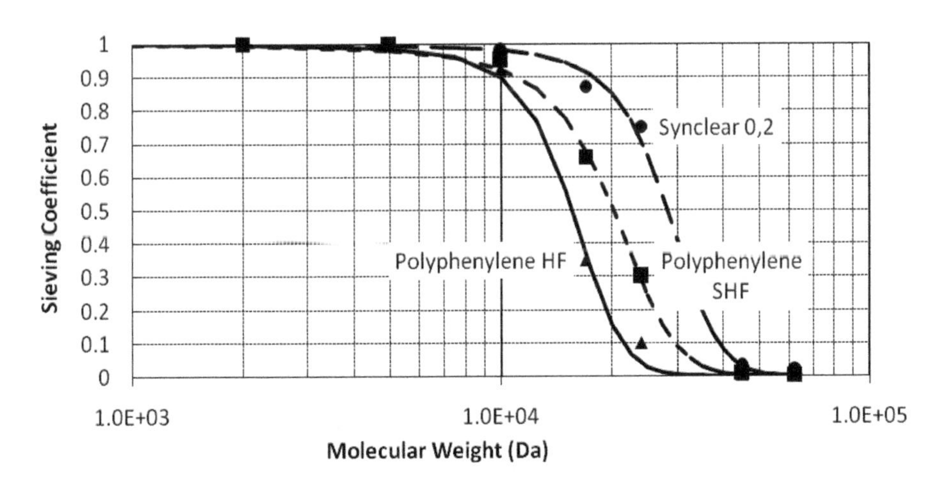


**Figure 5.** Sieving Coefficient calculated using *in vivo* data for the membrane Polyphenylene HF, Polyphenylene SHF, Synclear 02.

Through nephelometric quantification, (see Figure 6), it is clearly remarkable the high permeability of Synclear 0.2 membrane as shown by the different quantity of high molecular weight molecules which are present in the *uf*.

In particular, it is worth to note, that the membrane with higher pores dimension (Synclear 0,2) allows passage of a higher percentage of albumin with respect to the membrane with lowest pore size (pHF). Much more interesting is the extraction rate of a molecule as $\alpha$-1-acid glycoprotein despite it has a molecular weight lower than albumin (41-43 kDa vs 66.5 kDa). The different behaviour of such a peptide can be explained by introducing the concept of Stokes radii of a protein, its glycosylation and its subproducts.

The Stokes radius or hydrodynamic radius, is the radius of a hard sphere that diffuses at the same rate as the molecule. This is subtly different to the effective radius of a hydrated molecule in solution. The behaviour of this sphere includes hydration and shape effects. Since most molecules are not perfectly spherical, the Stokes radius is smaller than the effective radius (or the rotational radius). A more extended molecule will have a larger Stokes radius compared to a more compact molecule of the same molecular weight. [39]. For an unglycosylated polypeptide, a value to +l g/mol can be obtained from sequence information or from mass spectrometry. A similar precision cannot be obtained for glycosylated proteins because of polydispersity deriving from the variability of a cell's glycosylation process. Many proteins -and glycoproteins- contain more than one non-covalently linked protein chain, particularly at higher concentrations, and important roles of hydrodynamic methods for mass analysis in protein chemistry are to give the molar mass of the "intact" or "quaternary" structure and to provide an idea of the strength of binding of these non-covalent entities through measurement of association constants [40].

Finally, Table 1 compares the percentage extraction of the different solutes according to molecular weight and the Stokes radius.

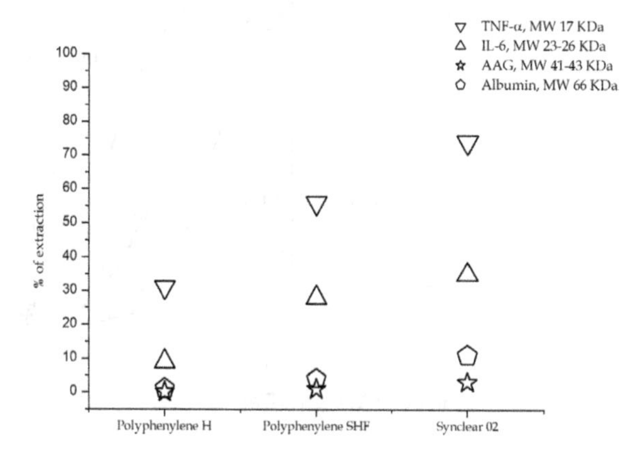


**Figure 6.** Extraction capability of three different membranes of four molecules.

| | TNF-α | IL-6 | Albumin | AAG |
|---|---|---|---|---|
| Molecular weight | monomer 17 KDa, trimer 51 KDa | 23-26 KDa | 41-41 KDa | 66,5 KDa |
| Stokes radii | monomer 1.9 nm / trimer 2,3 nm | 2 nm | 3,5 nm | 3,5 nm |
| Polyphenylene H | 31% | 9% | 1% | 0% |
| Polyphenylene SHF | 56% | 28% | 4% | 1% |
| Synclear 02 | 74% | 35% | 11% | 3% |

**Table 1.** Differences between molecular weight and Stokes radii of TNF-alpha, IL-6, AAG and Albumin. Stokes radii come from literature data: [41-44]. Extraction percentage of different molecules with different membranes.

## 6. Clinical experiences with HFR

Several studies have been published since the first introduction of filtration-adsorption therapies on the late 80's. Many of them showed that this technique is particularly suited for chronic patients at major risk of inflammation, malnutrition and with cardiovascular function impairment, such as diabetics, elderly, with high C-reactive protein (CRP) levels.

Table 2 shows the results observed in the main clinical trials comparing HFR against or standard HD or convective technique such as on-line HDF (OL-HDF). Most of the authors reported a significant reduction of pre-dialysis levels of β2-microglobulin, particularly marked when comparing the time pattern against standard HD. For instance Kim et al. found out a reduction of pre-dialysis plasma levels from 37.7 to 28.3 mg/L when patients were treated with HFR. Similar results were also observed from Bolasco et al (from 28.9±8.9 to 22.9±6.7 mg/L, $p=0.008$). Panichi et al did not find any significant reduction of the pre-dialysis β2-microglobulin over the time but the results were similar to those obtained with OL-HDF.

Pre-dialysis IL-6 significantly reduced over the time as shown by Panichi et al from 14.8±6.5 to 10.1±3.2 pg/mL and by Bolasco et al from 21.8±20.4 to 18.9±22.2 pg/mL. On the contrary Kim et al found out an increase of IL-6 even though the patients plasma levels were extremely low (1.69 to 2.48 pg/mL).

The results about CRP are in accordance to those on IL-6. In fact, CRP decreased by 30% to 50% over time respect to conventional HD. Similar results were obtained by Panichi in OL-HDF and the best results have been seen when patients presented high CRP plasma levels at the baseline.

It must be underlined that pre-dialysis albumin plasma levels did not changed significantly in all the studies reported (on average nearly 3.6 g/dL) even though Panichi reported a prealbumin levels increase more pronounced in HFR than in OL-HDF (from 30.5±3.5 to 34.0±3.9 mg/dL in HFR vs 30.6±3.9 to 32.3±3.5 mg/dL in OL-HDF). This result can be partly explained by the use of a sterile apyrogen substitution fluid (which is true for OL-HDF and particularly for HFR where the substitution fluid is regenerated by patient *uf*) and by the lower removal of essential and branched chain aa typical of HFR. In fact, as already mentioned, in addition to a good removal of uremic toxins and reduction of inflammation of the molecules, the HFR is also characterized by a considerable saving of aa and vitamins. Hemodialysis high flux and OL-HDF are associated with a depletion nearly of 25-30% of the aa concentration from the beginning of the dialysis session, which quantifies in a loss of about 5-10 g/treatment [7, 50-52].

Ragazzoni et al. [53] have firstly shown that HFR is associated with a significant saving of total aa (essential and branched chain), in comparison with OL- HDF. In a pilot study, 11 patients in conventional HD were randomized to HFR or OL-HDF, and the overall aa removal measured as pre to post-dialysis plasma levels were from 3122±578 μmol/L to 2395± 493in HFR and from 3030±578 to 1852±302 in post-dialysis respectively.

Borrelli [48] confirmed these results by comparing the HFR with acetate free biofiltration (AFB). In particular, the 48 patients recruited (24 in HFR and 24 in AFB), were observed in a single session as regard the AA loss. The authors reported a depletion of plasma total aa levels from 3176±722 to 3044±687 μmol/L in HFR more pronounced than in AFB from 3399±621 to 2551±428 μmol/L ($p<0.01$).

Morosetti M. [58] conducted a pilot study of patients treated with HFR and on-line HDF, measuring plasma levels of vitamin C at the beginning, the end of treatment and in the uf in pre-and post-cartridge. The results have documented that, in HFR, levels of vitamin C in the ultrafiltrate are lower than those detected in plasma, a phenomenon due to the partial oxidation of vitamin during the convection (removal of other species anti-oxidants such as proteins), but at the same time has been shown that the vitamin C contained in the uf is not adsorbed by the HFR cartridge and therefore is re-infused to the patient. Furthermore, the authors have demonstrated that plasma levels of vitamin C, are higher in patients treated with HFR compared to those with on-line HDF

Calò et al. [55] recently studied the plasma levels of inflammation and oxidative stress markers, and the long-term changes in mononuclear cell protein expression of heme-oxygenase-1 (HO-1) in a prospective longitudinal study trial comparing HFR versus standard HD. Patients in HD were recruited and assessed at the baseline and then they were treated for one year in HFR. Change of oxidized low-density lipoprotein(OxLDL) was significantly lower after 12 months on HFR compared with baseline: 475.4±110.8 ng/mL (time zero) versus 393.1±101.9 ng/mL (12 months), $p < 0.04$. Moreover, during treatment with HFR the protein expression of HO-1 over time increased ($p< 0.00001$) and it approached the statistical significance versus time zero at six months (0.27±0.10 vs. 0.17± 0.11, $P = 0.0527$) and became significantly different from time zero at 9 (0.48 ±0.20, $p < 0.043$) and 12 months (0.59±0.32, $p < 0.004$). This result is accompanied by the lack of any change of inducible Nitric Oxide Synthase (iNOS) protein expression over time (1.02±0.39 and 1.06±0.42 from 0 to 12 months, respectively, p= ns).

| Author | Patients | Study Design | Major Results on HFR | *p* |
|---|---|---|---|---|
| Panichi, 2006 [45] | Unselected<br>n=25 | Prospective randomized cross-over trial<br>OL-HDF(4ms) – HFR (4ms)<br>HFR(4ms) – OL-HDF(4ms) | β2-microglobulin no change in HFR while decreased by 7% in OL-HDF<br>IL-6 reduction by 32% in HFR vs 21% in OL-HDF (significant vs baseline)<br>CRP reduction by 30% in HFR vs 38% in OL-HDF(significant vs baseline)<br>No change in albumin (3.7±0.3 g/dl)<br>Prealbumin increase by 11.5 in HFR vs 5% in OL-HDF | ns<br><0.02<br><0.05<br>ns<br>ns |
| Bolasco, 2006 [46] | No severe cirrosis, no heart failure, no neoplasm or chronic inflammation<br>n=44 | Longitudinal<br>HD (3ms) – HFR (6ms) | β2-microglobulin decrease by 21%<br>CRP drecrease by 50%<br>PTH no changes (on average 318 pg/mL)<br>Phospates non change (on average 5 pg/mL) | 0.022<br>0.02<br>ns<br>ns |
| Kim, 2009 [47] | Unselected<br>n=11 | Longitudinal study<br>BHD(12wks) – HFR(12wks) | 72% reduction of plasma level of leptin<br>67% reduction of adiponectin<br>No change of IL-6<br>72% reduction of plasma level of β2-microglobulin | 0.014<br>0.001<br>ns<br>0.002 |
| Borrelli, 2010 [48] | No severe cirrosis, heart failure, neoplasm chronic inflammation<br>n=48 | Observational matched case-control study<br>HFR(1s) vs AFB(1s) | 17% less post-dialysis level of total AA in AFB than HFR<br>20% less post-dialysis level of essential AA in AFB than HFR | 0.0001<br><0.0001 |
| Bolasco, 2011 [49] | Patient with no chronic or acute recurrent inflammation<br>n=38 | Prospective randomized cross-over<br>AF HFR(3ms) – HFR(3ms) - AF HFR(3ms) | 25% reduction of pre-dialysis level of β2-microglobulin<br>IL-6 reduction by 13% vs baseline HD<br>CRP increase by 40% vs baseline HD<br>7% increase predialysis level Hgb<br>18% reduction of ESA consumption<br>No change in cytokine preedialysis level<br>No change in pre-dialysis serum albumin<br>No change in vitamin supplementation | 0.002<br><0.04<br>ns<br><0.04<br>ns<br>ns<br>ns<br>ns |

**Legend:** AF=Acetate Free, AA=AminoAcids, AFB=Acetate Free Biofiltration, OL-HDF=On Line Hemodiafltration, ms=months, s=session, wks=weeks, ns=not significant, CRP=C-Reactive Protein.

**Table 2.** Summary of clinical trials HFR in the last six years comparing inflammatory parameters and nutritional makers

Splendiani et al. [56] have shown that the styrenic resin HFR cartridge is able to adsorb significant amounts of homocysteine without simultaneous adsorption of vit. B12 and folate: this suggests an important mechanism for reducing cardiovascular risk. Cardiac troponin (cTnT) is a sensitive marker of cardiac hypertrophy and myocardial injury and correlates with left ventricular mass. There is evidence that the cTnT plasma concentration increases in chronic uremic patients in renal replacement therapies even without signs of heart disease [57, 58] and that cTnT is an independent predictor of cardiovascular events. De Filippi et al. [59] reported that cTnT can be elevated in 30% to 75% of uremic patients on hemodialysis, and that even small increases are associated with an increased likelihood of coronary heart disease. Lippi et al. [60] showed that variations of cTnT level after dialysis can be linked to blood hemoconcentration and membranes type. Sommerer at al. [61] reported the existence of a significant correlation between cTnT levels and non-native arteriovenous fistulae (implants and catheters), probably due to a state of chronic inflammation often associated with this type of vascular access.

Even though the recent scientific literature generally reports a diminished impact on inflammation and hyper-catabolism induced by extracorporeal dialysis [62] (maybe due to different types of membranes [63]), a further optimization of the various methods HDF must take into account also the buffer used in dialysis (Dialysis Solution DS) and reinfusion fluids. The use of large amounts of on line reinfusion fluid (pre-, post- or pre/post-dilution) exposes the patient to a risk of direct toxic effects or fluid hemo-compatibility with negative clinical consequences. It 's well known that accelerated atherosclerosis is the main risk factor for morbidity and mortality for dialyzed patients: in addition to traditional risk factors, some others play a key role, such as formation of non-enzymatic glycation products, hyper-homocysteinemia, alterations in calcium-phosphorus balance, hemo-incompatibility reactions. All this is due, not only to the dialysis membranes contact, but can be activated by components of the DS or substitution fluids.

Bolasco et al. [49] studied 25 patients in a cross-over longitudinal study. Patients were recruited and studied in a run-in period of three months in standard HD and they were subsequently treated with standard HFR and acetate free (AF) DS (Lympha ®), each period lasting three months. At the beginning and at the end of each period, blood samples were taken to analyse cTnT plasma levels while blood pressure and heart rate were recorded in all the sessions. The results showed a significant decrease in cTnT from standard HD, to HFR AF at the end of first period (from 1.32±0.35 to 1.12±0.31 ng/mL, $p < 0.05$), a subsequent rise in HFR with DS containing acetate (from 1.12±0.31 to 1.28±0.37 ng / mL, $p = < 0.05$) and a further decline (although not statistically significant) from 1.28±0.37 to 1.21±0.35 ng/mL in the last period of HFR AF. It was observed a significant systolic and diastolic pressure drop accompanied by a compensatory increase in heart rate during the sessions in standard HFR while arterial blood pressure did not significantly changed in HFR AF. No significant differences of acid-base recovery were observed in the two therapies.

Bolasco et al. [64] studied 16 patients, in a comparison of HFR with conventional HD, with regard erythropoiesis And erythropoiesis stimulating agents (ESAs) requirement. They demonstrated a statistically significant increase of Hb levels in HFR vs HD (from 11.22 to

11.66 g/dL, p <0.05), while for ESAs has been a simultaneous significant decrease from 29,188 to 16,750 IU/month (p = 0.01). The data showed that the HFR itself is able to determine an improvement of erythropoiesis.

Based on this study, the HFR seems therefore to be an HDF technique that can positively affect the level of Hb and the needs of ESAs. This favourable effect seems to be independent from the dialysis dose (Kt/V), the replacement fluid volume, and the presence or absence of acetate in the DS. This result could be attributed to a saving of useful substances such as aa and vitamins, and the lack of depletion of factors inhibiting erythropoiesis [60].

It must be pointed out that the reinfusion of the same closed-loop patient plasma water guarantees undoubtedly sterility and pyrogenicity that is not always assured in OL-HDF, then reducing the effects of micro-inflammation. In a study involving 166 patients, Axelsson et al. [65] have demonstrated, that there is a significant correlation between the indices of sensitivity to ESAs and levels of CRP and IL-6. Moreover, with a multivariate stepwise regression model they can concluded that ferritin (log), PTH, leptin (log), IL-6 (log)) are significantly associated with the ratio of ESAs/Hb.

The association between purity of dialysate solution and substitution fluid and ESA consumption or Hb levels in hemodialysis patients have shown that the ESA dose increases linearly as the plasma levels of IL-6. Patients in whom ultrapure dialysis fluid was used required less epoetin than those in whom standard dialysis fluid was used (64±22 vs 92±12 UI/Kg/week, p<0.05) [66].

Recently, Testa et al. [67] have published positive clinical results on the use of HFR for the removal of serum free light chains (Immunoglobulin Free Light Chains - FLCs). The FLCs are divided into two major classes κ and λ depending on the aa sequence in the constant portion of the polypeptide. Light chains k are usually monomers of the weight of 22 kD, those λ dimers of the weight of 44 kD. The production of light chains by plasma cells in the bone marrow is around 500 mg/day. They have a half-life of between two and six hours and are usually filtered and subsequently reabsorbed in the proximal tubule. It 'clear that the concentration of FLCs increases in two situations: increase in production (gammopathies) or reduced clearance, such as in renal failure. There is a direct correlation between serum creatinine and FLCs, and the increase of these units represents a reliable measurement of the progression of renal failure.

The highest rates of FLCs are typical of the uremic patients on hemodialysis, and this shows how the current methods of purification will not be able to offer an adequate clearance of these molecules, defined as true uremic toxins. By contrast, Hutchison et al. [68] have described an alternative strategy of HD intensive filters with membranes with high permeability (Poliariletersulfone with a cut-off of 45 kD), capable of removing significantly FLCs in excess, method, however, associated with an important loss of albumin of 20-40 g/session.

Testa et al. [67] have studied two different groups of patients treated with HFR: one with production of polyclonal light chains, the other with monoclonal antibodies; the results showed a significant reduction of FLCs in both groups (31% and 34% reduction rate of κ chains respectively in polyclonal and monoclonal FLCs group; 20% and 11% reduction rate of $\lambda$ chains again in polyclonal and monoclonal FLCs group). The analysis by *uf* at cartridge inlet and outlet confirmed the adsorptive capacity of FLCs.

In summary, it should be noted that the HFR can not be greater than the traditional HDF in the field of the elimination of toxic solutes, as the adsorption can not be more effective. The focal point is the best compromise between saving of essential elements and a satisfactory toxins removal in a wide spectrum.

## 7. Clinical experience with Couple Plasma-Filtration Adsorption (CPFA)

First animal experiments with CPFA were done to determine safety and efficacy, as well as whether CPFA could actually play a role in modulating the inflammatory response [69].

Table 3 reports the results obtained in the main clinical trials comparing CPFA with standard treatments. It can be seen that this therapy is in general able to ameliorate the hemodynamic response of septic shock patients highlighted by the general reduction or early interruption of vasopressors and amines in groups treated with CPFA. Moreover, the cytokines plasma levels seem to reduce faster in CPFA than standard treatments.

Ronco and co-workers studied haemodynamic parameters and the ability to restore leucocyte responsiveness in a cross-over trial of septic patients who underwent 10 h of CPFA followed by 10 h of continuous venovenoushaemodiafiltration (or vice versa)[70]. They also monitored leucocyte responsiveness to in vitro stimulation by endotoxin. At the beginning of the CPFA treatment the cells were not able to produce appropriate amounts of TNF-$\alpha$, whereas production was restored at the end of treatment. Cell hyporesponsiveness to secondary bacterial challenges is part of an overall immunosuppressive effect seen in septic patients and is frequently associated with worse outcomes [74].

These authors observed a significant improvement in hemodynamics with the use of CPFA compared with hemodiafiltration. They also observed a significant increase in leukocyte responsiveness after CPFA treatment. For these experiments, they monitored spontaneous and endotoxin-stimulated leukocyte TNF- $\alpha$ production after 10 h of treatment. At the beginning of the treatment, there was a marked leukocyte hyporesponsiveness to endotoxin stimulation (immunosuppression). As the treatment progressed, the responsiveness increased. Further support for the role of CPFA in the restoration of immune responsiveness was observed by incubating pre and post resin plasma with monocytes obtained from healthy donors. The pre-resin plasma at the beginning of treatment had a strong immunosuppressive effect – unless the plasma had first been incubated with monoclonal antibodies to IL-10. In contrast, the post-resin plasma (at the beginning of treatment) produced higher quantities of TNF- $\alpha$ after endotoxin challenge, and nearly normal quantities after 10-hour treatment. One of the interesting observations of this study was the absence of significant changes in circulating plasma levels of IL-10 or TNF- $\alpha$ even though there was almost complete adsorption of these cytokines by the resin cartridge. This suggests that there may still be other factors that are adsorbed by the cartridge that play a role in immunosuppression.

For this reason, the results presented in this study may be particularly relevant as the end point of the study was restoration of immune responsiveness, rather than a net increase or decrease in specific inflammatory mediators.

Formica and colleagues conducted one of the first trials of CPFA to include septic patients with and without renal insufficiency all of them with a high APACHE II score (24.8 B 5.6) and multiorgan failure. Six of the 10 patients had normal renal function. The authors performed 10 consecutive sessions and observed a net decrease in vasopressor requirement, increased mean arterial pressure, improved pulmonary function and a reduction in C-reactive protein. The patients treated with CPFA had a 70% survival [71].

Another study by Mariano and colleagues [77] evaluated CPFA in burn and polytrauma patients with septic shock and acute renal failure. Patients were divided into either heparin or citrate anticoagulation based on whether they had a high bleeding risk. The citrate anticoagulation was well tolerated and gave comparable results to the group with heparin anticoagulation. The previous CPFA studies included septic patients with acute renal failure that required renal support.

Recently, Berlot et al. [78] showed in septic shock a case report in which CPFA was able to ameliorate the microcirculation during the session. Sublingual microvascular perfusion was assessed using the orthogonal polarisation spectral imaging technique at three different times: pre-CPFA, at two hours during the treatment and two hours after the end of the session. During CPFA, the number of perfused vessels increased compared with the pre-treatment period, but decreased again after its termination. The author concluded that the elimination of septic mediators during the procedure could account for the observed microvascular perfusion variations.

Further case histories pointed out the effectiveness of CPFA in several other diseases such liver failure [79], Weil's syndrome [80] acute respiratory distress syndrome (ARDS) [81].

Caroleo et al. studied a case of a 70-year-old woman who developed hypoxic hepatitis secondary to cardiogenic shock after cardiac surgery [79]. CPFA was used primarily as an extracorporeal supportive therapy for multiple organ failure (MOF). The authors reported a significant reduction of the plasmatic concentration of conjugated bilirubin, achieving a mean reduction rate (RR) of 53% during treatment. CPFA proved to be a valid tool for concomitant hemodynamic support and organ replacement therapy.

Moretti and coworkes reported a case of a 27-year-old man with Weil's syndrome accompanied with hypotension, anuria refractory to fluid therapy, ARDS, and hepatic involvement [80]. CPFA was started early after the onset of shock and five treatments were performed. Each session lasted for 10 h with 14 h interval. Weaning from vasopressors was achieved during the second course of CPFA, while weaning from ventilation was achieved after 6 days.

Lucisano et al reporteda case of a 43-year-old male who developed ARDS secondary to pneumonia and acute kidney injury, whose clinical conditions rapidly improved after early CPFA therapy [81]. CPFA was performed for 6–8 h (daily, for three consecutive days).

Twenty-four hours after the first CPFA session CPAP was withdrawn. After 4 days, the oxygen saturation achieved 97% without ventilation. During the 3 days in which CPFA treatments were carried out, serum levels of pro-inflammatory cytokines, procalcitonin and CRP decreased progressively as well as APACHE II which achieved a score of 9 five days after the first CPFA session.

| Author | Patients | Study Design | Major Results | *P* |
|---|---|---|---|---|
| Ronco 2000 [70] | Septic pts N=unknown | Prospective Randomized Controlled Trial CPFA – CVVH CVVH - CPFA | Improvement of hemodynamic response<br>Reduction of norepinephrine dose | |
| Formica 2003 [71] | Septic shock pts N= 12 | Prospective Longitudinal CPFA | Improvement of MAP<br>Improvement of Cardiac Index<br>Increase of SystVasc Res Index<br>Improvement of PaO2/FiO2<br>No change extracvascular lung water<br>intra-thoracic blood index<br>Survival @ 28 days 90%, @90 days 70% | <0.001<br><0.001<br><0.001<br><0.001<br>Ns<br>Ns |
| Ronco 2002 [72] | Septic shock pts N= 10 | Prospective pilot CPFA (10h) – CVVHDF (10h) CVVHDF (10h) – CPFA (10h) | Increase of MAP by 11.8 vs 5.5 mmHg<br>Reduction of norepinephrine 0.08 vs 0.0049 ug/Kg/min | 0.001<br>0.003 |
| Lentini 2009 | Septic shock, AKI N=8 | Prospective Randomized Controlled Trial HVHF-CVVH-CPFA-CVVH CPFA-CVVH-HVHF-CVVH | No change MAP<br>No change Norepinephrine<br>No change Vasopressor<br>No change PaO2/FiO2 | 0.29<br>0.18<br>0.22<br>0.08 |
| Mao 2011 [74] | Septic shock, MOF N=7 | Prospective Randomized Controlled Trial CPFA (10h) – HVHF (10h) HVHF (10h) – CPFA (10h) | Increase MAP 120.75±20 vs 115.3±18.5 mmHg<br>paO2/FiO2 297.3±204 vs 265.45±173.7<br>reduction of Cytokines plasma levels | <0.05<br><0.05 |
| Hu D 2012 [75] | Septic patients or MODS N=14 | Prospective Randomized Controlled Trial CPFA HVHF | TNFa (pg/mL): 178±58 → 186.9±55.1 in HVHF; 229.8±44.2 → 151.8±29.4 in CPFA<br>Intercellular adhesion molecule-1 (ng/mL): 708.1±98.3 to 675.6±44.4 in HVHF vs 798.1±134.1 to 347.6±181.5 | <0.01<br><0.01 |

**Legend:** CVVH=Continuous Venous-Venous Hemofiltration; HVHF=High Volume HemoFiltration; MAP=Mean Arterial Pressure; MODS= Mutli Organ Distress Syndrome.

**Table 3.** Summary of the main clinical CPFA trials.

## 8. Conclusions

Although extracorporeal treatments have shown several developments over the years in the attempt to achieve better results in terms of survival both in acute and chronic patients, nevertheless they still remain poorly selective and with many limitations linked to the loss of nobles substances.

Filtration-adsorption architectures seems to be viable forms of extracorporeal blood purification systems which can enhance the capability to remove molecules in a wide range of molecular weight spectrum with the advantage of retaining molecules essential to the organs and subject life.

HDF has bee proven to obtain better clinical results in chronic dialysis population, even though renal replacement therapies still suffer from drawbacks related to inflammation, oxidative stress, morbidity and cardiovascular associated diseases. Diabetes, hypertension and age, often translate into clinical frailty and poor quality of life, often closer to survival than to cope with the disease. All these factors are extremely important in the choice of the convective therapy to adopt. HFR seems to combine a high removal of uremic toxins thus lowering the micro-inflammation status which can bring to benefits especially in cardiac compromised.

Further developments of this architecture could come from the use of super high-flux membranes with cut-off values much higher than the albumin limit and/or from the discovery of new adsorbent resins even more selective to specific molecules responsible for particular diseases.

In the meanwhile, we can take advantages of the clinical results gathered so far which can address the HFR to malnourished and inflamed patients and CPFA to septic ones.

Further studies are advocated to understand the potential of such architectures on high-end points like survival of both acute and chronic population as well as quality of life.

## Author details

Fabio Grandi[1], Piergiorgio Bolasco[2], Giuseppe Palladino[1], Luisa Sereni[1], Marialuisa Caiazzo[3], Mauro Atti[1] and Paolo Maria Ghezzi[1]

1 Bellco S.r.l., Mirandola, Italy

2 Territorial Department of Nephrology and Dialysis, ASL Cagliari, Italy

3 Laboratory Diagnostics and Forensic Medicine University of Modena and Reggio Emilia, Italy

## References

[1] Andrade, J., Hlady, V., Plasma, protein., adsorption, the., big, twelve., Ann, Ny., & Acad, Sci. (1987). 516, 158-172.

[2] Lagsdorf LJ, Zydney AL, Effect of blood contact on the transport properties of hemodialysis membranes: a two-layers model, Blood Purif,. (1994). 12, 292-307.

[3] Lutz, H., Ultrafiltration, fundamentals., engineering, in., Drioli, , Giorno, ., Ed., , Comprehensive, membrane., science, , & engineering, Elsevier. (2010). 2.

[4] Rockel, A., Hertel, J., Fiegel, P., et al., Permeability, , secondary, membrane., formation, of. a., high, flux., polysulfonehemofilter, , & Kidney, International. (1986). 30, 429-32.

[5] Kunitomo, T., Lowrie, E. G., Kumazawa, S., et al. Controlled ultrafiltration with hemodialysis: analysis of coupling between convective and diffusive mass tansfer in a new HD-uf system, Trans Am SocArtif Intern Organs (1977). , 23, 234-43.

[6] Leber, H. W., Wizemann, V., Goubeaud, G., et al., Simultaneous, hemodialysis/hemofiltration., an, effective., alternative, to., hemofiltration, , conventional, hemodialysis., in, the., treatment, of., uremic, patients., & Clin, . ClinNephrol (1978). , 9, 115-21.

[7] Navarro, J. F., Marcen, R., Teruel, J. L., et al. Effect of different membranes on amino-acid losses during hemodialysis. Nephrol Dial Transplant (1998).

[8] Sargent, J. A., Gotch, F. A., Principle, , biophysics, of., dialysis, Jacobs. C., Kjellstrand, C. M., Koch, K. M., Winchester, J. F., 4th, Ed., Replacement, of., renal, function., & by, dialysis. (1996). 34-102.

[9] Michaels AS, Operating parameters and performance criteria for hemodialyzers and other membrane-separation devices, Trans Am SocArtiflnt Organs,. (1966). 12, 387-392.

[10] Ghezzi, P. M., Frigato, G., Fantini, G. F., et al. Theoretical model and first clinical results of the Paired Filtration Dialysis (PFD),. Life Support Syst (1983). suppl 1) , 271 EOF-4 EOF.

[11] Botella, J., Ghezzi, P. M., Sanz-Moreno, C., et al. Multicentric study on paired filtration dialysis as a short efficient dialysis technique. Nephrol. Dial Transplant, (1991). , 6, 715-721.

[12] Gurland, H. J., Davison, A. M., Bonomini, V., et al. Definitions and terminology in biocompatibility. Nephrol Dial Transplant, (1994). Suppl 2), 4-10., 4 EOF.

[13] Winchester, JF: Hemoperfusion, in Maher JF, Dordrecht, Kluwer Academic Publishers (3rd ed), Replacement of Renal Function by Dialysis. (1989). 439-459.

[14] Muirhead, , Reid, A. F., Resin, artificial., kidney, J., & Lab, Clin. ClinMed,(1948). , 33, 841-844.

[15] Yatzidis, H. A., convenient, hemoperfusion., micro-apparatus, over., charcoal, for., the, treatment., of, endogenous., exogenous, intoxication., Proc, Eur., Dial, Transplant., & Assoc, . (1964). 1, 83-86.

[16] Chang, TMS: Semipermeable aqueous microcapsules (artificial cells): With emphasis on experiments in an extracorporeal shunt system.Trans Am SocArtif Intern Organs, (1966)., 12, 13-19.

[17] Chang, T. M. S., Chirito, E., Barre, B., Cole, C., Hewish, M., Clinical, evaluation., of, chronic., intermittent, , short, term., hemoperfusion, in., patients, with., chronic, renal., failure, using., semipermeable, microcapsules., (artificial, cells., formed, from., membrane, coated., & activated, charcoal. Trans Am SocArtif Intern Organs, (1971)., 17, 246-252.

[18] Gordon, A., Greenbaum, Marantz. L. B., Mc Arthur, Maxwell. M. H. A., sorbent-based, low., recirculating, dialysate., & system, . Trans Am SocArtiflnt Organs, (1969)., 15, 347-352.

[19] Branger, B., Ramperez, P., Marigliano, N., et al., Aluminium, transfer., in, bicarbonate., dialysis, using. a., sorbent, regenerative., system, an., in, vitro., & study, Proc. E. D. T. A. (1980). 17, 213-218.

[20] Randerson, D. H., Gurland, H. J., Schmidt, B., et al. Sorbent membrane dialysis in uremia. ContribNephrol, (1982)., 29, 53-64.

[21] Shaldon, S., Beau, M. C., Claret, G., et al. Haemofiltration with sorbent regeneration of ultrafiltrate: First clinical experience in end stage renal disease. ProcEur Dial Transplant Assoc, (1978)., 15, 220-227.

[22] Mion, C., Branger, B., Issautier, R., et al. Dialysis fracturing osteomalacia without hyperparathyroidism in patients treated with HCO3 rinsed Redy cartridge. Trans Am SocArtif Intern Organs, (1981)., 27, 634-638.

[23] Randerson, D. H., Gurland, H. J., Schmidt, B., et al. Sorbent membrane dialysis in uremia,. Contrib Nephrol, (1982)., 29, 53-64.

[24] Atti, M., Wratten, M. L., Sereni, A., et al. Contact phase activation can occur with certain types of activated carbon. G ItalNefrol. (2004). Suppl 30), S, 62-66.

[25] Wratten, M. L., Sereni, L., Lupotti, M., et al. Optimization of a HFR sorbent cartridge for high molecular weight uremic toxins. G ItalNefrol. (2004). Suppl 30), S, 67-70.

[26] Ghezzi, P. M., Dutto, A., Gervasio, R., Botella, J., Hemodiafiltration, with., the, separate., convection, , diffusion, Paired., filtration, dialysis., & Contrib, Nephrol. (1989). 69, 141-161.

[27] Botella, J., Ghezzi, P. M., Sanz-Moreno, C., et al. Multicentric study on paired filtration dialysis as a short efficient dialysis technique. Nephrol. Dial Transplant, (1991)., 6, 715-721.

[28] Aucella, F. Hemodiafiltration with endogenous reinfusion, G ItalNefrol, (2012). S55), SS82., 72.

[29] De Simone, W., De Simone, M., De Simone, A., et al. Aspetti dell'emodiafiltrazione online con rigenerazione e reinfusione dell'ultrafiltrato (HFR). Studio multicentrico. Giorn It Nefrol, (2004). Suppl 30), SS167., 161.

[30] Richter, R., Schulz-Knappe, P., Schrader, M., et al. Composition of the peptide fraction in human blood plasma: Database of circulating human peptides,. J Chromatogr B Biomed SciAppl, (1999)., 726, 25-35.

[31] Lefler DM, Pafford RG, Black NA, et al.Identification of proteins in slow continuous ultrafiltrate by reversed-phase chromatography and proteomics,. J Proteome Res, (2004)., 3, 1254-60.

[32] Weissinger, E. M., Kaiser, T., Meert, N., et al., Proteomics, a., novel, tool., to, unravel., the, patho-physiology., of, uraemia., Nephrol, Dial., & Transplant, . (2004). 19, 3068-77.

[33] Botella, J., Ghezzi, P. M., Sanz-Moreno, C., Adsorption, in., hemodialysis, Kidney., & Int, . (2000). SS65., 60.

[34] Ronco, C., Brendolan, A., d'Intini, V., et al. Coupled plasma filtration adsorption: rationale, technical development and early clinical experience,. Blood Purif, (2003).

[35] Winchester, J. F., Kellum, J. A., Ronco, C., et al. Sorbents in acute renal failure and the systemic inflammatory response syndrome. Blood Purif, (2003)., 21, 79-84.

[36] Wratten ML Therapeutic approaches to reduce systemic inflammation in septic-associated neurologic complications European Journal of Anaesthesiology,(2008). Suppl 42), 1-7.

[37] De Bock, M., de Seny, D., Meuwis, M., , A., Chapelle, J., , P., et al., Challenges, for., biomarker, discovery., in, body., fluids-T, using. S. E. L. D. I., & , O. F. M. S. Journal of biomedicine & biotechnology (2010).

[38] Caiazzo M., CuoghiA., Monari E., et al. STEPS Study: Superior Therapies for hEmodialysiS. A proteomic approach. Poster at 49 ERA-EDTA 2012 DOI:pso.eu.49era. (2012).

[39] Gert, R., & Strobl, . (1996). The Physics of Polymers Concepts for Understanding Their Structures and Behavior. Springer-Verlag. 3-54060-768-4

[40] Hardinc, S. H., & Protein, Hydrodynamic_. H. A. R. D. I. N. G. S. E. (1999). Protein hydrodynamics. In: ALLEN, G., ed., Protein: A Comprehensive Treatise 2. JAI Press Inc, Greenwich, USA. , 271-305.

[41] Kimmel, J. D., Gibson, G. A., Watkins, S. C., Kellum, J. A., Federspiel, W. J. I. L., Adsorption, Dynamics., in, Hemoadsorption., Beads, Studied., Using, Confocal., Laser, Scanning., Microscopy, Journal., of, Biomedical., Materials, Research., Part, B., & Applied, Biomaterials. (2009). B(2), 390-396.

[42] Narhi, L.O., Arakawa, T., Dissociation of recombinant tumor necrosis factor-$\alpha$ studied by gel permeation chromatography; Biochem and biopsy Res Communic,. (1978).

[43] Atmeh, R. F., Arafa, I. M., Al-Khateeb, M., Albumin, Aggregates., Hydrodynamic, Shape., Physico-Chemical, Properties., Jordan, Journal., & of, Chemistry. (2007).

[44] Sviridov, D., Meilinger, B., Drake, S. K., Hoehn, G. T., Hortin, G. L., Coelution, of., other, proteins., with, albumin., during, size-exclusion. H. P. L. C., Implications, for., analysis, of., & urinary, albumin. (2006). *Clinical Chemistry*, 389 EOF-97 EOF.

[45] Panichi, V., Manca-Rizza, G., Paoletti, S., et al. Effects on inflammatory and nutritional markers of hemodiafiltration with online regeneration of ultrafiltrate (HFR) vs. online hemodiafiltration: a cross-over randomized multicentre trial, Nephrol Dial Transplant (2006)., 21, 756-62.

[46] Bolasco, P. G., Ghezzi, P. M., Ferrara, R., et al. Effect of on-line hemodiafiltration with endogenous reinfusion (HFR) on the calcium-phosphorus metabolism: medium-term effects,. Int J Artif Organs, (2006)., 29, 1042-52.

[47] Kim, S., Oh, K. H., Chin, H. J., Na, K. Y., et al. Effective removal of leptin via hemodiafiltration with on-line endogenous reinfusion therapy, Clinical Nephrology, (2009).

[48] Borrelli, S., Minutolo, R., De Nicola, L., et al. Intradialytic changes of plasma amino acid levels: effect of hemodiafiltration with endogenous reinfusion versus acetate-free biofiltration. Blood Purif, (2010)., 166 EOF-171 EOF.

[49] Bolasco, P., Ghezzi, P. M., Serra, A., et, al. E., Effects, of., acetate-free, haemodiafiltration. . H. D. F., with, endogenous., reinfusion, . H. F. R., on, cardiac., & troponin, levels. Sardinian Polycentric Study on Acetate-Free Haemodiafiltration, Nephrol Dial Transplant, (2011).

[50] Ikizler TA, Flakoll PJ, Parker RA, Hakim RM.Amino acid and albumin losses during hemodialysis,. Kidney Int, (1994)., 830 EOF-7 EOF.

[51] Navarro, J. F., Mora, C., Leon, C., et al. Amino acid losses during hemodialysis with polyacrylonitrile membranes: effect of intradialitic amino acid supplementation on plasma amino acid concentrations and nutritional variables in nondiabetic patients. Am J ClinNutr (2000).

[52] Prado de, Negreiros., Nogueira, Maduro. I., Elias, N. M., & Nonino, Borges. C. B. Total nitrogen and free amino acid losses and protein calorie malnutrition of hemodialysis patients: do they really matter? Nephron Clin Pract, (2007). cc17., 9.

[53] Ragazzoni, E., Carpani, P., Agliata, S., et, al. H. F. R., on-line, H. D. F., valutazione della, perdita., & aminoacidica, plasmatica. Giorn It Nefrol (2004). suppl 30), 85-90.

[54] Morosetti, M. personal communication

[55] Calò, L. A., Naso, A., Devis, P. A., et al. Hemodiafiltration with on-line regeneration of ultrafiltrate: effect on Heme-Oxygenase-1 and inducible subunit of Nitric Oxide Synthase and implication for oxidative stress and inflammation.,Artif Org (2010).

[56] Splendiani, G., De Angelis, S., Tullio, T., et al. Selective adsorption of homocysteine using an HFR online technique, Artif Organs (2004)., 28, 592-95.

[57] Deléaval, P., Descombes, E., Magnin, J. L., Rossi, S., & Chiatto, M. Differences in cardiac troponin I and T levels measurement in asymptomatic hemodialysis patients with last generation immunoassays, NephrolTher, (2008)., 2, 75-81.

[58] Katerinis, I., Nguyen, Q. W., Magnin, J. L., & Descombes, E. (2008). Cardiac findings in asymptomatic hemodialysis patients with persistently elevated cardiac troponin levels, Ren Fail. 30, 357-62.

[59] De Filippi, C., Wasserman, S., Rosani, S., Cardiac, troponin. T., C-reactive, protein., for, predicting., progonosis, coronary., atherosclerosis, , cardiomyopathy, in., patients, undergoing., & long-term, hemodialysis. J. A. M. A. (2003). 290, 353-59.

[60] Lippi, G., Tessitore, N., Montagnana, M., et al. Influence of sampling time and ultrafiltration coefficient of the dialysis membrane on cardiac troponin I and T. ArchPathol Lab Med (2008)., 132, 72-76.

[61] Sommerer, C., Heckele, S., Schwenger, V., et al. Cardiac biomarkers are influenced by dialysis characteristics,. ClinNephrol, (2007)., 68, 392-400.

[62] Peruzzi, L., Camilla, R., Bonaudo, R., Coppo, R., & Amore, A. Bioincompatibility of acetate even at low concentrations. G ItalNefrol. (2011)., 289 EOF-95 EOF.

[63] Amore, A., Cirina, P., Bonaudo, R., et al., Bicarbonate, dialysis., unlike, acetate-free., biofiltration, triggers., mediators, of., inflammation, , apoptosis, in., endothelial, , smooth, muscle., cells, J., & Nephrol, . (2006). 57 EOF-64 EOF.

[64] Bolasco, P. G., Ghezzi, P. M., Serra, A., et al. Hemodiafiltration with endogenous reinfusion with and without acetate-free dialysis solutions: effect on ESA requirement. Blood Purif, (2011)., 235 EOF-242 EOF.

[65] Axelsson, J., Quereshi, A. R., Heimburger, O., et al. Body fat mass and serum leptin levels influence epoetin sensitivity in patients with ESRD. Am J Kidney Dis, (2005)., 46, 628-34.

[66] Sitter, T., Bergner, A., Schiffle, H., Dialysis-relate, cytokine., induction, , response, to., recombinant, human., erythropoietin, in., hemodiaysis, patients., Nephrol, Dial., & Transplant, . (2000). 15, 1207-1211.

[67] Testa, A., Dejoie, T., Lecarrer, D., et al. Reduction of free immunoglobulin light chains using adsorption properties of hemodiafiltration with endogenous reinfusion. Blood Purif, (2010)., 34 EOF-36 EOF.

[68] Hutchison, Cockwell. P., Reid, S., et al. Efficient removal of immunoglobulin free light chains by hemodialysis for multiple myeloma. J Am Soc Nephrol (2007). ; ., 18, 886-95.

[69] Tetta, C., Gianotti, L., Cavaillon, J. M., et al. Coupled plasma filtration-adsorption in a rabbit model of endotoxic shock,. Crit Care Med, (2000). , 1526 EOF-33 EOF.

[70] Ronco, C., Brendolan, A., Dan, M., et al., Adsorption, in., sepsis, Kidney., & Int, Suppl. (2000). Aug;76:S, 148-55.

[71] Formica, M., Olivieri, C., Livigni, S., et al. Hemodynamic response to coupled plasmafiltrationadsoprtion in human septic shock, Intensive Care Med, (2003). , 29, 703-708.

[72] Ronco, C., Brendolan, A., Lonnemann, G., et, al. A., pilot, study., of, coupled., plasma, filtration., with, adsorption., in, septic., shock, Crit., & Care, . (2002). 1250 EOF-5 EOF.

[73] Lentini, P., Cruz, D., Nalesso, F., et, al. A., pilot, study., comparing, pulse., high, volume., hemofiltration, (p. H. V. H. F., coupled, plasma., filtration, adsorption. . C. P. F. A., in, septic., shock, patients. G., & Ital, Nefrol. (2009).

[74] Mao, H., Yu, S., Yu, X., et al. Effect of coupled plasma filtration adsorption on endothelial cell function in patients with multiple organ dysfunction syndrome. Int J Artif Organs. (2011). , 288 EOF-294 EOF.

[75] Hu, D., Sun, S., Zhu, B., et al. Effects of coupled plasma filtration adsorption on septic patients with multiple organ dysfunction syndrome. Ren Fail. 2012; 34(7), Epub (2012). May 18., 834 EOF-839 EOF.

[76] Ronco, C., Tetta, C., Mariano, F., et al. Interpreting the mechanisms of continuous renal replacement therapy in sepsis: the peak concentration hypothesis. Artif Organs, (2003). , 27, 792-801.

[77] Mariano, F., Tetta, C., Stella, M., et al. Regional Citrate Anticoagulation in Critically Ill Patients treated with Plasma Filtration and Adsorption. Blood Purif, (2004). , 22, 313-9.

[78] Berlot, G., Bianco, N., Tomasini, A., et al. Changes in microvascular blood flow during coupled plasma filtration and adsorption Anaesth Intensive Care, (2011). , 39, 687-689.

[79] Caroleo, S., Rubino, Tropea. F., et al., Coupled, plasma., filtration, adsorption., reduces, serum., bilirubine, in. a., case, of., acute, hypoxic., hepatitis, secondary., to, cardiogenic., shock, Int. J., & Artif, Organs. (2010).

[80] Moretti, R., Scarrone, S., Pizzi, B., et al. Coupled Plasma Filtration Adsorption in Weil's syndrome: a case report. Minerva Anestesiol, (2011). , 77, 846-849.

[81] Lucisano, G., Capria, M., Matera, G., et al., Coupled, plasma., filtration, adsorption., for, the., treatment, of. a., patient, with., acute, respiratory., distress, syndrome., acute, kidney., injury, a., case, report., Nephrol, Dial., & Transplant, Plus. (2011). 4, 285-288.

# Chapter 8

# Push/Pull Based Renal Replacement Treatments

Kyungsoo Lee

Additional information is available at the end of the chapter

## 1. Introduction

The incidence of kidney disease is rapidly increasing worldwide [1], accompanied by widespread research and development resulting in remarkable improvements in the technologies used for treatment in end-stage renal disease (ESRD) patients. Polymeric membranes are better at preventing the transfer of pyrogenic substances into the blood stream and membrane biocompatibilities are much improved [2]. The sharp molecular cut-offs of these membranes also prevents further loss of albumin during high-dose convective treatment [3]. These membrane technology advancements have been accompanied by the evolution of varied choices for renal replacement treatment. Particularly, better outcomes achieved by convective treatment have encouraged the use of synthetic membranes with high water permeability and sieving characteristics in clinical setups worldwide [4, 5].

Maintenance hemodialysis (HD) nevertheless remains a standard protocol for treating ESRD patients, despite the development of renal replacement modalities. This process is a result of two physical phenomena that facilitate mass transfer in purifying blood. Diffusion caused by a concentration gradient between blood and dialysate contributes to the removal of uremic solutes, particularly small-sized, water-soluble molecules. Excess water and mid-sized molecules are removed primarily by convective mass transfer, resulting from the transmembrane pressure gradient [6]. Plasma water flow through a membrane leads to the simultaneous movement of a solute through the membranes. Thus, volume-controlled high-flux HD adequately clears mid-size solutes without sterile fluid infusion because forward filtration exceeding the desired volume removal is compensated for by backfiltration [7], and this modality can provide a simpler form of dialysis treatment than other treatment methods. However, although the convective dose delivered during high-flux HD has been shown to reduce mortality in patients at risk [8], overall patient survival remains comparable to that of low-flux HD [9]. This is presumably caused by the limited amount of internal filtration involved due to limitations imposed by fluid dynamics and the geometric nature of the hemodialyzer.

In contrast, hemodiafiltration (HDF) is characterized by a large filtration volume that far exceeds the desired volume removal. Given that, the dehydration must be corrected in real time by infusing exogenous sterile replacement fluid. HDF has been reported to deliver better dialysis outcomes than high-flux HD, because of the improved middle-to-large size molecular removal, better control of EPO and inflammation [10-13], resulting in less patient mortality [14, 15]. However, HDF use is limited globally because the requirement of exogenous fluid infusion raises concerns about water quality, safety and cost. This has led to modifications of HDF strategies to increase convective mass transfer without the need for exogenous replacement fluid infusion. This is achieved by spontaneous fluid reinfusion at a rate that matches convection. Backfiltration and regenerated ultrafiltrate can be the methods of spontaneous fluid restoration.

Push/pull strategies have also been examined to increase total filtration volumes without the exogenous replacement fluid infusion. The push/pull technique uses the entire membrane as the forward filtration domain for a period of time. However, backfiltration must accompany the forward filtration to compensate for the fluid depletion that occurred due to the forward filtration, and as a result, making it necessary to switch the membranes to a backfiltration domain. In other words, push/pull systems rely on alternate repetitions of forward and backward filtration during dialysis treatment and the repetitive filtration contributes to the increased total filtration volume.

In this chapter, the trials of push/pull-based renal supportive treatments are reviewed in terms of their technical description, hemodialytic efficacy and applicability for clinical use. In addition, the fluid management accuracy of the push/pull dialysis method will be discussed in depth.

## 2. Backfiltration and push/pull operation

Precise volume control is a crucial pre-requisite in renal replacement therapy. With kidney malfunction, the accumulation of uremic toxins and surplus water is a consistent fact in ESRD patients, and appropriate, timely renal supportive treatment must be conducted to avoid deadly uremic conditions. It has been recently reported that dialysis outcomes are considerably improved with enhanced convective mass transfer during hemodialysis, and techniques to maximize the convective volume exchange have been extensively explored. As the volume depletion exceeds the prescribed amount, it must be promptly compensated. A straightforward way is to infuse sterile fluid after calculating the desired fluid level. However, the external infusion of sterile dialysate raises concerns like high standard water quality and treatment-related cost. Reverse movement of dialysate within a hemodialyzer has been tried as an alternative approach.

Backfiltration is the phenomenon that dialysate moves into the blood stream across membranes, in the area where dialysate pressures are higher than hydraulic blood and osmotic pressures. A pressure drop is inevitable as fluid flows through a cylindrical tube, and blood and dialysate pressures decrease along the dialyzers. In a normal countercurrent dialysis setup, because blood and dialysate flow in opposite directions, these pressure drops occur with opposing gradients, and in some regions hydraulic blood and dialysate pressures overlap. Thus, the sum of hydraulic and osmotic pressures, termed transmembrane pressure (TMP), is positive in the proximal region of a hollow fiber dialyzer, and plasma moves to the dialysate compartment across the membranes (forward filtration). However, fluid movement occurs in the opposite direction in the distal region because TMP becomes negative, and backfiltration occurs. This backfiltration compensates for fluid loss in the proximal region (Figure 1) [16].

While backfiltration method could provide fluid restoration easily, the amount of forward filtration in the normal countercurrent dialysis setup is limited, because (1) a small area of the membranes is used for the filtration inside the hemodialyzer and (2) the increase of pressure gradients through the hemodialyzer is limited in a particular hemodialyzer geometry and flow conditions. These limitations have led to investigations for techniques to increase the blood-to-dialysate pressure gradients. As fluid pressure drop through a cylindrical tube is proportional to the tube length, but is inversely proportional to the 4th power of tube diameter, hemodialyzers with reduced fiber diameters or elongated hemodialyzers have been developed [17-19]. In addition, a unique design for the hemodialyzer was also introduced [20-22] in which forward and backward filtration regions are separated longitudinally, instead of horizontally, giving the independent control of blood or dialysate pressures in each region.

Additionally, push and pull actions were devised for an infusion-free HDF technique. Differently from other methods, forward filtration and backfiltration repeat in the push/pull technique. During a given period of time, the entire membrane is used as the forward filtration domain, as in the HDF method, by regulating blood pressure higher than dialysate. Thus, the filtration rates necessarily exceed prescribed rates. Immediately after the forward filtration, the pressure gradients through the hemodialyzer are reversed, the fluid movement is switched to the opposite direction. This opposite fluid movement compensates for the excessive fluid loss during the previous filtration phase. The alternate repetition of forward filtration and backfiltration constitutes a cycle of fluid movement and the difference of the forward and backward filtration rates, i.e., net-filtration rates, is regulated at the desirable level.

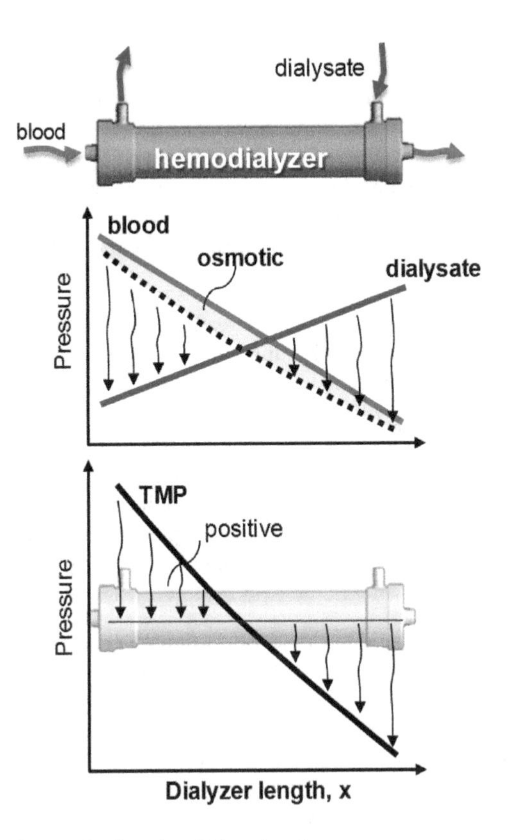


**Figure 1.** Transmembrane Pressure Gradient along Dialyzer Length.

## 3. Push/pull hemodiafiltration

The concept for repetitive use of forward and backward filtration during conventional dialysis treatments was first introduced in Japan in the early 1980's, in an effort to simplify the infusion-free HDF technique, using a serial arrangement of two hemodiafilters [23 25]. However, that system requires a means of repeating backfiltration [26]. Thus, a redundant dialysate bag is integrated downstream of the hemodialyzer and connected to the dialysate stream by a bidirectional peristaltic pump [27]. The push/pull action accomplished by this bi-directional pump alternates the evacuation and replenishment of the bag. During normal operation, dialysate flow rates upstream and downstream of the hemodialyzer are maintained in balance and the desired volume removal is achieved by a separate ultrafiltration pump. Therefore, when the bidirectional push/pull pump pulls a portion of dialysate into the bag (e.g., 70 ml/min for 3 minutes), hydrostatic pressures through the dialysate compartment decrease, because the dialysate compartment is closed and has a fixed volume, and water flux occurs from blood to the dialysate compartment (ultrafiltration) at the same rate as dialysate removal from the dialysate compartment. Soon after the ultrafiltration completes, the pump reverses and pushes the dialysate in the bag into the dialysate stream, causing a volume overload in the dialysate compartment. The surplus dialysate in the closed dialysate compartment is then moved to the blood compartment (backfiltration). Another bag and an additional bidirectional peristaltic pump is also integrated into the venous chamber, and conducts the pulling and pushing of blood, although in this case, the actions of the blood-side pump are $180^{O}$ out of phase with those of the dialysate side pump to keep blood flow returning to the patient constant.

When pure dialysate is pushed into the blood stream, solute concentrations in blood are immediately equilibrated and decreased by dilution. Soon after, the blood-to-dialysate pressure gradient reverses from negative to positive, and plasma fluid in blood is forced to move into the dialysate compartment, which removes various molecules from the plasma. This repetitive ultrafiltration contributes to convective mass transfer and increases the removal of small-sized (urea) or mid-sized (beta-2-microglobulin) molecules compared to hemofiltration (HF) or hemodialysis method, respectively [28]. On the other hand, repetitive backfiltration during push/pull HDF prevents volume depletion. In addition, the repetitive backflushing of dialysate also helps prevent membrane bindings of various blood components [26].

However, the disposable bags and separate bidirectional peristaltic pumps make this unit notably complicated. To overcome these shortcomings, a double-chamber cylinder pump was devised. The double cylinder pump includes two independent chambers and a reciprocal piston, and each chamber is connected to either dialysate or the blood stream [29], as seen in Figure 2. When the piston squeezes the chamber on the dialysate side, the dialysate compartment, which has a fixed volume, is pressurized and backfiltration begins. At this time, the chamber on the blood side expands and blood in the venous chamber starts flowing in the direction of the cylinder pump. Since the blood volume that returns to the blood-side chamber of the pump is equal to the backfiltration volume, blood flow returning to patients remains constant. The piston then moves in the opposite direction and squeezes the blood-side chamber, the dialysate compartment begins to expand, and the dialysate compartment is depressurized, leading to ultrafiltration. However, despite the large amount of ultrafiltration, blood flow in the venous line is maintained, because the ultrafiltrate removed in the hemodialyzer is replenished in the venous chamber.

The reciprocating movement of the piston is regulated by pressure differences between the two chambers of the cylinder pump (i.e., Pb-Pd). The rotation torque of the driving motor attached to the piston can be adjusted in accord with TMP (i.e., torque = TMPxSxLxsinθ). Voltage applied to the motor is adjustable, allowing the TMP to be set at 400 mmHg during forward filtration, but at -400 mmHg during the backward filtration phase. Pressure-controlled push/pull HDF can maintain transmembrane pressures at the maximum permissible level throughout treatment [30]. In addition, contrary to the original push/pull HDF, in which one cycle of filtration and backfiltration takes approximate 4~5 minutes, the pressure controlled push/pull HDF unit can repeat one cycle in1.5~1.7 seconds.

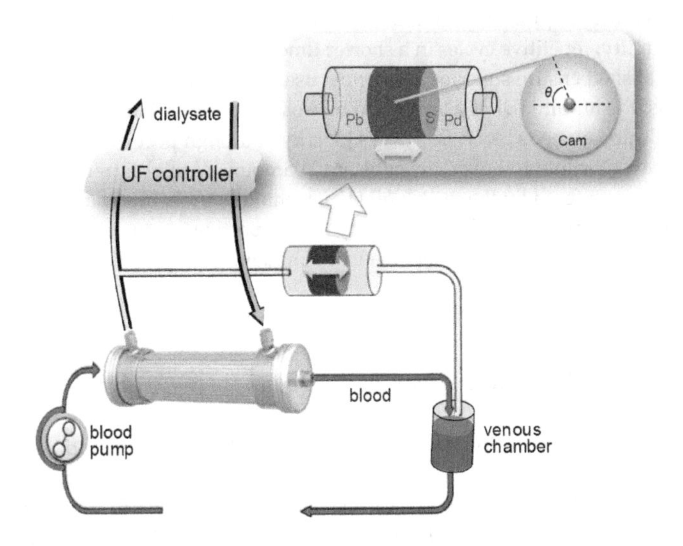


**Figure 2.** Push/Pull HDF and Double-Chamber Cylinder Pump

This optimized use of transmembrane pressure and more frequent alternations of forward and backward filtration in the revised push/pull HDF unit are obviously accompanied with a markedly larger total filtration volumes and higher solutes clearances [30]. The push/pull HDF unit tends to relieve symptoms like arthralgia (joint pain), irritability, pruritus, and insomnia more rapidly than conventional HD mode [27, 31, 32]. Furthermore, the optimal maintenance of membrane permeabilities by prompt backfiltration has the added benefit of considerably inhibiting albumin loss while increasing convection and diffusion [33]. Some albumin loss is unavoidable when using membranes with high water permeabilities and sieving characteristics [34]. Since convective therapy is based on larger amounts of fluid exchange and solvent drag during fluid exchange occurs randomly, albumin permeation becomes more worrisome during convective treatments [3]. In addition, filtration-induced elevated albumin concentration at the inner membrane wall also aggravates the albumin loss [35]. Protein concentration polarization develops quickly after sudden TMP development and the hydraulic permeabilities of the membrane decrease rapidly in about 2 seconds. However, during push/pull HDF, backward flushing of dialysate takes place within the time frame required for the protein layer to fully develop (i.e., 1.5~1.7 seconds), and thus, it can effectively wash out the inner lumen and inhibit excessive albumin leakage [33]. This dialysate backflushing eventually allows membrane hydraulic capabilities to be better maintained throughout the treatment.

In summary, push/pull HDF was developed in an effort to perform infusion-free, simultaneous HD and HF by using a single hemodialyzer. Thus, it alternates between ultrafiltration and backfiltration instead of dividing ultrafiltration and backfiltration regions. Pressure-controlled push/pull HDF can maintain TMPs at maximal levels and the total filtration volumes achieved are far greater than that of any other treatment modality. In addition to the filtration quantity, repetitive cycles in a shorter time than the time required for a protein layer to be established ensure superior membrane use throughout treatment, further inhibiting albumin loss. Push/pull HDF is assumed to be close to pre-dilution mode HDF because the repetitive dilution exceeds blood flow rates [36]. Even though post-dilution HDF is more efficient in terms of solute removal, the substantial amount of total filtration and the optimal use of membrane offered by the push/pull HDF technique probably translate to outstanding hemodialytic outcomes. Therefore, a prolonged prospective study on push/pull HDF may be worthwhile to determine the benefits of this modality versus other forms of convective renal replacement.

## 4. Pulse push/pull hemodialysis

Flow patterns have been an obvious research avenue for treatments requiring extracorporeal blood circulation. Blood pulsation has been accepted, although with controversy, as beneficial during cardiopulmonary bypass, because it achieves greater perfusion to peripheral vessels and end-organs [37, 38]. Blood pulsation in a pediatric CRRT animal model delivers adequate performance over a 2-hour period in terms of ultrafiltration rates and cross-filter blood pressure drops [39, 40]. It was further found that the pulsatile flow tends to enhance ultrafiltration rates versus non-pulsatile flow [41, 42], attributable to increased rheological power of pulsatile flow. However, little evidence is available clinically or experimentally that explains the efficacy of pulsatile flow on dialysis outcomes. Pulse push/pull HD (PPPHD) is a convection-enhanced dialysis treatment, using pulsatile devices for blood and dialysate to achieve the cyclic repetition of forward and backward filtration. During an early trial, a T-PLS pump (Twin Pulse Life Supporter, AnC Bio Inc., Seoul, Korea) was used as the pulsatile pump [43]. The T-PLS consists of blood and dialysate sacs, a reciprocating actuator and a motor-cam assembly [44], with the actuator between the blood and dialysate sacs (Figure 3). When the actuator squeezes the blood sac, blood can move forward due to one-way check valves. At the same time, the dialysate sac expands and is filled with fresh dialysate. In the same manner, dialysate also moves forward when the sac is squeezed and the blood sac is filled with blood. These reciprocating movements create pulsatile flow. By setting their phase difference at 180$^{o}$ degrees, the pushing phases of blood and dialysate pumps alternate, and TMPs cycle between positive and negative, driving consecutive periods of ultrafiltration and backfiltration.

The hemodialytic efficiencies of PPPHD have been demonstrated, and studies show that PPPHD substantially improves uremic marker molecules clearance, particularly for mid-sized molecules (Table 1) [43]. Increased filtration volumes in the PPPHD unit may also be due to reduced membrane fouling. In an *in vivo* setup on PPPHD, one cycle of ultrafiltration and backfiltration took 3 seconds at a pulse frequency of 20 bpm [45]. When ultrafiltration and backfiltration times were defined as the durations of positive and negative TMPs, respectively, ultrafiltration and backfiltration times for the PPPHD unit were approximately 1.7 and 1.3 seconds, respectively. Since protein concentration polarization on the blood-side membrane develops during forward filtration and is reduced by backfiltration, membrane convective capacity could be better maintained during PPPHD than during CHD, showing smaller reductions in post-dialysis hydraulic permeabilities [45].

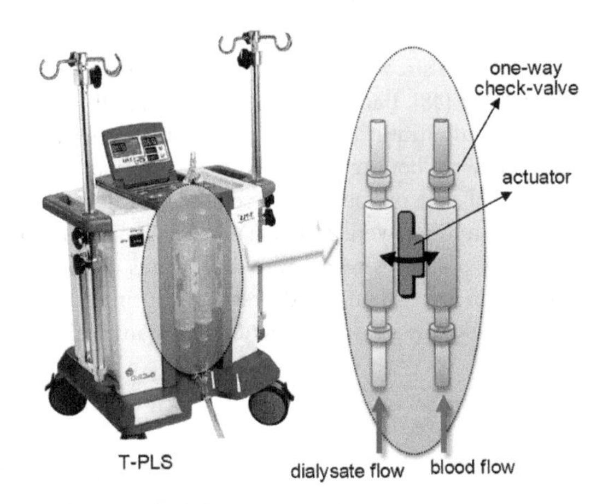


**Figure 3.** T-PLS pump for the original PPPHD

| Group | BPM | QB | QD | Clearance (ml/min) | | | |
|---|---|---|---|---|---|---|---|
| | | | | BUN | Creatinine | Vitamin b12 | Inulin |
| CHD | - | 236±3.6 | 420±3 | 161.1±4.3 | 127.2±3.9 | 37.5±6.3 | 25.3±5.1 |
| PPPHD | 40 | 234±3.1 | 419±3 | 166.2±3.8 | 136.9±4.2 | 55.7±5.0 | 37.8±3.9 |
| % Increase | | - | - | 3.2 | 7.6 | 48 | 49 |
| P-value | | NS | NS | 0.053 | <0.05 | <0.001 | <0.001 |

**Table 1.** Solutes Clearances. (CHD, conventional high-flux HD; PPPHD, pulse push/pull HD; BPM, beats per minute; QB, blood flowrate; QD, dialysate flowrate; BUN, blood urea nitrogen; NS, not significant) (Reproduction was permitted by a publisher)

## 5. Modified pulse push/pull hemodialysis

Pulsatile circulation of blood and dialysate offers a simple and efficient strategy for the repetitive cycle of filtration and backfiltration. However, blood pulsation during extracorporeal renal replacement treatment is potentially problematic. Specifically, instant suction generated by a pulse pump through a narrow catheter may cause blood damage, vessel narrowing, or vessel collapse. In addition, instantaneous negative pressures generated upstream of a pulsatile blood pump not only introduce the possibility of circuit aeration, but could lead to a failure to maintain predetermined blood flow rates [46, 47].

Hence, PPPHD unit was revised, and while many facets of the original PPPHD were retained, including the alternating water flux across the membrane, blood pulsation was excluded. This was achieved by employing dual pulsation in the dialysate stream, that is, pulsatile devices in the dialysate stream upstream (a dialysate pump) and downstream (an effluent pump) of the dialyzer [48]. Backfiltration occurs when the sum of the cross-membrane pressures is negative, but ultrafiltration when the sum is positive. The hydraulic pressures of blood and dialysate were both manipulated in the original PPPHD, but since blood pulsation was eliminated, dialysate pressure alone regulates TMP in the revised unit. Therefore, the following two assumptions were made; (1) dialysate compartment pressures must be far higher than blood-side pressures when pure dialysate is forced into the dialyzer, and (2) dialysate pressures drop to lower than blood pressures during effluent pump expansion. Given these assumptions, the dialysate and effluent pumps are replaced with a dual pulse pump [49].

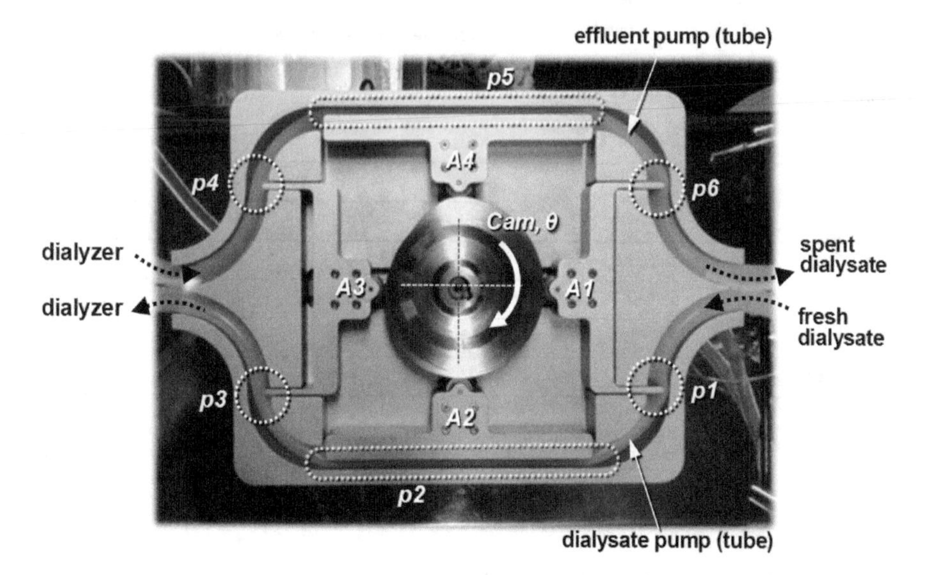


**Figure 4.** Dual Pulse Pump (DPP). DPP is composed of a base plate, a unidirectional electric motor, a cam, and four actuators. It contains two separate silicone tubes. Pulsatile flow is generated by squeezing each dialysate and effluent tubing segments. (A1~A4, actuators 1 to 4; p1~p6, silicone tubing segments at positions 1 to 6, respectively) (Reproduction was permitted by a publisher)

The dual pulse pump (DPP) is a pulsatile device that was developed to eliminate the one-way valves that are generally required for pulsatile devices to prevent retrograde flow. Instead, time-delayed tube openings and closings constitutes a cycle of pulse generation (Figure 4). In other words, two separate silicone tubes in the DPP are periodically opened or closed. Pulse generation with DPP can be described in terms of four phases as determined by cam rotation, which translates motor rotation to actuator linear displacement. As the cam rotates, the four actuators periodically push on the tubing segments at the positions shown in Figure 4. Actuator 1 pushes on the tubing segments at positions 1 and 6 (p1 and p6) simultaneously, and actuator 3 squeezes the tubing segments at positions 3 and 4. Actuators 2 and 4 squeeze tubing segments at p 2 and p5, respectively, and cause the dialysate in the tube to move in the required direction. For pulse generation by the dialysate pump, as the cam rotates from θ=0° to 90°, the p2 tubing segment opens and p1 closes, and these processes overlap such that pure dialysate fills p2 tubing. While p2 expands, p3 remains closed, acting as an upstream valve to prevent retrograde dialysate. These tube openings and closings are depicted diagrammatically in Figure 5. During the first phase, with p3 closed, p2 tube openness increases whereas p1 tube openness decreases. During the 2nd phase (θ=90°~180°), with p1 closed, p2 begins to be squeezed and simultaneously p3 begins to open, and pure dialysate is driven into the hemodialyzer. Closure of p1 fulfills the same function as atrioventricular valve closure during left ventricular systole, which prevents retrograde flow. Likewise, during the 3rd phase (θ=180°~270°), p3 is closed, while p1 and p2 remain closed and in the final phase (θ=270°~360°), p1 is open, and p2 and p3 remain closed in preparedness for the next filling phase. These time-delayed tube openings and closures constitute one cycle of pulse generation. In the same manner, effluent pulsations were also generated through the effluent tube, although in this case, the actions of actuators 1 and 3 were reversed, and the pulsatile flow pattern was 180° out of phase with that in the dialysate tube.

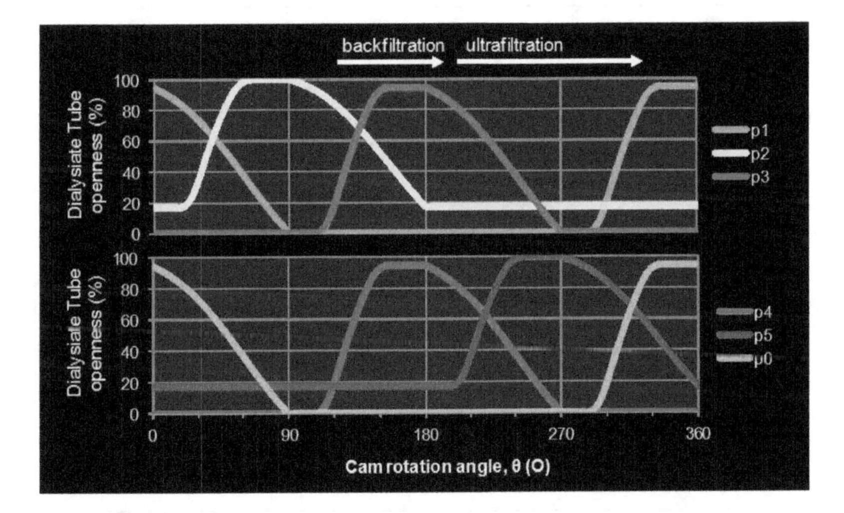


**Figure 5.** Changes in DPP Tube Openness at p1~p3 for Dialysate Pump (top) and at p4~p6 for Effluent Pump (bottom). Tube openness is defined as the ratio of compressed to original tube cross-sectional area. Tube openness at p1 (p6) and p3 (p4) during cycles ranged between 94% and 0%, corresponding to fully opened and completely closed, respectively. The p2 and p5 had an openness that ranged from 99% to 17%. (p1~p6, tubing segments at positions 1 to 6, respectively, as shown in Figure 4) (Reproduction was permitted by a publisher)

Theoretically, forward and backward filtration rates during one cycle of PPPHD are identical to effluent and dialysate flow rates, respectively. The moment when pure dialysate is driven to the dialyzer (i.e., during p2 squeezing), the effluent dialysate path is closed at p6. At the same time, p1 is also closed, and thus, the pure dialysate pushed into dialyzer moves into the blood stream (backfiltration), because the whole dialysate compartment is fixed and closed. Immediately after the backfiltration is completed, the effluent tubing (p5) begins to expand (i.e., p5 expansion during the 3rd phase), and since the dialysate and effluent pathways are still closed at p1 and p6, respectively, dialysate pressures in the hemodialyzer drop steeply and ultrafiltration takes place at a rate determined by effluent stroke volume.

During experiments using the revised PPPHD, the animals remained stable without any procedurally related complications. Molecular removals were satisfactory while total protein levels, albumin concentrations, and glucose levels were preserved uniformly throughout sessions (Table 2) [50]. As stated before, the DPP is additionally characterized by a lack of valves, which makes the pulsatile device simple and inexpensive, and thus, any medical-grade silicone tubes can be used as dialysate and effluent sacs. With the exception of small tubing sections at p1, p3, p4, and p5, most of the tubing is operated non-occlusively, reducing the chances of tubing rupture and spallation [51, 52].

| | | | | | PPPHD | | | | | |
|---|---|---|---|---|---|---|---|---|---|---|
| (h) | aPTT | PT | WBC | Hct | TP | ALB | Glu | Ca2+ | Na+ | K+ |
| 0 | 16±14 | 6.0±2.6 | 10.5±6.1 | 28.5±4.6 | 5.3±0.4 | 3.1±0.1 | 119±7 | 12.4±0.8 | 136±5.7 | 5.7±0.6 |
| 1 | 48±48 | 3.9±2.1 | 6.9±2.6 | 27.8±4.0 | 5.3±0.4 | - | - | - | - | - |
| 2 | 166±149 | 4.8±1.9 | 8.0±3.1 | 28.0±3.6 | 5.6±0.7 | 3.1±0.2 | 111±4 | 11.5±0.8 | 134±4.2 | 5.1±0.6 |
| 3 | 317±220 | 4.4±1.3 | 8.7±2.8 | 28.5±2.9 | 5.6±0.7 | - | - | - | - | - |
| 4 | 205±69 | 3.8±0.7 | 9.2±2.7 | 27.3±3.5 | 5.3±0.4 | 3.1±0.2 | 126±44 | 10.8±0.5 | 132±3.1 | 4.3±0.5 |
| | CHD | | | | | | | | | |
| (h) | aPTT | PT | WBC | Hct | TP | ALB | Glu | Ca2+ | Na+ | K+ |
| 0 | 16±6 | 3.2±1.1 | 9.3±4.1 | 30.3±6.8 | 5.7±0.4 | 3.2±0.3 | 124±10 | 11.7±0.4 | 138±4.9 | 5.9±0.2 |
| 1 | 170±93 | 3.8±0.6 | 6.9±4.4 | 27.3±5.5 | 5.7±0.1 | - | - | - | - | - |
| 2 | 232±125 | 4.5±0.5 | 7.8±4.8 | 28.3±6.1 | 5.6±0.2 | 3.2±0.3 | 111±8 | 11.3±0.3 | 136±5.5 | 4.2±2.4 |
| 3 | 154±50 | 4.3±2.3 | 7.5±4.2 | 28.0±5.6 | 5.5±0.3 | - | - | - | - | - |
| 4 | 248±150 | 6.0±1.6 | 9.1±4.7 | 26.3±5.1 | 5.2±0.3 | 3.1±0.3 | 108±10 | 10.7±0.2 | 137±5.2 | 4.9±0.7 |

**Table 2.** Physiologic Parameters and Electrolytes Balance during PPPHD and CHD. (aPTT, activated partial thromboplastin time in sec; PT, prothrombin time in sec; WBC, white blood cell in $10^3/\mu l$; Hct, hematocrit %; TP, total protein in g/dl; ALB, albumin in g/dl; Glu, glucose in mg/dl) (Reproduction was permitted by a publisher)

## 6. Pulse push/pull hemodialysis with dual piston pump

Pulse push/pull HD is conceptually similar to the push/pull HDF method. Both modalities were devised to increase total filtration level by alternating forward and backward filtration. However, the underlying design of PPPHD significantly differs from push/pull HDF. The supplementary component required to switch from ultrafiltration to backfiltration phases or vice versa used in push/pull HDF is not needed for PPPHD because the alternating bimodal pulsation in the dialysate stream creates the cyclic repetition. In addition, the dual pulsatile device in the PPPHD unit serves as a flow equalizer.

Maintaining pre-determined flow rates and precise volume control are pre-requisites of extracorporeal renal replacement treatments for ESRD patients, particularly when using membranes with high-water permeability. Accordingly, the dual pulsatile pump integrated into the dialysate stream has been remarkably improved to achieve substantially more accurate fluid balancing, and the dual pulsation system acting on the PPPHD dialysate compartment was replaced with a dual piston pump. Figure 6 is a schematic diagram for the PPPHD system as combined with the dual piston pump. This modification allows pulse generation and push/pull actions to be achieved, not only by the novel design of the piston pump, but also by the unique control of piston movements offered. As the dialysate piston compresses the cylinder, pure dialysate is forced into the dialyzer, but at this time, the effluent stream is functionally closed at the effluent piston pump, thereby increasing dialysate compartment pressures rapidly and backfiltration occurs (a→b in Figure 7).The effluent piston then begins to expand and dialysate moves into the effluent cylinder, while the dialysate supply line remains closed at the dialysate pump. Because of effluent suction, dialysate compartment pressures fall sharply and water flux from blood lumen to dialysate occurs (b→c). During the final step (c→a), pure dialysate fills the dialysate cylinder, and simultaneously used dialysate is drained.

In an *in vitro* test of PPPHD with the dual piston pump, in which bovine blood was circulated, the phenomena of push (backfiltration) and pull (ultrafiltration) were well sustained throughout, and their levels perfectly balanced those of stroke volumes of the dialysate and effluent pumps. In addition, dialysate and effluent piston pumps served as a means of controlling isovolumetic dialysate flow rates upstream and downstream of the dialyzer. Results showed the balancing error between dialysate and effluent piston pumps was less than 0.09% of total dialysate volume. During the 4-hour session, total dialysate volume supplied to the dialyzer is 95.8L, and 95.7L of the used dialysate was collected during the same period. Furthermore, TMPs clearly cycled positive and negative due to huge fluctuations in hydraulic dialysate pressures (Figure 8). Despite the use of a peristaltic roller pump for blood, the blood pressures acquired during PPPHD showed an obvious fluctuation which was perfectly synchronized with dialysate pressure pulsation. Generally, peristaltic roller pumps create small fluctuations in flow and pressure because of the way they squeeze tubing. However, the blood pressure fluctuations acquired during PPPHD were much larger than that observed with peristaltic roller pumps during conventional HD, providing clear evidence of dialysate flux to the blood stream. Hydrostatic dialysate pressures were approxi-

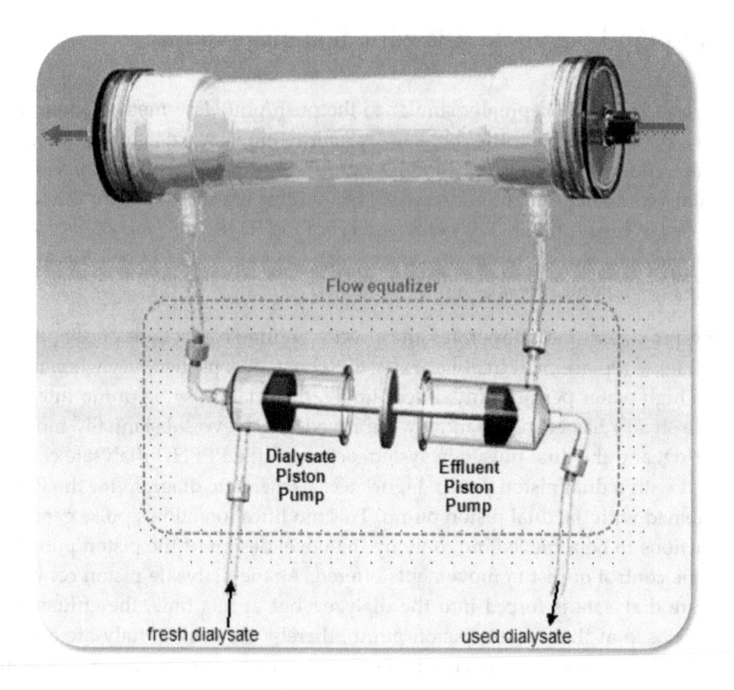


**Figure 6.** Circuit Diagram for PPPHD with Dual Piston Pump.

mately 620~660 mmHg during the backfiltration phase and -480~-520 mmHg during the ultrafiltration phase, which correspond to the positive and negative TMPs of 400~420 mmHg and -460~-506 mmHg, respectively.

In addition, the optimal use of transmembrane pressures and enhanced convective mass transfer translates into a significant increase of molecular removal. Even though no significant difference was observed with respect to clearances of low molecular weight substances, the inulin clearances were increased significantly for the PPPHD versus the conventional high-flux HD (CHD) mode. In addition, there is a clear tendency that the proportionate increase (%increase) of solutes clearances between the PPPHD and CHD was increased as the molecular weights increase.

PPPHD with the dual piston pump is also versatile and can be easily converted to conventional high-flux HD mode. Time-controlled piston operations perform the push and pull operations, but when the two piston movements are synchronized alternately (that is, dialysate piston compression and effluent piston expansion or dialysate piston expansion and effluent piston compression occur simultaneously), dialysate passes through the hemodialyzer without significant volume exchange. In this situation, the two piston pumps serve as a flow equalizer only and dialysis is largely achieved by diffusive mass transfer.

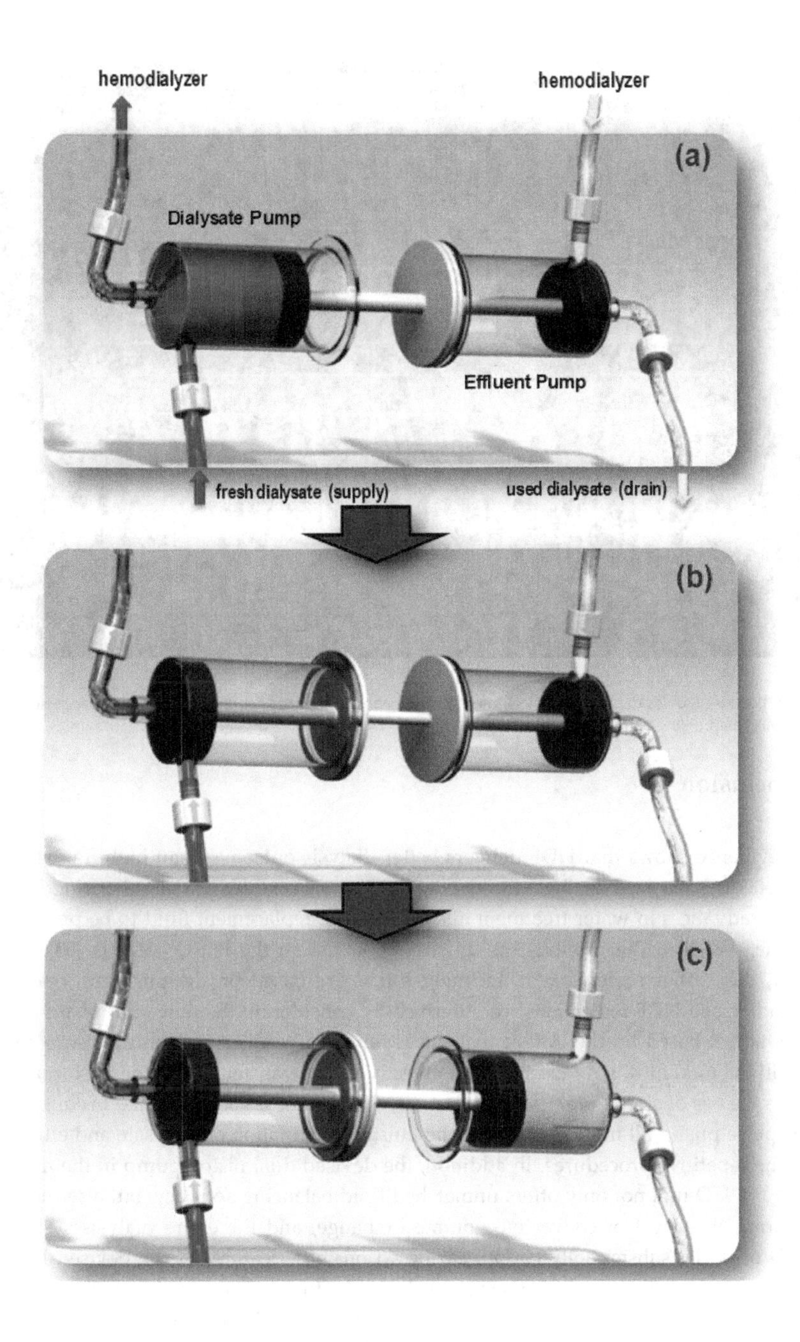


**Figure 7.** Three Phases for Push/Pull Generation for the PPPHD with Dual Piston Pump.

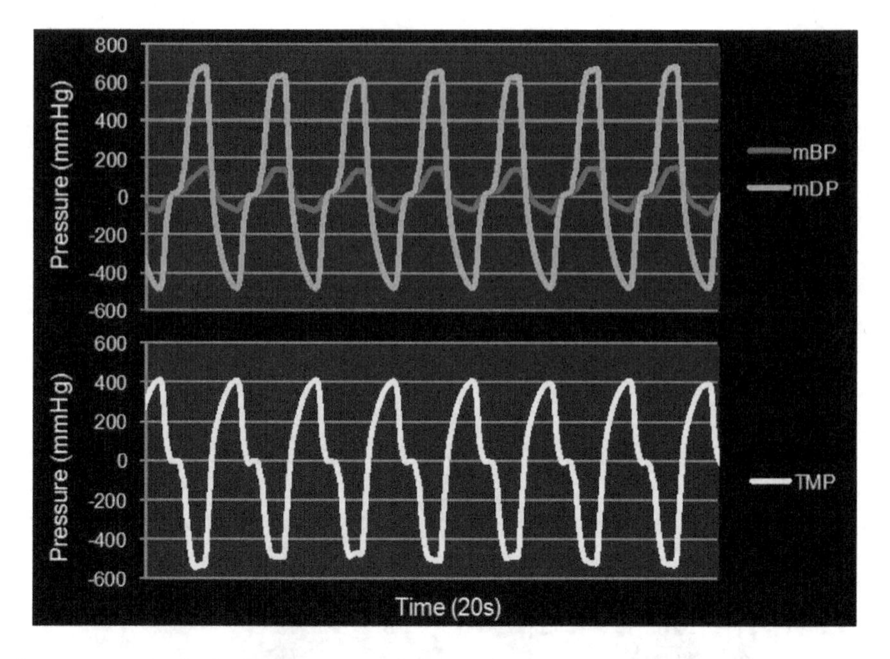


**Figure 8.** Pressure Profiles during PPPHD treatment (mBP, mean blood pressure; mDP, mean dialysate pressure; TMP, transmembrane pressure defined by mBP-mDP)

## 7. Conclusion

Much evidence shows that HDF delivers better dialysis outcomes than high-flux HD, and these benefits have been attributed to the higher convective doses permitted during HDF. In addition, advances in water treatment allow ultrapure replacement fluid to be prepared in real time, which further inhibits the inflammation risk in the ESRD patients [53]. In this chapter, the author reviews HDF techniques that are based on the push/pull operation. Push/pull based HDF techniques were derived by considering the time-split phase separation, which is based on the notion that the repetitive ultrafiltration contributes to the increase in the total filtration volume and convective mass transfer. While the push/pull HDF requires the use of a separate device so that dialysate pressures are regulated instantaneously, the pulse push/pull method employs the pulsatile circulation of dialysate and effluent to effect the repetitive procedures. In addition, the devised dual piston pump in the most advanced PPPHD unit not only offers unmatched fluid balancing accuracy, but also the maximal permissible level of convective volume exchange, and the entire dialysis system for PPPHD could be substantially simplified. Based on these features of the devised PPPHD, the author believes that the PPPHD system should be further improved by being equipped with features that simplify overall dialysis treatment and enable dialysis to be performed in free-standing clinics. A dialysis unit equipped with these features may also provide treatment alternatives beyond the current thrice weekly 4-hour practice, and perhaps allow even daily home dialysis for ESRD patients.

## Author details

Kyungsoo Lee[1,2*]

1 Nephrology Division, Department of Internal Medicine, University of Michigan, Ann Arbor, Michigan, USA

2 AnC Bio Inc., Seoul, Korea

## References

[1] The United States Renal Data System (USRDS).(2010). Part , 2252-66.

[2] Weber, V., Linsberger, I., Rossmanith, E., Weber, C., & Falkenhagen, D. (2004). Pyrogen transfer across high- and low-flux hemodialysis membranes. *Artificial organs*, 28(2), 210-7.

[3] Ahrenholz, P. G., Winkler, R. E., Michelsen, A., Lang, D. A., & Bowry, S. K. Dialysis membrane-dependent removal of middle molecules during hemodiafiltration: the beta2-microglobulin/albumin relationship. Clin Nephrol (2004). , 62(1), 21-8.

[4] Merello, Godino. J. I., Rentero, R., Orlandini, G., Marcelli, D., Ronco, C., Results, from., Eu, Cli. D. ., European, Clinical., Dialysis, Database., impact, of., shifting, treatment., & modality, . (2002). *The International journal of artificial organs*, 25(11), 1049-60.

[5] Woods, H. F., & Nandakumar, M. Improved outcome for haemodialysis patients treated with high-flux membranes. Nephrol Dial Transplant (2000). Suppl , 136-42.

[6] Daugirdas JT, Van Stone JC.Physiologic principles and urea kinetic modeling. In: Daugirdas JT, Blake PG, Ing TS, eds. Handbook of Dialysis: Lippincott Williams & Wilkins (2000). , 2000, 15-45.

[7] Ofsthun NJ, Leypoldt JK. (1995). Ultrafiltration and backfiltration during hemodialysis. *Artificial organs*, 19(11), 1143-61.

[8] Locatelli, F., Martin-Malo, A., Hannedouche, T., Loureiro, A., Papadimitriou, M., Wizemann, V., Jacobson, S. H., Czekalski, S., Ronco, C., & Vanholder, R. Effect of membrane permeability on survival of hemodialysis patients. J Am Soc Nephrol (2009). , 20(3), 645-54.

[9] Effect of dialysis dose and membrane flux in maintenance hemodialysis. N Engl J Med 2002;, 347(25), 2010-9.

[10] Vaslaki, L. R., Berta, K., Major, L., Weber, V., Weber, C., Wojke, R., Passlick-Deetjen, J., & Falkenhagen, D. (2005). On-line hemodiafiltration does not induce inflammatory response in end-stage renal disease patients: results from a multicenter cross-over study. *Artificial organs*, 29(5), 406-12.

[11] Vaslaki, L., Major, L., Berta, K., Karatson, A., Misz, M., Pethoe, F., Ladanyi, E., Fodor, B., Stein, G., Pischetsrieder, M., Zima, T., Wojke, R., Gauly, A., & Passlick-Deetjen, J. (2006). On-line haemodiafiltration versus haemodialysis: stable haematocrit with less erythropoietin and improvement of other relevant blood parameters. *Blood purification*, 24(2), 163-73.

[12] Lornoy, W., Becaus, I., Billiouw, J. M., Sierens, L., Van Malderen, P., D'Haenens, P., & On-line, haemodiafiltration. Remarkable removal of betamicroglobulin. Long-term clinical observations. Nephrol Dial Transplant (2000). Suppl 149-54., 2.

[13] Ward, R. A., Schmidt, B., Hullin, J., Hillebrand, G. F., Samtleben, W. A., comparison, of., on-line, hemodiafiltration., high-flux, hemodialysis. a., prospective, clinical., & study, . J, Hillebrand GF, Samtleben W. ((2000). A comparison of on-line hemodiafiltration and high-flux hemodialysis: a prospective clinical study. J Am Soc Nephrol 2000;, 11(12), 2344-50.

[14] Mortality risk for patients receiving hemodiafiltration versus hemodialysis: European results from the DOPPS. Kidney Int 2006;, 69(11), 2087-93.

[15] Jirka, T., Cesare, S., Di Benedetto, A., Perera, Chang. M., Ponce, P., Richards, N., Tetta, C., & Vaslaky, L. Mortality risk for patients receiving hemodiafiltration versus hemodialysis. Kidney Int (2006). author reply-5., 1524 EOF-5 EOF.

[16] Ronco, C., Brendolan, A., Feriani, M., Milan, M., Conz, P., Lupi, A., Berto, P., Bettini, M., La Greca, G. A., new, scintigraphic., method, to., characterize, ultrafiltration., in, hollow., & fiber, dialyzers. Kidney Int (1992). , 41(5), 1383-93.

[17] Ronco, C., Brendolan, A., Lupi, A., Metry, G., & Levin, N. W. Effects of a reduced inner diameter of hollow fibers in hemodialyzers. Kidney Int (2000). , 58(2), 809-17.

[18] Dellanna, F., Wuepper, A., & Baldamus, . Internal filtration--advantage in haemodialysis? Nephrol Dial Transplant (1996). Suppl , 283-6.

[19] Sato, Y., Mineshima, M., Ishimori, I., Kaneko, I., Akiba, T., & Teraoka, S. (2003). Effect of hollow fiber length on solute removal and quantification of internal filtration rate by Doppler ultrasound. *The International journal of artificial organs*, 26(2), 129-34.

[20] Lee, K., Mun, C. H., Min, B. G., Won, Y. S. A., Dual-Chambered, Hemodialyzer., for-Enhanced, Convection., & Hemodialysis, . Artificial organs(2012). E, 78-82.

[21] Lee, J. C., Lee, K., & Kim, H. C. Mathematical analysis for internal filtration of convection-enhanced high-flux hemodialyzer. Computer methods and programs in biomedicine (2012).

[22] Lee, K., Jeong, J. H., Mun, C. H., Lee, S. R., Yoo, K. J., Park, Y. W., Won, Y. S., Min, B. G., Convection-enhanced, high-flux., hemodialysis, Artificial., & organs, . (2007). 31(8), 653-8.

[23] Cheung, A. C., Kato, Y., Leypoldt, J. K., & Henderson, L. W. Hemodiafiltration using a hybrid membrane system for self-generation of diluting fluid. Trans Am Soc Artif Intern Organs (1982)., 2861-5.

[24] Shinzato, T., Sezaki, R., Usuda, M., Maeda, K., Ohbayashi, S., Toyota, T., Infusion-free, hemodiafiltration., simultaneous, hemofiltration., dialysis, with., no, need., for, infusion., & fluid, . (1982). *Artificial organs*, 6(4), 453-6.

[25] von, Albertini. B., Miller, J. H., Gardner, P. W., Shinaberger, J. H., High-flux, hemodiafiltration., under, six., & hours/week, treatment. Trans Am Soc Artif Intern Organs (1984)., 30227-31.

[26] Usuda, M., Shinzato, T., Sezaki, R., Kawanishi, A., Maeda, K., Kawaguchi, S., Shibata, M., Toyoda, T., Asakura, Y., Ohbayashi, S., New, simultaneous. H. F., with, H. D., no, infusion., & fluid, . Trans Am Soc Artif Intern Organs (1982)., 2824-7.

[27] Maeda, K., Kobayakawa, H., Fujita, Y., Takai, I., Morita, H., Emoto, Y., Miyazaki, T., & Shinzato, T. (1990). Effectiveness of push/pull hemodiafiltration using large-pore membrane for shoulder joint pain in long-term dialysis patients. *Artificial organs*, 14(5), 321-7.

[28] Shinzato, T., Kobayakawa, H., & Maeda, K. (1989). Comparison of various treatment modes in terms of beta 2-microglobulin removal: hemodialysis, hemofiltration, and push/pull HDF. *Artificial organs*, 13(1), 66-70.

[29] Tsuruta, K., Andoh, F., Kurahara, I., Kaku, T., Fukushima, J., Shimada, H. A., simple, method., for, clinical., application, of., & push/pull, hemodiafiltration. Contrib Nephrol (1994)., 10871-8.

[30] Shinzato, T., Fujisawa, K., Nakai, S., Miwa, M., Kobayakawa, H., Takai, I., Morita, H., & Maeda, K. Newly developed economical and efficient push/pull hemodiafiltration. Contrib Nephrol (1994)., 10879-86.

[31] Maeda, K., Shinzato, T., Push/pull, hemodiafiltration., technical, aspects., & clinical, effectiveness. (1995). *Nephron*, 71(1), 1-9.

[32] Shinzato, T., Miwa, M., Kobayakawa, H., Morita, H., Nakai, S., Miyata, T., & Maeda, K. Effectiveness of new push/pull hemodiafiltration for arthralgia in long-term hemodialysis patients. Contrib Nephrol (1995)., 112111-8.

[33] Shinzato, T., Miwa, M., Nakai, S., Takai, I., Matsumoto, Y., Morita, H., Miyata, T., & Maeda, K. Alternate repetition of short fore- and backfiltrations reduces convective albumin loss. Kidney Int (1996)., 50(2), 432-5.

[34] Combarnous, F., Tetta, C., Cellier, C. C., Wratten, M. L., Custaud De, Catheu. T., Fouque, D., David, S., Carraro, G., & Laville, M. (2002). Albumin loss in on-line hemodiafiltration. *The International journal of artificial organs*, 25(3), 203-9.

[35] Miwa, M., Shinzato, T., Push/pull, hemodiafiltration., technical, aspects., & clinical, effectiveness. (1999). *Artificial organs*, 23(12), 1123-6.

[36] Shinzato, T., Maeda, K., Push/pull, hemodiafiltration., & Contrib, . Nephrol (2007). , 158169-76.

[37] Dapper, F., Neppl, H., Wozniak, G., Strube, I., Zickmann, B., Hehrlein, F. W., & Neuhof, H. Effects of pulsatile and nonpulsatile perfusion mode during extracorporeal circulation--a comparative clinical study. Thorac Cardiovasc Surg (1992). , 40(6), 345-51.

[38] Orime, Y., Shiono, M., Hata, H., Yagi, S., Tsukamoto, S., Okumura, H., Nakata, K., Kimura, S., Hata, M., Sezai, A., & Sezai, Y. (1999). Cytokine and endothelial damage in pulsatile and nonpulsatile cardiopulmonary bypass. *Artificial organs*, 23508-12.

[39] Ruperez, M., Sanchez, C., Garcia, C., Garcia, E., Lopez-Herce, J., Del Canizo, F. J., & Vigil, D. Continuous venovenous renal replacement therapy using a pulsatile blood pump. Pediatr Nephrol (2003). , 18(1), 29-32.

[40] Lopez-Herce, J., Ruperez, M., Sanchez, C., Garcia, C., Garcia, E., Rodriguez, D., & Del Canizo, J. F. (2006). Continuous venovenous renal replacement therapy with a pulsatile tubular blood pump: analysis of efficacy parameters. *Artificial organs*, 30(1), 64-9.

[41] Lim KM, Park JY, Lee JC, Kim JC, Min BG, Kang ET, Shim EB. (2009). Quantitative analysis of pulsatile flow contribution to ultrafiltration. *Artificial organs*, 33(1), 69-73.

[42] Runge, T. M., Briceno, J. C., Sheller, Moritz., Sloan, L., Bohls, F. O., Ottmers, S. E., Hemodialysis, evidence., of, enhanced., molecular, clearance., ultrafiltration, volume., by, using., & pulsatile, flow. (1993). *The International journal of artificial organs*, 16(9), 645-52.

[43] Lee, K., Lee, S. R., Min, B. G., Pulse, push/pull., hemodialysis, in., vitro, study., on, new., dialysis, modality., with, higher., & convective, efficiency. (2008). *Artificial organs*, 32(5), 406-11.

[44] Lee, J. J., Lim, C. H., Son, H. S., Kim, H. K., Hwang, C. M., Park, Y. D., Moon, K. C., Kwak, Y. T., & Sun, K. In vitro evaluation of the performance of Korean pulsatile ECLS (T-PLS) using precise quantification of pressure-flow waveforms. Asaio J (2005). , 51(5), 604-8.

[45] Lee, K., Min, B. G., Mun, C. H., Lee, S. R., & Won, Y. S. (2008). Pulse push/pull hemodialysis in a canine renal failure model. *Blood purification*, 26(6), 491-7.

[46] Depner, T. A., Rizwan, S., & Stasi, T. A. Pressure effects on roller pump blood flow during hemodialysis. ASAIO Trans (1990). M, 456-9.

[47] Teruel, J. L., Fernandez, Lucas. M., Marcen, R., Rodriguez, J. R., Lopez, Sanchez. J., Rivera, M., Liano, F., & Ortuno, J. (2000). Differences between blood flow as indicated by the hemodialysis blood roller pump and blood flow measured by an ultrasonic sensor. *Nephron*, 85(2), 142-7.

[48] Lee, K., Lee, D. W., Min, B. G., Lee, K. K., & Yun, Y. M. Development of a New Method for Pulse Push/Pull Hemodialysis. ASME J Medical Devices (2011). pages).

[49] Lee, K., Mun, C. H., Lee, S. R., Min, B. G., Yoo, K. J., Park, Y. W., & Won, Y. S. Hemodialysis using a valveless pulsatile blood pump. Asaio J (2008). , 54(2), 191-6.

[50] Lee, K., Min, B. G., Lee, K. K., Yun, Y. M., & Blagg, C. R. Evaluation of a new method for pulse push/pull hemodialysis: comparison with conventional hemodialysis. ASAIO J (2012). , 58(3), 232-7.

[51] Kim WG, Yoon CJ. (1998). Roller pump induced tubing wear of polyvinylchloride and silicone rubber tubing: phase contrast and scanning electron microscopic studies. *Artificial organs*, 22(10), 892-7.

[52] Leong AS, Disney AP, Gove DW.Spallation and migration of silicone from blood-pump tubing in patients on hemodialysis. N Engl J Med (1982). , 306(3), 135-40.

[53] Lonnemann, G. (2000). Chronic inflammation in hemodialysis: the role of contaminated dialysate. *Blood purification*, 18(3), 214-23.

Chapter 9

# Select Ion and Preparation of Patients for Dialysis

Pierpaolo Di Cocco, Antonio Famulari,
Francesco Pisani, Linda De Luca, Vinicio Rizza and
Katia Clemente

Additional information is available at the end of the chapter

## 1. Introduction

The prevalence of chronic kidney disease (CKD) is increasing [1]. This rise is probably attributable to the progressively aging population and to the increased prevalence of comorbid conditions namely obesity, diabetes, and hypertension. According to the data from the National Health and Nutrition Examination Surveys, the prevalence of CKD in participants 70 years old and older is 46.8% compared to 6.7% in those between 40–59 years of age [1]. Many patients with CKD are unlikely to exhibit sufficient progressive decline in renal function to require renal replacement therapy (RRT), in fact according to the findings present in literature only a small percentage of CKD patients ultimately require RRT [2-5]. In part, this low rate is explained by the increased risk of death from cardiovascular causes before progression to end-stage renal disease (ESRD) can occur [6]. In part, it is secondary to the earlier referral than in the past to nephrologists with improvement of nondialytic maximum conservative management (MCM) focused on quality of life and patient comfort (i.e. maximizing renoprotective therapies, additional dietary interventions) [7,8]. In 2008, more than 110,000 Americans were started on maintenance RRT, a life-saving therapy for patients with ESRD [6]. Ideally, when patients begin RRT they should meet the following conditions: firstly, they should not require hospitalization for the management of untreated acute or chronic complications of uraemia; secondly, they should have a thorough understanding of the different treatment options; and thirdly, they should have a functioning, permanent access for the RRT of their choice [9].

Unfortunately still a sizable proportion of patients in the USA are not adequately prepared for starting RRT. In 2008, 44% of patients received no predialysis nephrology care and only 25% had received ongoing care by a nephrologist for more than 12 months prior to initiating dialysis [6]. Despite the critical importance of lifestyle management fewer than 10% of patients receive dietary counselling prior to starting RRT [6]. Furthermore, many patients newly diagnosed with ESRD are not offered alternatives to RRT (such as home dialysis or preemptive transplantation), even in the absence of medical contraindications [10,11]. More than 80% of patients in the USA initiate RRT with a central venous catheter (CVC), a type of access associated with significantly higher rates of infectious complications and of long-term non-infectious complications compared with a permanent vascular access [6, 12-14]. Inadequate preparation for RRT in the USA can only partially be accounted for delayed referral to nephrologists; as a considerable number of patients who have received more than 1 year of specialist care prior to initiating RRT are also inadequately prepared for this treatment [6]. In 2006, the annualized mortality in the first 3 months of starting RRT for patients in the USA was approximately 45%, which was in part due to inadequate preparation and education [15]. The available data on RRT preparation practices outside the USA are limited but seem highlight the same challenge, the need of a better selection and preparation to RRT [16]. Analyses from the Dialysis Outcomes and Practice Patterns Study (DOPPS) and findings from studies conducted in the 1980s and 1990s indicate a high rate of delayed referrals to a nephrologist in Europe, and contemporary data from Canada also demonstrate a high incidence of suboptimal RRT initiation [1,16-19].

Although dialysis prolongs the lives of many individuals with ESRD, the burden of RRT might not justify the potential benefits of treatment in certain patients, such as the elderly [20]. However, as illustrated by the North Thames Dialysis Study and by one Canadian study, judgment on the appropriateness for RRT should not depend solely upon chronological age but should instead be based on a composite assessment of the health and functional status of the individual [21,22]. Results from other studies suggest that there are subgroups of patients who have a low likelihood of benefiting from RRT [23-25]. For example, initiating RRT does not reverse the progressive decline in functional status; instead this decline seemingly accelerates after RRT initiation [23]. For selected individuals with advanced CKD, nondialytic MCM might, therefore, be superior to initiating RRT [24] this suggestion highlights the importance of considering the appropriateness of RRT for individuals with CKD early in the disease course. Assessment of disease management requires shared decision-making between patients, their family members, and the treating physicians [25]. Most of the data on the principles of management and outcomes of patients with advanced CKD who elect to have MCM are derived from the United Kingdom [24,26,27]. In most of the published studies to date, the life expectancy of patients with advanced CKD who choose MCM is shorter than that of patients with matching characteristics who choose RRT; the median life expectancy of patients with ESRD who forgo RRT has been reported to range from 14 months to 23 months [24,26,27]. However, the primary goal of care in patients who opt for MCM should be focused on symptom management to enhance quality of life and ensure patient comfort [9].

## 2. How is the choice made between hemodialysis and peritoneal dialysis?

Global comparisons show interesting differences between countries in the proportion of patients with ESRD treated by peritoneal dialysis and hemodialysis. The wide discrepancy between countries such as UK [45% of patients treated by peritoneal dialysis), and its neighbour France, where only 10% are so treated, indicates strong non-medical influences on the choice of dialysis modality [28].

Economic reasons: the reimbursement to the physicians and the dialysis facilities for the cost of providing treatment varies widely around the world. There are also large differences between the levels of payment for hemodialysis and peritoneal dialysis in many countries. For example in French the facility is not reimbursed for peritoneal dialysis and the physicians receive no fee. Conversely in countries such as Hong Kong, where dialysis is only available in the private sector, more patients are treated by peritoneal dialysis than by hemodialysis, as the former is less expensive. If the physician has a financial interest in the hemodialysis facility, this may directly influence the decision on which modality of treatment to recommend.

Physician preference: there is a strong preference for hemodialysis among some influential nephrologists on both sides of the Atlantic. This is supported by data from USRDS [29]. In a large US-based survey reported in 1997, only 25% of patients remembered having peritoneal dialysis discussed with them. In contrast 68% of patients on peritoneal dialysis had had discussions on hemodialysis. Interestingly, a much greater proportion of patients on hemodialysis felt that the choice had been made by the medical team rather than by either themselves or by joint decision [29].

Geography and sociocultural influences: home dialysis, peritoneal dialysis or hemodialysis, is a much more attractive proposition if the alternative is a long journey to the dialysis facility. For example in New Zealand, in 1990 only 58% of dialysis patients lived in cities with dialysis facilities. As a result, 50% of patients received peritoneal dialysis and 32% home dialysis. In countries, such as Japan, most patients prefer to receive their medical care in a hospital setting [27]. They feel that is not appropriate for treatment to be done in the home and are often reluctant to take responsibility for delivering their own care, as a result only 6% of Japanese dialysis patients are on continuous ambulatory peritoneal dialysis.

## 3. Medical indications for peritoneal dialysis and hemodialysis

The majority of patients with ESRD are suitable for treatment with either peritoneal dialysis or hemodialysis. There are no completely reliable data comparing mortality or morbidity for these treatments and it is difficult to envisage an ethically acceptable trial where patients are allocated randomly to different dialysis modalities [30,31].

### 3.1. Contraindications to dialysis modalities

#### *3.1.1. Peritoneal dialysis*

There are few situations where there is a consensus that peritoneal dialysis is contraindicated. The consensus panel of the NKKF-DOQI has agreed the following relative contraindications to peritoneal dialysis [32]:

- Fresh intra-abdominal foreign body (e.g. aortic graft, ventriculo-peritoneal shunt): patients with prosthetic aortic grafts have been successfully treated with peritoneal dialysis. Hemodialysis is usually used initially for up to 16 weeks to allow the graft to be covered with epithelium and so avoid the risk of graft infection via peritoneal dialysate. However this risk must be balanced against that of bacterial seeding from the patient's hemodialysis access.
- Body size limitations and intolerance of intra-abdominal fluid volume: body size can be a problem at both ends of spectrum. The effect of increased intra-abdominal pressure can be particularly marked in patients with chronic respiratory disease, with low back pain and with large polycystic kidneys. In general, it is hard to predict a patient's tolerance of intra-abdominal fluid and so these limitations usually appear after a patient has started peritoneal dialysis.
- Bowel disease and other sources of infection: the presence of ischemic bowel disease, inflammatory bowel disease or diverticulitis is likely to increase the incidence of peritonitis due to organisms passing through the bowel wall into the peritoneum. Abdominal wall infection may lead to peritonitis via the exit site and catheter tunnel.
- Severe malnutrition or morbid obesity: patients should ideally commence peritoneal dialysis in an adequate nutritional state. Severe malnutrition may lead to poor wound healing and to leakage from the catheter tunnel. In addition peritoneal protein losses during dialysis may exacerbate hypoalbuminenia. At the other end of the spectrum it may prove difficult to satisfactorily place a catheter through the abdominal wall in patients with morbid obesity. Thereafter absorption of glucose from the dialysate may contribute to further weight gain.

#### *3.1.2. Hemodialysis*

Contraindications to hemodialysis are few. Access to the circulation can usually be obtained even in patients with extensive vascular disease or previous surgery. An aversion to needle puncture of the arteriovenous (A-V) fistula is common in the early stages but can usually be overcome by careful use of local anaesthetic and nursing encouragement. Some patients with severe cardiac disease may not tolerate the shifts in volume and electrolytes that occur during hemodialysis treatment. However, there are no objective measurements that will reliably identify such patients. Severe coagulopathy may make management of anticoagulation for the extracorporeal circuit difficult.

## 4. Vascular access for hemodialysis: Surgical considerations

The maintenance of adequate, durable vascular access for hemodialysis is essential for the wellbeing of the patient with ERSD. The provision of hemodialysis requires repetitive vascular access that can achieve a blood flow in excess of 350 mL/min. If vascular access cannot be achieved for even short period of time the patient will die from uraemia. Hemodialysis is employed in chronic maintenance hemodialysis, acute renal failure and elimination of poisons from the body. For the provision of chronic maintenance hemodialysis the requirements for vascular access are very different from those for acute hemodialysis.

## 5. Vascular access for acute hemodialysis

### 5.1. Dual-lumen cuffed catheters

The vascular access requirements for acute hemodialysis are best served by the use of dual lumen, non-cuffed, temporary catheters. These catheters are made of a variety of materials including polyurethane or polytetrafluoroethylene. These materials have the useful property that a room temperature they are rigid, which facilitates their insertion, but when in place, they achieve body temperature and become much more flexible. Dialysis catheters are most commonly placed in the femoral, subclavian or jugular vein. Each of these sites has advantages and disadvantages depending on specific clinical circumstances. The femoral vein is in most patients the easiest site to insert a catheter and is associated with the lowest risk of life threatening complications. The major disadvantages of using the femoral vein are that the patient must remain recumbent while the catheter is in place and the high rate of infection if the catheter is left in place for more than 72 hours. It is preferable to use femoral catheters of 24 cm length as the recirculation in these catheters has been shown to be considerably lower than in the shorter 15 cm catheters. For patients who require longer periods of renal replacement (>72 hours and <3 weeks), a dialysis catheter placed in the jugular vein is preferable. The acute complications associated with both jugular and subclavian line insertion are similar. However subclavian line insertions are associated with the longer-term complication of subclavian vein stenosis, thus compromising the use of ipsilateral limb for long term vascular access. Catheters placed under aseptic conditions in either the jugular or subclavian vein may be left in place for up to 3 weeks. Complications associated with subclavian or jugular catheters include pneumothorax and arterial or great vein puncture with associated mediastinal, pleural or pericardial haemorrhage. The risk of great vein perforation is probably greatest in patients who have previously had multiple line insertions and have developed subclavian vein stenosis. Patients with a previously documented subclavian vein stenosis should never have a temporary catheter inserted on that side. It is imperative that a chest X ray is taken prior to the initiation of hemodialysis after either jugular or subclavian lines are inserted. This is to exclude the development of either a pneumothorax or hemothorax and to confirm that the catheter is in a position compatible with the desired vessel. If there is any doubt that the tip of the catheter is within a great vein, a small amount of contrast should be injected into the catheter under fluoroscopic control.

Although a far inferior choice for vascular access than a primary artero-venous (A-V) fistula or polytetrafluoroethylene (PTFE) graft, dual-lumen cuffed catheters have assumed an important role in the provision of vascular access for ESRD patients. Whenever possible some form of vascular access other than a cuffed catheter should be sought for a patient who has a prognosis of more than 6 months. In our opinion the cuffed catheter is best used as a bridge between failed access and the establishment of permanent access.

## 6. Permanent vascular access

There is no doubt that a pre-emptively placed forearm primary A-V fistula is the most effective form of long-term vascular access for the uremic patient. It is important for physicians caring for patients with renal insufficiency to begin making plans for the provision of renal replacement therapy at an early stage and this usually begin when creatinine clearance is < 25 mL/min or serum creatinine> 4 mg/dL. Pre-emptive planning for the provision of vascular access is certainly cost-effective; it avoids emergency placement of femoral or subclavian catheters and also reduces hospital admissions for infection and temporary access failure.

## 7. Types of permanent vascular access

### 7.1. Primary fistula

In 1962 Cimino and Brescia described the technique of anastomosing the radial artery to the adjacent veins [33]. This technique allowed repeated puncturing of veins for dialysis access. The most frequent problem associated with A-V fistula is a failure to mature, as manifested by early thrombosis or inadequate blood flow rates. For patients in whom it is not possible to create a primary radio cephalic A-V fistula, an upper arm brachiocephalic fistula is a second best alternative and preferable to the use of a polytetrafluoroethylene (PTFE) graft. An upper arm brachiocephalic fistula takes few weeks to mature. Up to 80% of primary A-V fistulae will be functioning 3 years after creation.

### 7.2. PTFE grafts

PTFE was introduced in 1976 as a material for vascular bypass grafts. Since that time this material has become the mainstay for vascular access in dialysis when autologous A-V fistula is either technically impossible or has failed to mature. Using PTFE as a conduit, a fistula is created between an upper limb artery and vein.

More than 80% of the vascular procedures performed in the US [34]. Recent studies have demonstrated that the use of PTFE grafts is actually increasing rather than decreasing. These discrepancies between the US and other parts of the world have been attributed to the increased age of the dialysis population in the US and the increased proportion of ESRD patients with diabetes and with poor quality vessels that provide inadequate vascular access, as well as to the surgical practices that have evolved. More than 40% of patients who present ESRD in the US have not had vascular access created prior to the initiation of hemodialysis. Studies looking at the survival of PTFE grafts have noted cumulative patency rates for PTFE grafts of between 63-90% at 1 year and 50-77% at 2 years; fewer than 50% survive beyond the third year. Newly inserted PTFE grafts should not be needled for at least 14 days because adhesions of the subcutaneous tunnel and graft has not yet occurred; potential bleeding into the graft tunnel and hematoma thereof may ruin the access site.

Prior to the creation of a new vascular access route, it is important to evaluate the patient for possible central vein stenosis. Clinical clues that should raise suspicion include oedema in the extremities, collateral vein development, differential size of the extremities, and current or previous placement of a cardiac pacemaker. If any of these findings are present the patient should undergo venography or duplex ultrasound. If venous stenosis is identified, it is preferable to plan access for the contralateral side if possible, although we have had occasional success in performing angioplasty on proximal veins and then proceeding with A-V fistula or PTFE graft insertion.

## 8. The importance of preparation for dialysis

Every patient would make an informed choice between peritoneal and hemodialysis after a period of counselling and preparation, unfortunately RRT is frequently started in less than ideal circumstances. Reports from both Europe and US clearly document the excess of morbidity and mortality associated with patients presenting late in ESRD and requiring RRT as an emergency procedure [14,15]. In fact patients starting RRT as an emergency usually receive hemodialysis and require a temporary CVC. Compared with non-emergency patients, their length of hospital stay is significantly greater and during this time there is a higher incidence of major complications and death. Data from USRD report [1997] showed that 25% of hemodialysis and 16% of peritoneal dialysis patients stated that a nephrologist first saw them less than one month before starting RRT; many of these patients would not have sought any medical attention prior to their presentation but it is clearly important that GPs promptly refer these patients for a specialist opinion.

Predialysis care by the nephrologist is focused on preventing or treating complications of CKD, preserving residual renal function, ensuring that the patient has sufficient understanding of his condition to chose between different RRT, and then arranging for appropriate access to be created in time before dialysis is required. In addition to the nephrologist giving advice, further benefits may be gained if patients are offered a multidisciplinary educational program.

Although few clinical trials have been conducted, there is enough evidence of clear benefits of CKD education [35-41]. Early patient education is highly effective when focused on health promotion, shared decision-making and discussion of treatment options [36]. In one randomized, controlled trial on patient education, a one-on-one educational session followed by phone calls every 3 weeks significantly extended the time to requiring dialysis [38]. *Post hoc* analyses from this clinical trial, as well as findings from other observational studies, demonstrate a variety of additional benefits from patient education, including the following: reduced patient anxiety; reduced number of hospitalizations; reduced numbers of emergency room and physician visits; increased likelihood that the patient will remain employed in work and be more adherent to therapy; and reduced mortality [37,39,40]. Furthermore, results from several studies have demonstrated a substantially reduced need for CVCs following patient education [40,41]. Consequently, it is important to maximize these benefits by engaging patients in CKD education prior to planning dialysis access placement. Patient education involves messengers, messages, receivers and a process. Before patient education can begin, the physician must initiate the discussion of what is often called breaking the bad news [42,43]. Patients do not want insensitive truth telling but prefer for the truth to be told with support to assist them in decision-making [44]. It is estimated that it takes an average of five encounters before individuals actually understand the message; therefore, patient education on CKD should be iterative [45]. The initial message should be delivered in a private room that is free of interruptions, and preferably when the patient has a supportive friend or relative with them [45]. Components of successful CKD education programs have also included individualized and ongoing education throughout the course of the disease, tours of dialysis facilities, meeting patients who are undergoing treatment with different dialysis modalities, use of videos and written materials, and behaviour changing protocols with small group problem-solving activities [37,46,47]. These and other strategies can be incorporated into any CKD education program. The educator needs to possess skills in patient communication and to understand the nature of the patient's barriers to receiving the information.

Presenting treatment options to the patient is a major undertaking for the educator, and offering decision support is an important goal of successful CKD education. There is a large variability in the uptake of home dialysis options (peritoneal dialysis or hemodialysis) between centres, regions, and different countries [6]. Data from the USA indicate that the low uptake of peritoneal dialysis in the country does not reflect patient choice but is instead more often a reflection of the choice not being offered to patients by healthcare providers [10,11]. Results from recent studies indicate that the 5-year and 10-year survival rates of patients treated with in centre hemodialysis are equivalent to survival rates with peritoneal dialysis [48]. Accordingly, for the vast majority of patients with CKD, decisions about dialysis modality should be based on what fits best with their lifestyle a decision that patients and their families must make for themselves [49]. Widespread, comprehensive CKD education will also empower patients to assume responsibility for their dialysis care, thereby increasing the uptake of home dialysis options. Expansion of home dialysis therapy is likely to be safe as the equivalency of outcomes of home peritoneal dialysis with in centre hemodialysis are maintained even when much larger proportions of patients are treated with the former therapy [48]. This therapy is also potentially more cost-effective given the lower societal costs for providing peritoneal dialysis, compared with in centre hemodialysis, in many countries[50].

The discussion about treatment options should begin with open questions and can be followed by introducing the two choices available to patients, dialysis or MCM. If the patient's preference is for dialysis, the choice of home dialysis versus in centre dialysis should be discussed next. Notably, fear and/or lack of knowledge of home dialysis has been shown to dissuade many patients from selecting this option [51]. One of the goals of patient education should be to offer patient support and help overcome such fear. Regular contact between the educator and the patient over the weeks to months after starting education is important in the process of decision-making. However, it is should be noted that the patient's choice of dialysis modality is simply the treatment with which they begin RRT, as many patients will actually transition between different therapies (for example, changing dialysis modalities, or from dialysis to transplantation and possibly back to dialysis again).

## 9. When RRT should be started?

In the 1990s, expert groups recommended that initiation of dialysis be considered when renal function declines to a predetermined level (mean of urea and creatinine clearance of ≤10.5 ml/min/1.73 m2] [52]. Over the past years, however, the mean estimated Glomerular Filtration Rate (eGFR) of patients starting dialysis in the USA has progressively increased [6,53]. Notwithstanding this change over time, there is no relationship between the duration of pre- dialysis nephrology care and eGFR at the time of starting dialysis [54]. Furthermore, patients who start dialysis with a high eGFR are as likely as patients with a lower eGFR to use CVCs as the first dialysis access [54]. These observations suggest that nephrologists might be recommending patients for dialysis for the same general reasons, irrespective of eGFR. For example, individuals with low levels of serum creatinine (and a high eGFR) might need to start dialysis if they are likely to have poor tolerance for the consequences of renal function decline. Findings from several observational studies demonstrate that patients who start dialysis with a high eGFR are substantially more likely to have characteristics associated with an increased mortality (such as older age, male sex, white ethnicity, diabetes mellitus and other cardiovascular comorbidities). Concerns about the rising trend of starting RRT in patients with a high eGFR have been raised, particularly since many studies now show a direct association between a high eGFR at the time of RRT initiation and subsequent risk of death [54-64]. This risk persists even after statistical adjustment for potential confounders and also when analyses are restricted to the healthiest subgroup; however, there is always the issue of residual confounding in observational studies [57,58]. Furthermore, with decreasing renal function, muscle mass becomes a more important determinant of serum creatinine level than is eGFR [65]. It follows then that the association between high eGFR and an increased risk of death might, in part, be a reflection of the effect of cachexia (muscle loss causing lower levels of serum creatinine at any given level of eGFR) on mortality [56]. Given the limitations of observational studies, it is fortuitous that the importance of renal function at RRT initiation has been tested in a randomized controlled clinical trial. In the IDEAL study, there was no difference in terms of survival between patients randomly assigned to begin dialysis early (at a creatinine clearance of 10–14 ml/min) or late (at a creatinine clearance of 5–7 ml/min) [66]. It is important to note that three-quarters of patients randomly assigned to starting dialysis late actually needed to begin treatment earlier, primarily owing to the development of uremic symptoms [66]. These data suggest that initiation of dialysis simply when renal function approaches a predetermined threshold, as measured by eGFR, is not appropriate. Indeed, it seems that dialysis can be safely delayed in otherwise asymptomatic individuals with advanced CKD. This is particularly important in patients in whom a permanent dialysis access is not ready for use, and deferring dialysis might mitigate the need for CVCs. However, findings from the IDEAL study also indicate that it might not be universally possible to defer initiation of dialysis until patients reach an eGFR<7 ml/min/1.73 m2 as many patients with advanced CKD can develop uremic symptoms at high levels of renal function [66]. In addition to the indications for emergent dialysis (hyperkalaemia, volume overload, pericarditis and encephalopathy), dialysis therapy has been shown to be effective in ameliorating uremic anorexia and is associated with improvement in measures of protein energy wasting [67]. Hence, it is important to observe patients with advanced CKD for the early development of symptoms and/or uremic complications and begin dialysis at an appropriate time such that it precludes the development of complications that might require hospitalization or emergency intervention.

## 10. Conclusions

It is extremely important to ensure that the resources dedicated to ESRD treatment are used to best effect. If the greatest benefit is to be gained from RRT, the importance of selection and preparation of patients reaching ESRD must be recognised and addressed. Educating these individuals about CKD might, nevertheless, facilitate their participation in selection of RRT modality and might also result in an earlier transition to a permanent RRT. Several studies show that those measures lead to a reduction of the proportion of patients who start RRT as an emergency procedure (higher incidence of major complications and death) [14,15] and to an increasing number of patients that actively participate in developing their care plan and who start dialysis with a permanent access [68,69].

## Author details

Pierpaolo Di Cocco, Antonio Famulari, Francesco Pisani, Linda De Luca, Vinicio Rizza and Katia Clemente

The Royal London Hospital, University of L'Aquila, United Kingdom

## References

[1] Coresh J, Selvin E, Stevens LA. Prevalence of chronic kidney disease in the United States. JAMA 2007; 298: 2038-2047

[2] Keith, D. S., Nichols, G. A., Gullion, C. M.,
Brown, J. B. & Smith, D. H. Longitudinal follow-up and outcomes among a popula-

tion with chronic kidney disease in a large managed care organization. Arch. Intern. Med. 2004; 164, 659–663

[3] Levin, A., Djurdjev, O., Beaulieu, M. &Er, L. Variability and risk factors for kidney disease progression and death following attainment of stage 4 CKD in a referred cohort. Am. J. Kidney Dis. 2008; 52, 661–671

[4] O'Hare, A. M. et al. When to refer patients with chronic kidney disease for vascular access surgery: should age be a consideration? Kidney Int. 2007; 71, 555–561

[5] Demoulin, N., Beguin, C., Labriola, L. &
Jadoul, M. Preparing renal replacement therapy in stage 4 CKD patients referred to nephrologists: a difficult balance between futility and insufficiency. A cohort study of 386 patients followed in Brussels. Nephrol. Dial. Transplant. 2011; 26, 220–226

[6] US Department of Public Health and Human Services, Public Health Service, National Institutes of Health, Bethesda. United States Renal Data System [online], http://www.usrds.org/atlas08.aspx - 2008

[7] Carson, R. C., Juszczak, M., Davenport, A. & Burns, A. Is maximum conservative management an equivalent treatment option to dialysis for elderly patients with significant comorbid disease? Clin. J. Am. Soc. Nephrol. 2009; 4: 1611–1619

[8] Murtagh,F.E.,Addington-Hall,J.M.,Donohoe,P. & Higginson, I. J. Symptom management in patients with established renal failure managed without dialysis. EDTNA ERCA J. 2006; 32, 93–98

[9] Harward, D. H. The Kidney Education Outreach Program: hey doc, how are my kidneys? N. C. Med. J. 2008; 69, 228

[10] Mehrotra, R., Marsh, D., Vonesh, E., Peters, V. &Nissenson, A. Patient education and access of ESRD patients to renal replacement therapies beyond in-centerhemodialysis. Kidney Int. 2005; 68, 378–390

[11] Kutner, N. G., Zhang, R., Huang, Y. &Wasse, H. Patient awareness and initiation of peritoneal dialysis. Arch. Intern. Med. 2011, 171, 119–124

[12] Ethier, J. et al. Vascular access use and outcomes: an international perspective from the Dialysis Outcomes and Practice Patterns Study. Nephrol. Dial. Transplant. 2008; 23, 3219–3226

[13] Ishani, A., Collins, A. J., Herzog, C. A. & Foley, R. N. Septicemia, access and cardiovascular disease in dialysis patients: the USRDS Wave 2 study. Kidney Int. 2005, 68, 311–318

[14] Agarwal, A. K. Central vein stenosis: current concepts. Adv. Chronic Kidney Dis. 2009; 16, 360–370

[15] US Department of Public Health and Human Services, Public Health Service, National Institutes of Health, Bethesda. United States Renal Data System [online], http://www.usrds.org/atlas09.aspx 2009

[16] Jungers, P. et al. Detrimental effects of late referral in patients with chronic renal failure: a case-control study. Kidney Int. Suppl. 1993; 41, S170–S173

[17] Jungers, P. et al. Late referral to maintenance dialysis: detrimental consequences. Nephrol. Dial. Transplant. 1993; 8: 1089–1093

[18] Ratcliffe, P. J., Phillips, R. E. & Oliver, D. O. Late referral for maintenance dialysis. Br. Med. J. (Clin. Res. Ed.) 1984; 288: 441–443

[19] Mendelssohn, D. C. et al. Suboptimal initiation of dialysis with and without early referral to a nephrologist. Nephrol. Dial. Transplant. 2011; 26: 2959–2965

[20] Kurella, M., Covinsky, K. E., Collins, A. J. &Chertow, G. M. Octogenarians and nonagenarians starting dialysis in the United States. Ann. Intern. Med. 2007; 146: 177–183

[21] Lamping, D. L. et al. Clinical outcomes, quality of life, and costs in the North Thames Dialysis Study of elderly people on dialysis: a prospective cohort study. Lancet 2000; 356: 1543–1550

[22] Barrett BJ, Parfrey PS, Morgan J et al. Prediction of early death in end stage renal disease patients starting dialysis. Am J Kidney Dis. 1997; 29: 214-22

[23] Kurella Tamura, M. et al. Functional status of elderly adults before and after initiation of dialysis. N. Engl. J. Med. 2009; 361, 1539–1547

[24] Carson, R. C., Juszczak, M., Davenport, A. & Burns, A. Is maximum conservative management an equivalent treatment option to dialysis for elderly patients with significant comorbid disease? Clin. J. Am. Soc. Nephrol. 2009; 4: 1611–1619

[25] Renal Physicians Association. Shared decision- making in the appropriate initiation and withdrawal from dialysis (Renal Physicians Association, Rockville, 2010).

[26] Wong, C. F., McCarthy, M., Howse, M. L. & Williams, P. S. Factors affecting survival in advanced chronic kidney disease patients who choose not to receive dialysis. Ren. Fail. 2007; 29: 653–659

[27] Ellam, T., El-Kossi, M., Prasanth, K. C., El-Nahas, M. &Khwaja, A. Conservatively managed patients with stage 5 chronic kidney disease-—outcomes from a single center experience. QJM 2009; 202: 547–554

[28] Nissenson AR, Prichard SS, Cheng IKP, et al. Non medical factors that impact on ESRD modality selection. Kidney Int. 1993; 43 (Suppl. 1): S120-27

[29] USRDS 1997 Annual Data Report. Am J Kidney Dis. 1997; 30 (Suppl. 1): www.med.umich.edu/usrds

[30] Fenton SS, Schaubel DE, Desmeules M, et al. Hemodialysis versus peritoneal dialysis: a comparison of adjusted mortality rates. Am J Kidney Dis. 1997; 30: 334-42

[31] Held PJ, Port FK, Turenne MN, et al. Continuous ambulatory peritoneal dialysis and hemodialysis: comparison of patient mortality with adjustment for comorbid conditions. KidnedyInt 1994; 45: 1163-9

[32] NKF-DOQI Clinical Practice Guidelines for Peritoneal Dialysis Adequacy. Am J Kidney Dis. 1997; 30 (Suppl. 2): S101

[33] Cimino JE, Brescia MJ. The early development of the arteriovenous fistula needle technique for hemodialysis. ASAIOJ. 1994; 40: 923-7

[34] Lazarus JM, Denker BM, Owen WF. Hemodialysis. In Brenner BM, ed. The Kidney, 5th edition. Philadelphia: Saunders, 1996: 2424-506

[35] Mehrotra, R. Bridging the care gap around dialysis initiation: is CKD education part of the solution? Am. J. Kidney Dis. 2011; 58, 160–161

[36] Hain D, Calvin DJ & Simmons DE Jr. CKD education: an evolving concept. Nephrol. Nurs. J. 2009; 36, 317–319

[37] Golper T. Patient education: can it maximize the success of therapy? Nephrol. Dial. Transplant. 2001; 16 (Suppl. 7), 20–24

[38] Devins GM, Mendelssohn DC, Barre PE et al. Predialysispsychoeducational intervention and coping styles influence time to dialysis in chronic kidney disease. Am. J. Kidney Dis. 2003; 42, 693–703

[39] Latham CE. Is there data to support the concept that educated, empowered patients have better outcomes? J. Am. Soc. Nephrol. 1998; 9, S141–S144

[40] Wu IW. et al. Multidisciplinary predialysis education decreases the incidence of dialysis and reduces mortality - a controlled cohort study based on the NKF/DOQI guidelines. Nephrol. Dial. Transplant. 2009; 24, 3426–3433

[41] Lacson E Jret al. Effects of a nationwide predialysis educational program on modality choice, vascular access, and patient outcomes. Am. J. Kidney Dis. 2011; 58, 235–242

[42] Rayner HC et al. Creation, cannulation and survival of arteriovenous fistulae: data from the Dialysis Outcomes and Practice Patterns Study. Kidney Int. 2003; 63, 323–330

[43] Shah BV &Levey AS. Spontaneous changes in the rate of decline in reciprocal serum creatinine: errors in predicting the progression of renal disease from extrapolation of the slope.
J. Am. Soc. Nephrol. 1992; 2, 1186–1191

[44] Buckman R. Breaking Bad News: A guide for Health Care Professionals - Johns Hopkins University Press, Baltimore, 1992

[45] Ptacek JT &Eberhardt TL. Breaking bad news. A review of the literature. JAMA 1996; 276, 496–502

[46] Owen JE et al. Implementation of a pre-dialysis clinical pathway for patients with chronic kidney disease. Int. J. Qual. Health Care 2006; 18, 145–151

[47] Manns BJ et al. The impact of education on chronic kidney disease patients' plans to initiate dialysis with self-care dialysis: a randomized trial. Kidney Int. 2005; 68, 1777–1783

[48] Chiu YW et al. An update on the comparisons of mortality outcomes of hemodialysis and peritoneal dialysis patients. Semin. Nephrol. 2011; 31, 152–158

[49] Mehrotra R. Choice of dialysis modality. Kidney Int. 2011; 80, 909–911

[50] Just PM et al. Economic evaluations of dialysis treatment modalities. Health Policy 2008; 86, 163–180

[51] McLaughlin K et al. Why patients with ESRD do not select self-care dialysis as a treatment option. Am. J. Kidney Dis. 2003; 41, 380–385

[52] National Kidney Foundation. NKF-DOQI clinical practice guidelines. Am. J. Kidney Dis. 1997

[53] Rosansky SJ et al. Initiation of dialysis at higher GFRs: is the apparent rising tide of early dialysis harmful or helpful? Kidney Int. 2009; 76, 257–261

[54] Wright S et al. Timing of dialysis initiation and survival in ESRD. Clin. J. Am. Soc. Nephrol. 2010; 5, 1828–1835

[55] Fink JC et al. Significance of serum creatinine values in new end-stage renal disease patients. Am. J. Kidney Dis. 1999; 34, 694–701

[56] Beddhu S et al. Impact of timing of initiation of dialysis on mortality. J. Am. Soc. Nephrol. 2003; 14, 2305–2312

[57] Kazmi WH et al. Effect of comorbidity on the increased mortality associated with early initiation of dialysis. Am. J. Kidney Dis. 2005; 46, 887–896

[58] Rosansky SJ et al. Early start of hemodialysis may be harmful. Arch. Intern. Med. 2011; 171, 396–403

[59] Traynor JP et al. Early initiation of dialysis fails to prolong survival in patients with end-stage renal failure. J. Am. Soc. Nephrol. 2002; 13, 2125–2132

[60] Sawhney S et al. Survival and dialysis initiation: comparing British Columbia and Scotland registries. Nephrol. Dial. Transplant. 2009; 24, 3186–3192

[61] Stel VS et al. Residual renal function at the start of dialysis and clinical outcomes. Nephrol. Dial. Transplant. 2009; 24, 3175–3182

[62] Evans M et al. No survival benefit from early- start dialysis in a population-based, inception cohort study of Swedish patients with chronic kidney disease. J. Intern. Med. 2011; 269, 289–298

[63] Hwang SJ et al. Impact of the clinical conditions at dialysis initiation on mortality in incident haemodialysis patients: a national cohort study in Taiwan. Nephrol. Dial. Transplant. 2010; 25, 2616–2624

[64] Lassalle M. et al. Age and comorbidity may explain the paradoxical association of an early dialysis start with poor survival. Kidney Int. 2010; 77, 700–707

[65] Grootendorst DC et al. The MDRD formula does not reflect GFR in ESRD patients. Nephrol. Dial. Transplant. 2011; 26, 1932–1937

[66] Cooper BA et al. A randomized, controlled trial of early versus late initiation of dialysis. N. Engl. J. Med. 2010; 363, 609–619

[67] Pupim LB et al. Improvement in nutritional parameters after initiation of chronic hemodialysis. Am. J. Kidney Dis. 2002; 40, 143–151

[68] CovicAet al. Educating end-stage renal disease patients on dialysis modality selection: clinical advice from the European Renal Best Practice (ERBP) Advisory Board. Nephrol. Dial. Transplant. 2010; 25: 1757–1759

[69] Tattersall J et al. When to start dialysis: updated guidance following publication of the Initiating Dialysis Early and Late (IDEAL) study. Nephrol. Dial. Transplant. 2001; 26: 2082–2086

Chapter 10

# Reduction of Heparin and Oxidative Potential by Means of Citrasate® in High-Flux Dialysis (HFD) and Online Hemodiafiltration (olHDF) in Pre and Postdilution

Roland E. Winkler, Peter Ahrenholz,
Wolfgang Paetow, Grit Waitz and Hartmut Wolf

Additional information is available at the end of the chapter

## 1. Introduction

Citrasate® is a new innovative dialysis acid concentrate, in which 3 mmol/l of acetic acid have been replaced by 0.8 mmol/l of citric acid along with 0.3 mmol/l of acetate.

Using citrate-containing dialysate, a reduction of the heparin dose by up to 55% was described in the literature (Kossmann et al., 2006, 2009). At the same time, the efficacy of dialysis was found to be increased. A local anticoagulation inside the dialyzer was supposed to be the reason, caused by a strong decrease of free calcium ions. A diminished thrombus formation inside the dialyzer should allow a higher mass transport across the membrane. The reduction of acetate concentration in the dialysate was found to increase the hemodynamic stability of hypertensive patients (Gabutti et al., 2009). So far, the question has not been investigated whether the reduction of acetate diminishes the inflammatory potential of acetate in such a way that the activation of thrombocytes and leucocytes as well as the release of cytokines will be reduced. Until now, a reduction of beta-2-microglobulin (beta-2-m) was observed, which could be attributed to an improved permeability of the membrane (Kossmann et al., 2009). The possible reduction of heparin by means of Citrasate® during chronic hemodialysis could lead to an economical benefit. The clinical benefit for patients would consist of the reduction of described side effects of acetate and heparin. Because of the small number of publications, it makes sense to verify the previous results and to check if the observed reduction of beta-2-m could be caused also by a reduction of oxidative potential in case of Citrasate® application.

Therefore the following questions should be answered:

- Is it possible to reduce the dosage of heparin by means of Citrasate® for chronic dialysis treatments remaining the efficacy of treatment (Kt/V), and without increasing clotting events in dialyzer and extracorporeal circuit?
- Which impact of Citrasate® can be found on the reduction of inflammatory and oxidative potential measured by the following parameters: plasma concentration of beta-2-m, hsCRP, prealbumin and myeloperoxidase (MPO)? Recently, MPO was described as a suitable marker for oxidative stress during acute dialysis treatment (Maruyama et al., 2004).
- Which influence can be observed on the plasma level of phosphate and ionized calcium as a result of application of Citrasate®?

In addition to the High-flux Dialysis study (HFD), it should be investigated if Citrasate® concentrate can be used also for on-line hemodiafiltration (olHDF). Because the infusate for olHDF will be prepared directly from the dialysate, the use of Citrasate® dialysate means the infusion of a considerable amount of citrate directly into the blood. Using olHDF in predilution mode, the substitution fluid will be infused into the blood stream before the dialyzer, meaning citrate will be included in the mass transfer processes of the dialyzer. During olHDF in postdilution mode, the citrate- containing fluid is infused into the peripheral blood behind the dialyzer. Since the effects of Citrasate® on free calcium ion concentration and coagulation system cannot predicted precisely, Citrasate® should be applied at first in the predilution mode of olHDF, and only later in the postdilution mode.

During the Citrasate® application in olHDF, the focus should be directed to the following questions:

- Is it possible to maintain a reduced heparin dose?
- Can the influence of Citrasate® on coagulation processes inside the dialyzer increase the efficacy of dialysis?
- Is it possible to reduce MPO activation?
- Will the plasma concentrations of calcium and phosphate stay in the physiologically optimal range?

## 2. Materials and methods

### 2.1. Time schedule

The HFD part of the investigation was conducted with the following time schedule:

Weeks 1-2: Measurement of parameters specified below, with standard dialysate and heparin dosage (baseline).

Weeks 3-6: Change to Citrasate® without any change in other treatment conditions.

Weeks 7-10: Dialysis with Citrasate® and 50% reduction of heparin bolus.

Weeks 11-14: Dialysis with Citrasate® and 50% reduction of bolus and maintenance amount of heparin resulting in 50% total reduction of heparin.

Afterwards, the investigation was continued with olHDF:

Week 1: Measurement of parameters mentioned below during HFD with Citrasate® ($Ca^{2+}$:1.5 mmol/l) using the reduced 50% heparin dose (bolus – 50% and maintenance dose -50 %).

Weeks 2-3: Change to olHDF predilution (substitution rate: 150 ml/min) with Citrasate® ($Ca^{2+}$: 1.5 mmol/l).

Weeks 4-5: olHDF predilution as described above, but with standard concentrate ($Ca^{2+}$:1.25 mmol/l).

Weeks 6-7: Change to olHDF postdilution (substitution rate: 60 ml/min) with Citrasate® ($Ca^{2+}$: 1.5 mmol/l).

Weeks 8-9: olHDF postdilution as described above, but with standard concentrate ($Ca^{2+}$:1.25 mmol/l).

## 2.2. Materials

The following types of standard concentrate were used, differing only in the $K^+$-concentration (3.0 or 4.0 mmol/l, respectively): Concentrations of final mixed dialysate:

| $Na^+$ | $K^+$ | $Ca^{2+}$ | $Mg^{2+}$ | $Cl^-$ | Acetate | $HCO_3^-$ | Glucose |
|---|---|---|---|---|---|---|---|
| mmol/l | mmol/l | mmol/l | mmol/l | mmol/l | mmol/l | mmol/l | g/l |
| 138 | 3.0/4.0 | 1.25 | 0.75 | 110.0 | 2.00 | 33 | 1.0 |

**Table 1.**

The following types were used for treatments with Citrasate®:

| Type | $Na^+$ | $K^+$ | $Ca^{2+}$ | $Mg^{2+}$ | $Cl^-$ | Acetate | Citrate | $HCO_3^-$ | Glucose |
|---|---|---|---|---|---|---|---|---|---|
| MTN | mmol/l | mmol/l | mmol/l | mmol/l | mmol/l | mmol/l | mmol/l | mmol/l | g/l |
| 413 | 135.3 | 3.0 | 1.25/1.50 | 0.50 | 107.0 | 0.30 | 0.80 | 32.60 | 1.0 |
| 415 | 135.3 | 4.0 | 1.25/1.50 | 0.50 | 111.0 | 0.30 | 0.80 | 32.60 | 1.0 |

**Table 2.**

The treatments were performed with dialysis machines of type FMC 5008 (autoflow deactivated for olHDF treatments).

The following FMC-high-flux dialyzers were used for hemodialysis: FX60, FX80 and FX100. The blood flow was equal to $Q_B$= 300 ml/min. Unfractionated heparin brand "Heparin sodium 5000 ratiopharm" was applied for anticoagulation.

### 2.3. Patients and heparin dosages

Ten patients were selected from the running dialysis program fulfilling sufficient inclusion and exclusion criteria. All specific data of patients and used heparin dosages are included in the table "patient's data" (see table 1).

| No. | Sex | Age | Time h | Dialyzer | **Body mass/kg** | Hep.bolus IU | Hep./h IU | **Total hep./IU** | Hep.bolus theor.*) | Hep.rate theor.* | Total hep. theor*/IU |
|---|---|---|---|---|---|---|---|---|---|---|---|
| 1 | f | 68 | 4.0 | FX60 | 50.0 | 4000 | 1000 | **7500** | 1340 | 1750 | **7465** |
| 2 | f | 79 | 4.0 | FX80 | 58.0 | 2000 | 250 | **2875** | 1420 | 1750 | **7545** |
| 3 | m | 78 | 4.0 | FX60 | 8.,0 | 3000 | 750 | **5625** | 1430 | 1750 | **7555** |
| 4 | f | 65 | 4.0 | FX60 | 61.5 | 2000 | 500 | **3750** | 1455 | 1750 | **7580** |
| 5 | f | 75 | 5.0 | FX100 | 76.5 | 2500 | 500 | **4750** | 1605 | 1750 | **9480** |
| 6 | m | 68 | 4.5 | FX60 | 82.0 | 3000 | 750 | **6000** | 1660 | 1750 | **8660** |
| 7 | f | 87 | 4.0 | FX60 | 65.5 | 2500 | 625 | **4688** | 1195 | 1750 | **7320** |
| 8 | m | 76 | 5.0 | FX80 | 75.0 | 2500 | 500 | **4750** | 1290 | 1750 | **9165** |
| 9 | f | 57 | 5.0 | FX60 | 68.5 | 2500 | 500 | **4750** | 1225 | 1750 | **9100** |
| 10 | m | 87 | 4.0 | FX60 | 62.5 | 2500 | 625 | **4688** | 1465 | 1750 | **7590** |

**Table 3.** Enrolled patients and administered heparin dosages, compared with theoretically proposed dosages (Ouseph/Ward formula)

The heparin dosages before study start were optimized by regarding bleeding time and clotting behavior. The theoretical heparin doses were calculated by means of the Ouseph/Ward-formula (Ouseph et al., 2000):

$$\text{Heparin-Bolus}\,(\text{IU}) = 1600 + 10^*(\text{BW} - 76) - 300^*\text{Fd} - 100^*\text{Fs} \quad (1)$$

Infusion Rate (IU/h) = 1750

BW: body mass (kg), Fd =1 diabetic, Fd = 0 non diabetic, Fs = 1 smoker, Fs = 0 non smoker.

The applied heparin doses during the baseline treatments were lower than theoretically proposed.

Two patients had to be excluded from the study after 7 weeks because of hospitalization. Another patient dropped out during the olHDF postdilution phase.

### 2.4. Measured parameters

Based on the HFD results, during the olHDF investigations some changes regarding the measured parameters were used:

No measurements of blood cell counts, albumin, hsCRP, but addition of iPTH measurements. Beta-2-microglobulin (beta-2-m) was measured before and after treatment, because the reduction rate of beta-2-m can be used as a measure for the efficacy of medium-sized molecule clearance. Instead of ACT, the activated prothrombin time (aPTT) was measured because of its higher reliability.

| Parameter | Period of measurement |
|---|---|
| Ionized Calcium | before and after each treatment |
| Total Calcium | before and after each treatment – 1x per week |
| Bicarbonate | before and after each treatment |
| pH | before and after each treatment |
| $Na^+$ | before and after each treatment |
| $K^+$ | before and after each treatment |
| Thrombocyte count | 1x per week , before, after 15 min and after treatment |
| Leucocyte count | 1x per week , before, after 15 min and after treatment |
| Phosphate | before and after each treatment – 1x per week |
| ACT | 1x per week , before, after 15 min and after treatment |
| Kt/V | once per month |
| beta-2-microglobulin pre-dialysis | once per month |
| Albumin pre-dialysis | once per month |
| hsCRP pre-dialysis | once per month |
| Weekly EPO [TN: please define] dose | each week |
| Weekly iron dose | each week |
| Myeloperoxidase (MPO) | 2x during each period of study before, after 15 min and after treatment [TN: isn't that rather 3x than 2x?] |

**Table 4.** Parameters to be measured

### 2.5. Analysis of data and statistical methods

The analysis of data was performed by means of Microsoft-Excel-Software.WinStat for Excel and SigmaStat were used for descriptive statistics. All parameters are shown as mean values and with standard error of the mean (SEM).

Differences between measured values during different treatment modes were evaluated by t-test for paired samples. The Mann-Whitney test (U-test) was used in case normal distribution was lacking. A p-value < 0.05 was considered statistically significant. Since the investigation had to be discontinued for 2 patients, their measured values were not included in the analysis.

Because of the change on hematocrit values during treatment, the measured plasma values ($Ca^{2+}$, phosphate, MPO) had to be corrected according to the following formula (van Beaumont, 1972):

$$C_{corr} = c_* \left(Hcto/Hctn\right) * \left(1\text{-}Hctn\right) / \left(1\text{-}Hcto\right) \tag{2}$$

Hcto = hematocrit before treatment

Hctn = hematocrit during sampling time n

Measured values related to total blood volume (thrombocyte and leucocyte count) were corrected to reflect the change in hematocrit value:

$$c_{corr} = c_* \left(Hcto/Hctn\right) \tag{3}$$

According to the manufacturer's information (Radiometer), the ionometer values (pH, $Ca^{2+}$, $Na^+$ und $K^+$) do not have to be corrected because ion activities are measured (Christiansen, 1991).

If Hct-values were not available (olHDF treatments), post-treatment concentrations (Total-Ca, phosphate, beta-2-m, MPO) were corrected using the plasma volume reduction by ultrafiltration by means of the Bergström-formula:

$$c_{corr} = c_* (1/(1+\Delta BW/0.2BW_{post}) \tag{4}$$

$\Delta BW$: change of body mass, $BW_{post}$ : body mass after treatment

## 3. Results and discussion

### 3.1. High-Flux Dialysis (HFD)

#### *3.1.1. Efficacy of dialysis in dependence on the heparin dose*

When performing hemodialysis with Citrasate®, it is assumed that the citrate causes a local anticoagulation inside the dialyzer because of chelation of ionized calcium. This process should be reflected by measurements of coagulation parameters like the "activated clotting time (ACT)". In fig. 1, the mean values of ACT measurements are shown before dialysis but after heparin bolus, after 15 min and after the end of treatment during the different periods of study (baseline: HD with standard concentrate, 50 % heparin reduction in the bolus, 50 % reduction of total heparin dose). Obviously, the influence of citrate-containing concentrate is not strong enough to achieve significant ACT changes in comparison to standard dialysate. After reduction of heparin in the bolus and in the maintenance dose, however, the changes in ACT are significant.

The possibility to reduce the heparin dose by using Citrasate® without incurring clotting events was in agreement with results of other authors (Kossmann et al., 2006: -55 %; Ahmad et al., 2006: -30 %, Sands et al., 2012: -33 %). An improvement of efficacy, especially concerning the value of

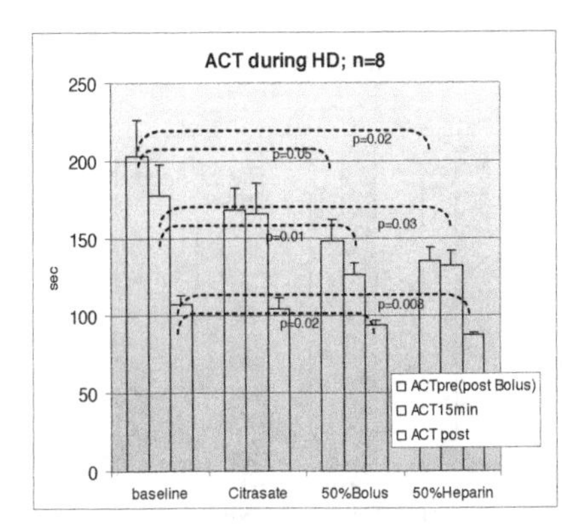


**Figure 1.** Activated clotting time pre dialysis, after 15 min and post dialysis during the different study phases: baseline (standard concentrate), Citrasate® instead of standard concentrate (treatment conditions unchanged), Citrasate® with reduction of the heparin bolus by 50 %, Citrasate® with total heparin dose reduced by 50 %.

Kt/V and elimination of beta-2-m, was detected as well (Kossmann et al., 2009, Sands et al., 2012). These results could not be confirmed in our investigations. Fig. 2 illustrates the values of spKt/V and eqKt/V (calculated using the Daugirdas formula) for the different study periods. The change from standard concentrate to Citrasate® has shown constant efficacy of dialysis, whereas the reduction of heparin dosage resulted in a non-significant decrease of Kt/V. This result was in agreement with data of Ahmad et al. (2006) while the investigations of Kossmann et al. (2009) and Ahmad et al. (2000) resulted in a significant increase of Kt/V using Citrasate® even after the reduction of heparin. These investigations, however, were performed with reuse of dialyzers. The increase of Kt/V was found to be dependent on the number of reuses. The smaller the number of reuses the smaller the increase of Kt/V. Exact data, however, were not given.

Also, the values of beta-2-m do not indicate an improvement of treatment efficacy due to use of Citrasate® (see fig. 3), in contrast to the results of Kossmann et al. (2009).

With regard to the $HCO_3^-$ concentrations before and after dialysis, it was found that both values were somewhat lower (4...5%) if Citrasate® was applied. This is due to the slightly smaller $HCO_3^-$ concentration in the Citrasate® concentrate (32.6 mmol/l instead of 33.0 mmol/l for standard concentrate).

Changes in the electrolytes $Na^+$ and $K^+$ before and after treatment could not be observed during the different periods of investigation.

### *3.1.2. The influence of Citrasate® on inflammatory and oxidative potential*

The typical temporary drop in leucocyte count after start of dialysis treatments was found to be associated with the activation of complement factors C3a and C5a (Craddock et al., 1977). A decrease of iCa inside the dialyzer should be followed by a smaller complement activation and smaller leucocyte drop because of the importance of ionized calcium (iCa) in the cascade of complement activation. This effect, however, was not observed under the conditions of pure

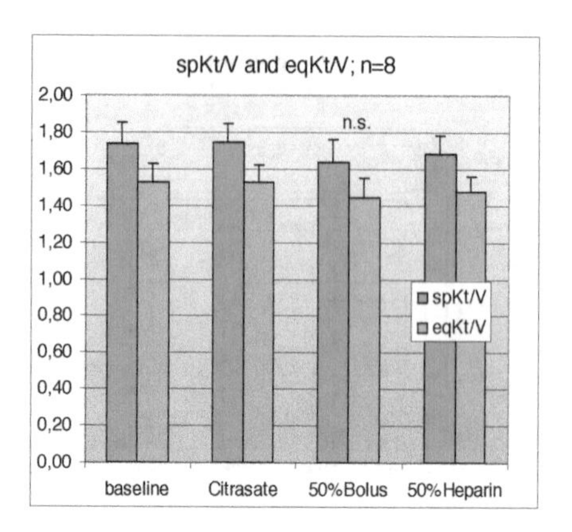


**Figure 2.** Single pool and equilibrated Kt/V during the different study phases.

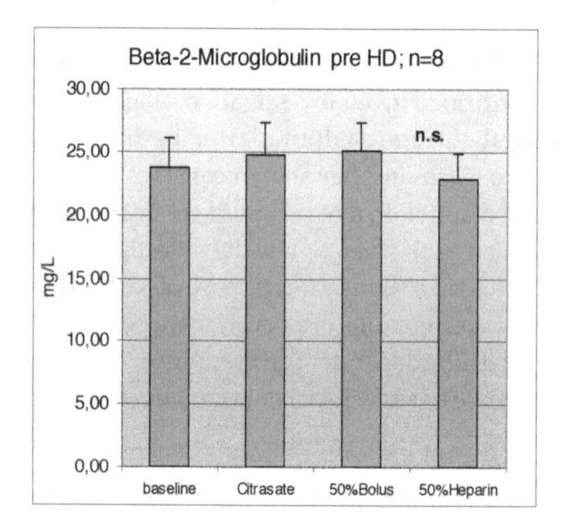


**Figure 3.** Pre dialysis beta-2-microglobulin during the different study phases.

citrate anticoagulation (Opatrný et al., 2007). A significant reduction of complement activation can be expected if the iCa concentration decreases to < 0.2 mmol/l (Hartmann et al., 2006). According to Opatrný, the iCa concentration of 0.4 mmol/l, which is usually found during citrate anticoagulation, does not guarantee a decrease of thrombogenicity and complement activation. Therefore, a distinct influence on the decrease in leucocytes cannot be expected during dialysis with Citrasate®. Nevertheless, according to Polakovic et al. (2010), a significant decrease of leucocyte count was observed during application of Citrasate®. In our investigations a similar trend was visible, which was not significant, however. After decrease of heparin dosage this trend disappears (fig. 4):

The likewise measured levels of albumin and hsCRP were stable during all study phases. However, with regard to myeloperoxidase (MPO), a significant influence was found.

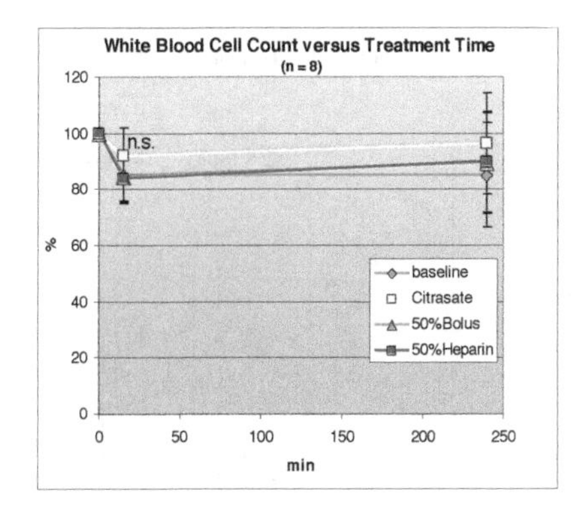


**Figure 4.** Leucocyte drop during HFD treatments in different study phases

MPO is considered an important parameter of biocompatibility and mortality during dialysis treatment (Borawski et al., 2006, Hörl, 2008, Gritters et al., 2006). MPO is part of the family of heparin-binding proteins. Additionally, MPO is contained in granulocytes, monocytes, macrophages and is also located along the vessel walls (e.g. Hörl, 2008). MPO is considered to be a marker of degranulation of neutrophils and, therefore, also as a parameter of biocompatibility of dialysis and oxidative stress (Borawski et al., 2006). During hemodialysis, the value of MPO increases by more than 100% (Gritters et al., 2006). MPO release can be inhibited by regional citrate anticoagulation, which suggests a strong influence of heparin on the degranulation of neutrophils. According to a review of Hörl (2008), MPO induces vascular complications by a variety of mechanisms:

- Inhibition of NO-dependent vasorelaxation.
- Production of endogenous NO-inhibitors.
- Oxidation of LDL with consecutive increased absorption in local macrophages.
- Production of reactive species.

The plasma levels of MPO are associated with atherosclerotic vascular complications as well as with the mortality of hemodialysis patients and the general population (Hörl, 2008).

The measured values of MPO show a strong increase 15 min after start of treatment (fig.5). After the change from standard dialysate to Citrasate®, no significant changes can be observed, but a tendency can be seen towards lower values after 15 min. The reduction of heparin dosage, however, causes a significantly smaller increase of MPO values as well as a tendency towards lower values before and after dialysis.

### *3.1.3. The influence of Citrasate® on the plasma levels of calcium and phosphate*

The complex formation between Ca-ions and citrate causes a decrease of ionized calcium (iCa) in the plasma. After the metabolization of citrate, one part of iCa returns into the blood plasma.

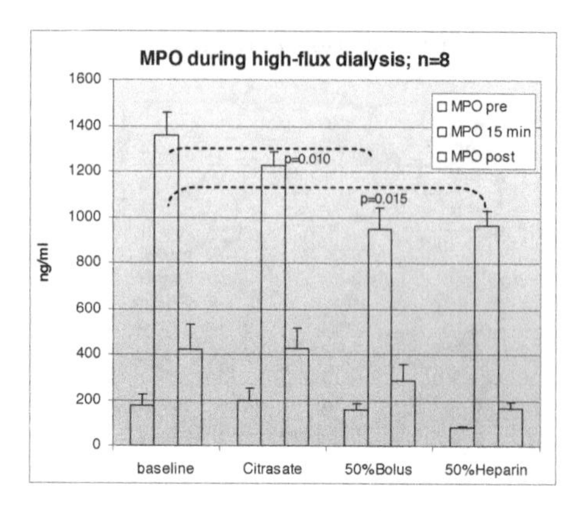


**Figure 5.** Myeloperoxidase during different study phases of HFD

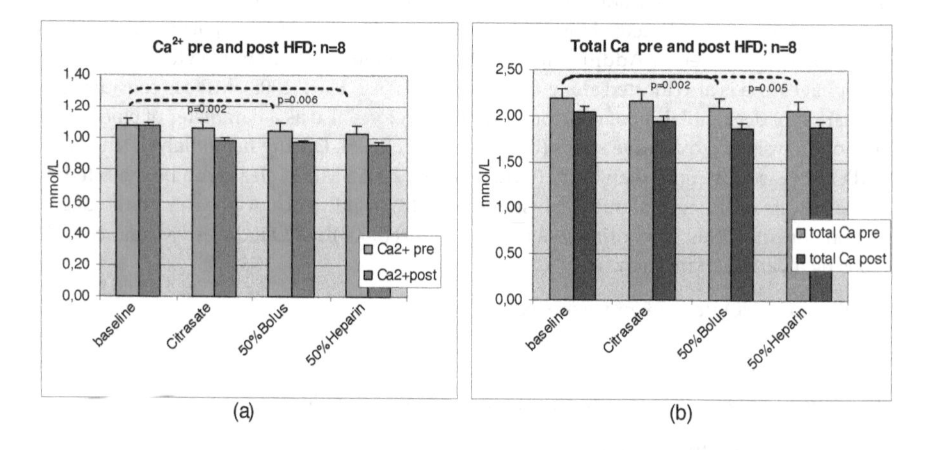


**Figure 6.** a, b. iCa and total calcium before and after dialysis during the different study phases of HFD

The other part of calcium-citrate-complex will be removed by means of dialysis. Therefore, a decrease of iCa can be observed during dialysis treatment, as shown in fig.6a.

The mean decrease of iCa amounts to 7 % for all treatments with Citrasate®, as can be seen in fig. 6a. The decrease of total calcium is shown in fig.6b. A decrease of total calcium can be observed also during treatments with standard concentrate, but it is more pronounced for treatments with Citrasate® (baseline: - 7%; Citrasate®: -9…-11 %).

The drop of iCa was also observed in the same magnitude from other users of Citrasate® (Sands et al., 2012), at least if the concentration of calcium was 1.25 mmol/l. With a calcium concentration of 1.5 mmol/l in Citrasate®, the iCa drop was smaller (e.g. Leimbach et al., 2011, Polacovic et al, 2010).

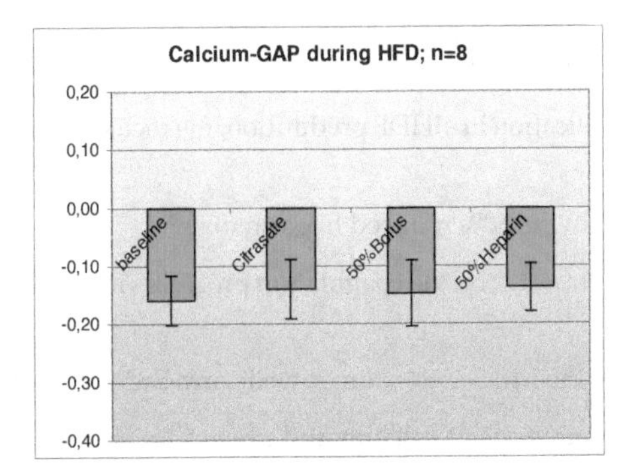


**Figure 7.** Calcium GAP during different study phases of high-flux dialysis

Compared with values of standard dialysis (baseline), the statistically significant decrease of pre-dialysis total Ca (see fig. 6b) results in values below the standard values (2.2…2.65 mmol/l). Because of a possible hypocalcemia, it is recommended to perform treatments with Citrasate® with a calcium concentration of 1.5 mmol/l in the dialysate (see also Polacovic et al., 2010).

The danger of an accumulation of citrate during the dialysis treatment does not exist under the given conditions. The accumulation of citrate can be expressed by the Ca-GAP:

$$\text{Ca-GAP} = (\text{totalCa post} - \text{totalCa pre}) - (\text{iCa post} - \text{iCa pre}) \quad (\text{Gabutti et al., 2009}) \tag{5}$$

If the metabolization of citrate is quick, the Ca-GAP becomes < 0.2 (Gabutti et al., 2009). As fig. 7 shows, this condition was fulfilled in case of dialysis with Citrasate®:

Regarding the likewise measured phosphate, it can be stated that the phosphate elimination was effective with approx. 70% and did not differ between the different periods of the study.

## 3.2. Online hemodiafiltration in pre- and postdilution mode

### *3.2.1. olHDF in predilution mode*

#### *3.2.1.1. Objectives*

In addition to the study with high-flux dialysis (HFD), it should be investigated if Citrasate® concentrate can be used also for on-line hemodiafiltration (olHDF). Since the infusate for olHDF will be prepared directly from the dialysate, the use of Citrasate® dialysate means the infusion of a considerable amount of citrate directly into the blood. Using olHDF in predilution mode, the substitution fluid will be infused into the blood before the dialyzer, which means citrate will be included in the mass transfer processes of the dialyzer. During olHDF in postdilution mode, the infusion of citrate containing fluid takes place behind the dialyzer into the peripheral blood of patients. Since the effects of Citrasate® on free calcium ion concentration and coagulation system cannot be precisely predicted, Citrasate® was applied at first in the predilution mode of olHDF.

During the Citrasate® application in olHDF predilution, the focus was directed to the following questions:

- Is it possible to maintain the 50% reduced heparin dose?
- Can the influence of Citrasate® on the coagulation processes inside the dialyzer increase the efficacy of dialysis?
- Is it possible to reduce the MPO activation as well, as found in high-flux hemodialysis?
- Will the plasma concentrations of calcium and phosphate stay within the physiologically optimal range?

Time schedule, materials, methods, patients and parameters were as described in section 2.

*3.2.1.2. Results and discussion*

The olHDF study was started with reduced doses of heparin (-50 % for bolus and -50% for maintenance dose) determined in the previous HFD study. This was possible without any problems for the baseline treatments (week 1 with HD and Citrasate®). After transition to olHDF in predilution with Citrasate® and a dialyzer FX100 with a larger surface area, it was necessary to increase the heparin dose for some patients. For one patient, the baseline dose had to be restored. For all other patients, the heparin dose remained –20…-50 % lower even if the predilution HDF was performed with acetate-containing standard concentrate.

Figures 8 and 9 show the results regarding the impact of olHDF in predilution on treatment efficacy. For small molecular substances such as urea or creatinine, an increase of efficacy cannot be expected after transition from HFD to olHDF especially for the predilution mode (Ahrenholz et al., 1997). Therefore, the determination of dialysis dose (spKt/V or eqKt/V) in fig. 8a shows no significant changes between the different treatment modes of study.

For medium-sized molecules such as beta-2-microglobulin, the treatment with olHDF is more effective than with HFD because of the larger part of convective transport. Accordingly, the reduction rate of beta-2-m increases from 66.6% to 70.5% after changing from HFD to olHDF. However, because of the large spread of HFD values, this change does not become significant. After changing from HFD with Citrasate® to olHDF with standard concentrate, a significant decrease of the beta-2-m reduction rate by 2% was observed ($p=0.03$) despite the small sample size. From this result, it can be presumed that the Citrasate® dialysate and -infusate perhaps reduces thrombus formation inside the hollow fibers of the dialyzer.

The time course of the myeloperoxidase (MPO) concentration during treatments with Citrasate® corresponds to the one of the HFD study baseline period (see fig. 5). Compared with this result, figure 10 shows an increase of the 15 min value during predilution olHDF with Citrasate® and, once more, during predilution olHDF with standard concentrate, which was not statistically significant. The stepwise increase in the heparin dose seems to be the reason for this observation (see fig. 11). A correlation between activation of MPO and heparin

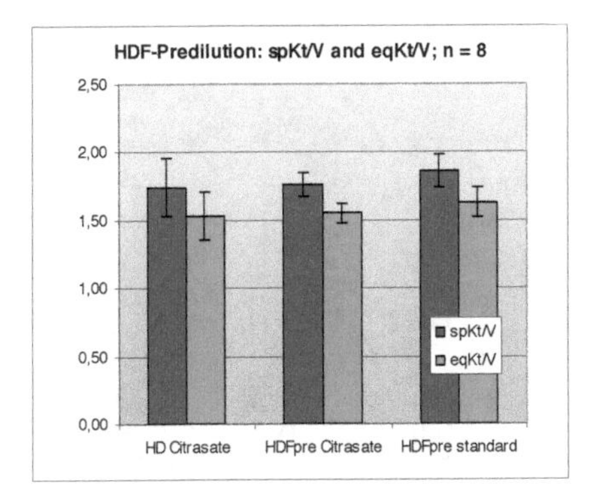


**Figure 8.** Single-pool and equilibrated Kt/V for treatments with HFD with Citrasate® and predilution olHDF treatments with Citrasate® and standard concentrate

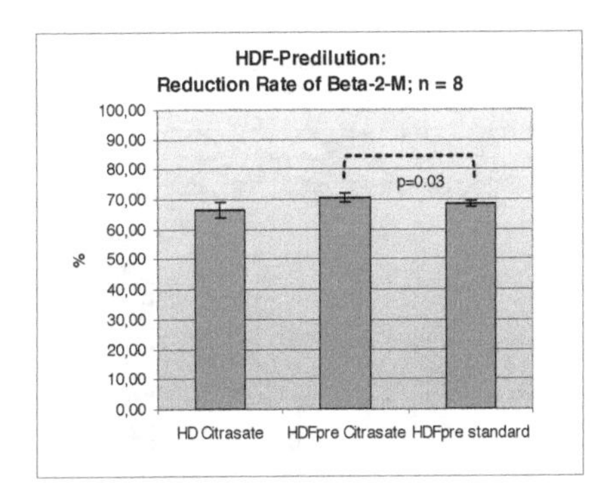


**Figure 9.** Reduction rate of beta-2-m for HFD treatments with Citrasate® and predilution olHDF treatments with Citrasate® and standard concentrate

concentration in blood was found also in some other investigations addressing extracorporeal blood purification (Hörl, 2008, Gritters et al., 2006, Daphna et al., 1998).

As a result of the HFD study with 1.25 mmol/l calcium in the citrate-containing dialysate, the calcium concentration had to be raised to 1.50 mmol/l (concentrate MTN 413/415). As shown in fig.12, the calcium concentrations reach a mean level of 1.09 mmol/l after treatment. The same observations could be made in case of predilution olHDF with standard dialysate ($Ca^{2+}$: 1.25 mmol/l). Patients usually treated with standard concentrate with 1.25 mmol/l $Ca^{2+}$ should obtain 1.50 mmol/l $Ca^{2+}$ after changing to Citrasate®. This increase becomes necessary to compensate for the iCa-losses resulting from calcium-citrate complex formation.

As shown in fig. 13, the total calcium concentration stays constant at 1.50 mmol/l-$Ca^{2+}$-Citrasate® during HFD and predilution olHDF, whereas the values after treatment with standard concentrate ($Ca^{2+}$: 1,25 mmol/l ) are reduced by about 9%. This phenomenon can be

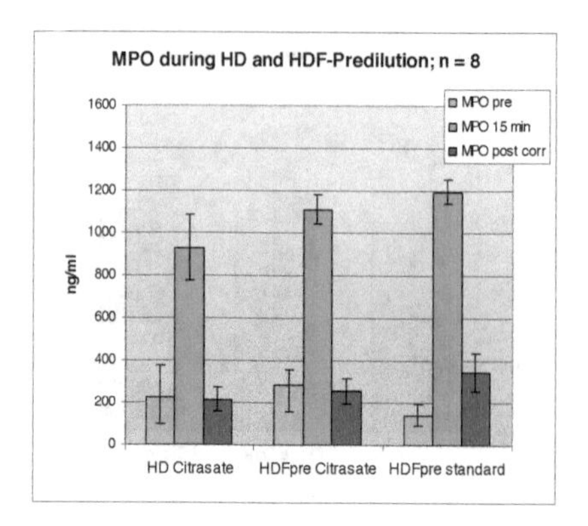


**Figure 10.** Myeloperoxidase concentrations pre-treatment, after 15 min and post-treatment for HFD and olHDF with Citrasate® and olHDF with standard concentrate

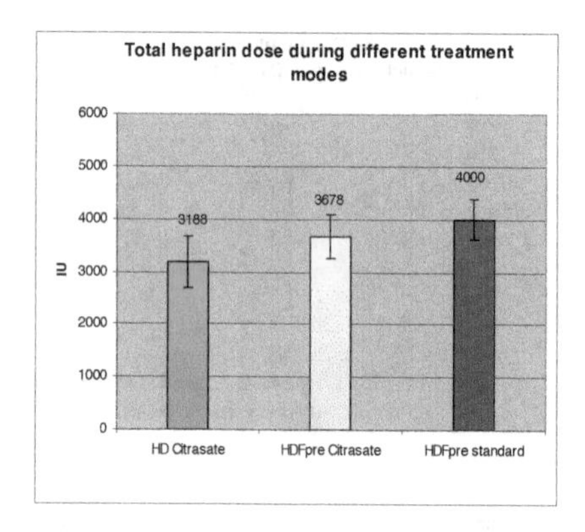


**Figure 11.** Total heparin dose for HFD and olHDF with Citrasate® and olHDF with standard concentrate

explained by the release of free calcium ions from the calcium-citrate complex due to citrate metabolism inside the bloodstream.

The balance between changes of total Ca and iCa during treatments can be expressed as Ca-GAP (see equation 5). The value of Ca-GAP should be less than +0.2. Fig. 14 shows that on average, this condition was fulfilled.

### *3.2.2. olHDF in postdilution mode*

#### *3.2.2.1. Objectives*

Following previous studies on the suitability of Citrasate® concentrate for high-flux hemodialysis (HFD) and online hemodiafiltration in pre-dilution mode (olHDF-pre), it should now

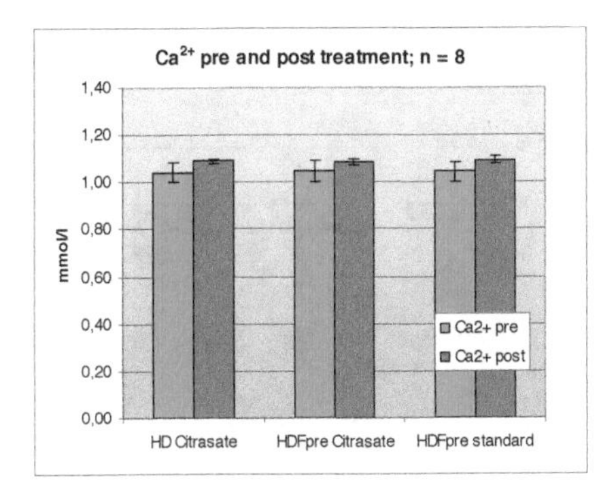


**Figure 12.** iCa concentrations pre and post treatment for different treatment modes with and without Citrasate®

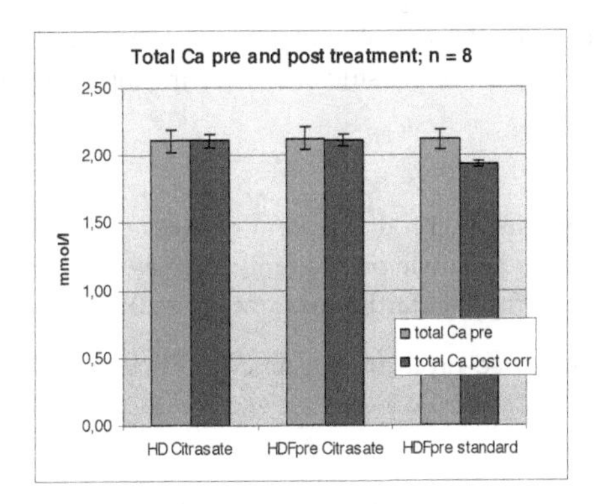


**Figure 13.** Total Ca concentrations pre and post treatment for different treatment modes with and without Citrasate®

be investigated whether the use of citrate-containing dialysate can cause problems during olHDF in postdilution mode (olHDF-post).

In contrast to olHDF-pre, the infusion of citrate-containing solution with olHDF-post occurs *behind* the dialyzer, i.e. directly into the peripheral blood of the patient, so that the physiological effects are more difficult to assess.

As with olHDF-pre, the main focus of Citrasate® application for olHDF-post should be whether:

- The reduced dose of heparin can be maintained,
- The influence on coagulation processes in the dialyzer leads to improved effectiveness,
- The MPO activation can be reduced in the same way as was possible with HFD,
- The plasma concentrations of calcium and phosphate can remain within the physiologically optimal range.

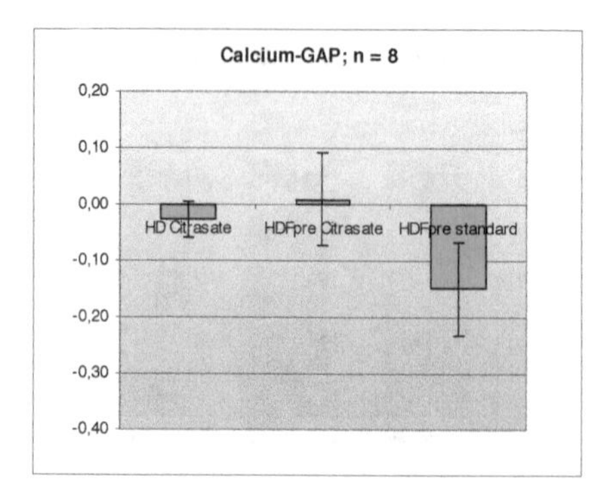


**Figure 14.** Ca-GAP for different treatment modes with and without Citrasate®

Time schedule, materials, methods, patients and parameters were as described in section 2. One patient dropped out after the olHDF-pre study (n = 7 during the olHDF-post investigations).

### *3.2.2.2. Results and discussion*

The investigation was continued with the heparin dosages from the prior olHDF-pre study (the baseline dose was reached again in one patient, whereas with the remaining patients, the dose even for olHDF employing standard concentrate was 20... 50% lower; see section 3.1.1.2).

The comparison of the activated prothrombin time (aPTT) between olHDF-post with Citrasate® and olHDF-post with standard concentrate showed that Citrasate® had no influence on systemic coagulation.

While with olHDF employing predilution, there was no significant difference regarding the removal of low molecular weight substances such as urea compared to HFD, olHDF employing post-dilution was more effective than HFD. However, a difference in effectiveness between the olHDF post-treatment with Citrasate® and standard concentrate could not be found (see Fig. 15). Regarding the removal of beta-2-microglobulin, an improvement in effectiveness compared to HFD could be seen, but a difference between the olHDF-post with Citrasate® and standard concentrate, as was seen in the predilution treatments, could not be determined here (see Fig. 16).

MPO is one of the most important predictors for compatibility and mortality for dialysis treatments. In the previous HFD study, there were significant differences between the individual study phases. Therefore, MPO was measured again at different time points (before treatment, after 15 min of treatment, and after treatment). As with the olHDF in predilution, there was no significant difference in MPO activation for treatments with Citrasate® or standard concentrate. The MPO values after treatment start tended to be somewhat larger for olHDF-post treatments (probably not significant due to the small number of cases). This is most likely due to the much greater ultrafiltration and therefore, also to the greater dilution of blood with infusion solution employing olHDF-pre (150 ml/min versus 60 ml/min).

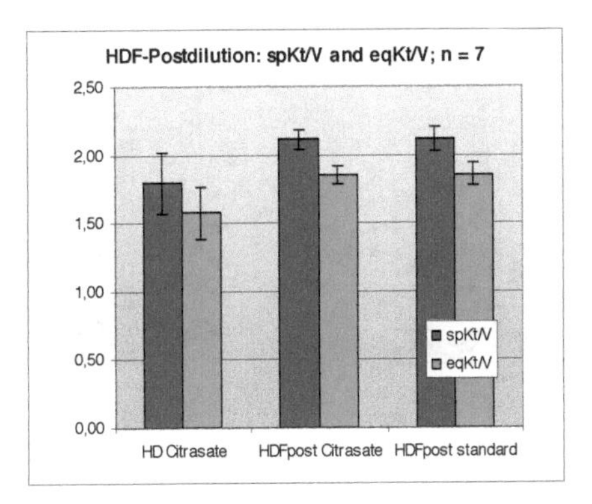


**Figure 15.** Single-pool and equilibrated Kt/V for treat-ments with HFD with Citrasate® and olHDF-post treatments with Citrasate® and standard concentrate

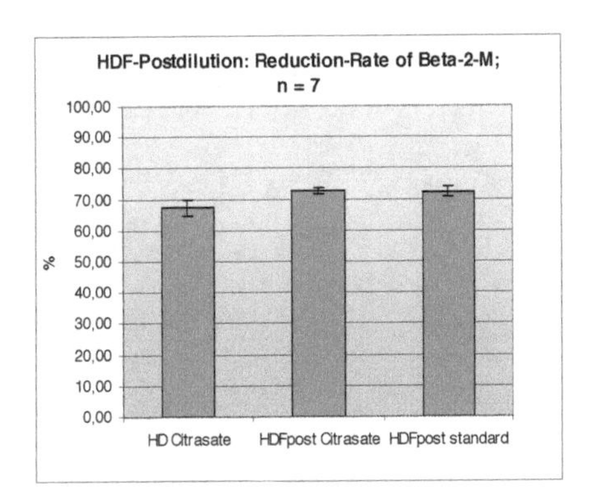


**Figure 16.** Reduction rate of beta-2-m for HFD treatments with Citrasate® and olHDF-post treatments with Citrasate® and standard concentrate

Since the heparin dose was constant for all olHDF treatments, an effect of heparin concentration on MPO activation as the one seen in the previous olHDF-pre study could not be observed (comparison MPO during olHDF-pre and –post: see fig. 17a, b.).

As a result of the HFD study with 1.25 mmol/l $Ca^{2+}$ in the dialysate, the $Ca^{2+}$ concentration was raised to 1.50 mmol/l (concentrate MTN 413/415). As shown in Fig 18a, b., the $Ca^{2+}$ concentrations of the individual patients level out to values of about 1.10 mmol/l after treatment, just as in the case of olHDF treatments with normal dialysate ($Ca^{2+}$ : 1.25 mmol/l). Losses of ionized calcium by chelation were adequately compensated by choosing a higher dialysate $Ca^{2+}$ for olHDF both in pre- or post-dilution.

The balance between the changes in total calcium and the iCa during treatment can be expressed by the Ca GAP (see equation 5, sections 3.1.3 and 3.1.1.2):

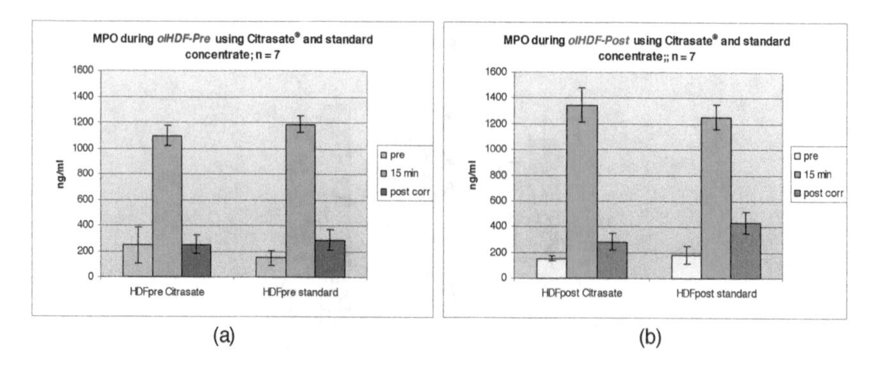


**Figure 17.** a, b. Comparison of the MPO values during olHDF with pre- and postdilution (same patient group, constant heparin dose)

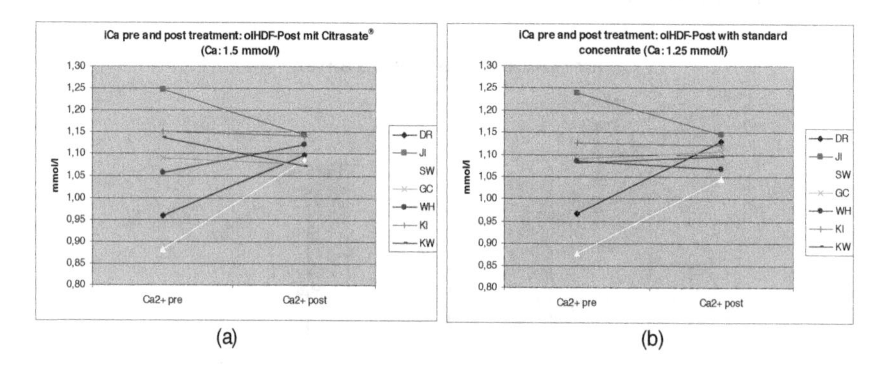


**Figure 18.** a, b. Comparison of the individual plasma $Ca^{2+}$ concentrations during olHDF-post with Citrasate® (1.5 mmol/l $Ca^{2+}$) and standard concentrate (1.25 mmol/l $Ca^{2+}$)

Figure 19 shows that with olHDF-post, there is no positive balance for total calcium. Accordingly, no surplus amount of bound Ca remains in the bloodstream, which would indicate an incomplete metabolism of the calcium citrate. According to studies by Bauer et al. (2005), this is also not to be expected. In that study, citrate kinetics during citrate anticoagulation were investigated both in patients with normal renal function and those on hemodialysis. It was found that citrate is also metabolized adequately with renal failure, as well as with mild hepatic dysfunction. Only in patients with severe liver failure is citrate anticoagulation not indicated. If one considers that with citrate anticoagulation the citrate infusion rate is about 0.3 mmol/kg/h, while with olHDF in post dilution with Citrasate® dialysate it is only about 0.04 mmol /kg /h, then problems arising from incomplete citrate metabolism are not to be expected (example: olHDF-post: 0.8 mmol/l citrate, infusion rate 3.6 l/h, 70 kg patient).

The calcium-phosphate balance is determined largely by parathyroid hormone. Disruptions of the balance due to non-physiological treatment conditions would therefore be reflected in

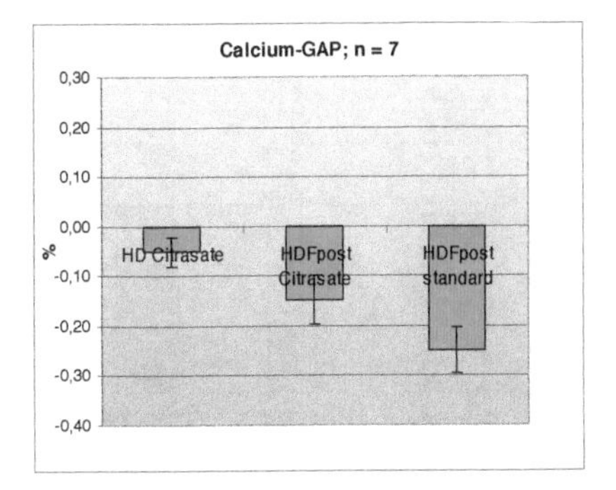


**Figure 19.** Calcium GAP for the different study phases HFD, olHDF-post with Citrasate® and standard concentrate

the concentrations of $Ca^{2+}$, phosphate and PTH. As shown in Figures 20 and 21, however, no significant differences between olHDF-post treatments with Citrasate® and standard concentrate were observed.

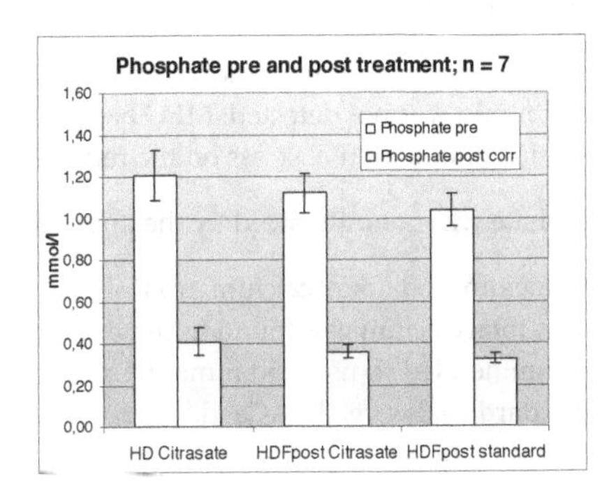


**Figure 20.** Plasma phosphate concentrations pre and post treatment for different treatment modes: HFD with Citrasate®, olHDF-postdilution with Citrasate® and standard concentrate

Regarding other measured parameters such as bicarbonate ($HCO_3^-$), $Na^+$, $K^+$, there were no significant differences in the individual study phases. The mean ESA (Aranesp®) and iron intake (Ferrlecit) remained constant during all study phases.

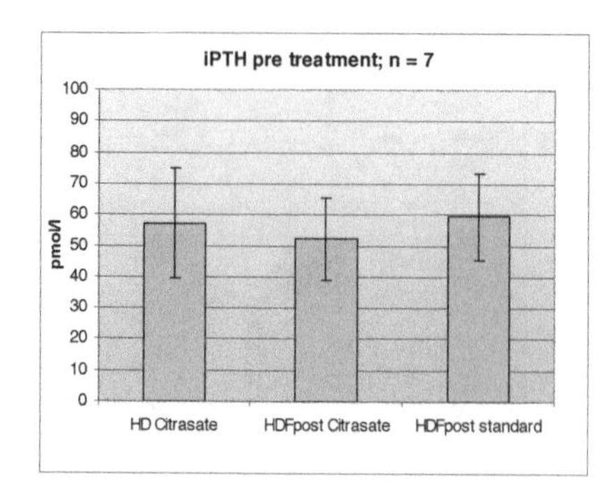


**Figure 21.** iPTH pre treatment for different treatment modes: HFD with Citrasate® and standard concentrate Citrasate®, olHDF-postdilution with

# 4. Summary

## 4.1. High-flux dialysis (HFD)

Using Citrasate® for HFD treatments, the results can be summarized as follows:

- A reduction of total heparin dose by 50% was possible (50% bolus and 50% maintenance amount) without increase of clotting events in the dialyzer or extracorporeal circuit and without change of treatment efficacy (Kt/V).
- An influence of Citrasate® on sensitive inflammation parameters such as beta-2-microglobulin, hsCRP and serum albumin was not detected. MPO has reacted sensitively as marker for granulocyte degranulation and oxidative stress on the reduction of heparin dosage.
- The plasma level of phosphate was not influenced by the application of Citrasate®.
- A reduction of ionized calcium and total calcium was observed during application of Citrasate®. The reduction of total calcium was found to be partially below the normal range. Therefore, it has to be recommended to use 1.50 mmol/l $Ca^{2+}$ instead of 1.25 mmol/l $Ca^{2+}$, which is common for standard dialysate. The Ca-GAP was found to be sufficient small, therefore a quick metabolization of citrate can be assumed.

In conclusion, the study has demonstrated that Citrasate® can be applied for high-flux dialysis, saving heparin and increasing the biocompatibility of treatment by reduction of oxidative stress.

## 4.2. Online hemodiafiltration with predilution (olHDF-pre)

The results can be summarized as follows:

- Several patients could be treated in this investigation with the 50% reduced total heparin dose, just as during the previous HFD study. This reduced total heparin dose, however, could not be maintained for all patients under the conditions of larger surface areas for dialyzers (FX100) during olHDF predilution.

- The beta-2-microglobulin elimination was slightly, but significantly, increased in comparison to standard concentrate. For urea, however, the efficacy could not be improved by olHDF predilution as expected.
- The activation of myeloperoxidase (MPO) corresponded to the values of the previous HFD study with Citrasate®. An increase in mean heparin dosage was connected with an increase in MPO concentration.
- The course of ionized Ca during HD and olHDF predilution with Citrasate® corresponds to the one of standard dialysate with 1.25 mmol/l $Ca^{2+}$ after raising dialysate calcium from 1.25 to 1.50 mmol/l.
- The mean plasma concentrations of phosphate and iPTH remained at the same level during all periods of study. The small size of Ca-GAP means that disturbance of Ca-phosphate balance did not occur because of the high infusion rate of citrate-containing infusion fluid and because of the sufficiently quick metabolism of citrate.

In conclusion, the study has demonstrated that Citrasate® can be applied also for online Hemodiafiltration (olHDF) with predilution mode. As found during high-flux dialysis as well, Citrasate® saves heparin and increases the biocompatibility of treatment by reduction of oxidative stress.

### 4.3. Online hemodiafiltration with postdilution (olHDF-post)

In summary, it can be stated that:

- The doses of heparin from the previous olHDF-pre study could be maintained also with olHDF-post. The baseline dose at the beginning of all three studies had to be re-administered in one case; with the remaining 6 patients, a 20...50% reduced total heparin dose could be administered. However, this was also possible with the olHDF post-treatment using standard concentrate.
- As expected, the treatment effectiveness was improved both in terms of the Kt/V values and the beta-2-m removal rate compared to HFD. However, no differences between the olHDF-post treatments with either Citrasate® or standard concentrate could be identified.
- Regarding the activation of myeloperoxidase (MPO), there were no significant differences between treatments with Citrasate® and standard concentrate. Compared to the treatments with olHDF-pre, with postdilution olHDF the MPO values tended to be somewhat larger, which is presumably due to the higher dilution of the blood with HDF-pre.
- After increasing the dialysate calcium from 1.25 to 1.50 mmol/l compared to the first study (HFD), the course of the ionized Ca during Citrasate® HFD and olHDF-post with Citrasate® corresponded to the one of olHDF-post with normal dialysate and 1.25 mmol/l $Ca^{2+}$.
- The mean plasma concentrations of phosphate and iPTH were at about the same level in all study phases. As with the significant shortfall of the Ca-GAP at 0.2, this means that

disruptions of the Ca-phosphate balance by the high infusion rate of citrate containing substitute infusions did not occur and that there was a sufficiently rapid metabolism of citrate.

## Author details

Roland E. Winkler[1], Peter Ahrenholz[2], Wolfgang Paetow[1], Grit Waitz[2] and Hartmut Wolf[3]

1 Praxisverbund für Dialyse und Apherese, Rostock, Germany

2 BioArtProducts GmbH, Rostock, Germany

3 Biomedical Consulting, Hohen Neuendorf, Germany

## References

[1] Kossmann, R. J, & Callan, R. Ahmad S: Fifty five percent heparin reduction is safe with citrate dialysate in chronic dialysis patients, *ASN's 39th Annual Renal Week meeting* November (2006).

[2] Kossmann, R. J, Gonzales, A, & Callan, R. Ahmad S: Increased Efficiency of hemodialysis with Citrate Dialysate, a prospective Controlled study, *JASN*, (2009)., 4(9)

[3] Gabutti, L, Lucchini, B, Marone, C, & Alberio, L. Burnier M: Citrate vs. Acetate based Dialysate in Bicarbonate Haemodialysis: Consequences on Haemodynamics, Coagulation, Acid-base status and Electrolytes. *BMC Nephrology* (2009)., 10

[4] Ouseph, R. Ward RA: Anticoagulation for Intermittent Hemodialysis. *Seminars in Dialysis*, (2000)., 13(3)

[5] van Beaumont W: Evaluation of hemoconcentration from hematocrit measurements *Journal of Applied Physiology*, May (1972)., 32(5)

[6] Christiansen TF: Determination of Sodium and Potassium in PlasmaA Comparison between Direct Potentiometry and Flame Photometry. *Radiometer Publication*, 0000-0906Denmark (1991).

[7] Leimbach, T, Jütterschenke, M, Czerny, J, & Aign, S. Kron J: Heparin-Einsparung durch Verwendung von citrathaltigem Dialysat? *Poster, Kongress für Nephrologie*, Berlin (2011)., 10-13.

[8] Ahmad, S, & Callan, R. Kossmann RJ: Heparin reduction with citrate dialysate. Presented at the *European Renal Association- European Dialysis and Transplant Association*

*congress*, Glasgow, Scotland, July (2006). and published in *Nephrology Dialysis Transplantation*, Supplement 4, 2006, 21

[9] Sands, J. J, Kotanko, P, Segal, J. H, Ho, C-H, Usvat, L, Young, A, Carter, M, Sergeyeva, O, Korth, L, Maunsell, E, Zhu, Y, & Krishnan, M. Diaz-Buxo JA: Effects of Citrate Acid Concentrate (Citrasate® on Heparin N Requirements and Hemodialysis Adequacy: A Multicenter, Prospective Noninferiority Trial. *Blood Purif* (2012). , 199-204.

[10] Craddock, P. R, Fehr, J, Dalmasso, A. P, & Brighan, K. L. Jacobs HS: Hemodialysis leukopenia. Pulmonary vascular leukostasis resulting from complement activation by dialyzer cellophane membranes. *J. Clin. Invest* (1977). May; , 59(5), 879-888.

[11] Opatrný Jr KRichtrová P, Polanská K, Wirth J, Sefrna F, Brandl M, Falkenhagen D: Citrate Anticoagulation Control by Ionized Calcium levels Does Not Prevent Hemostasis and Complement Activation During Hemodialysis. *Artificial Organs* 31(2), (2007).

[12] Hartmann, J, Strobl, K, & Fichtinger, U. Falkenhagen D: Citrate anticoagulation and activation of the complement system.*Poster, ESAO 2006*Umea, Sweden

[13] Polakovic, V, & Lopot, F. Svara F: Citrasate dialysis concentrate. General University Hospital and 1th Medical Faculty of the Charles University, Dept. of Medicine, Prague, *Research Report*,(2010).

[14] Locatelli, F, & Manzoni, C. Del Vecchio L, Di Filippo S, Pontoriero G, Cavalli A: Management of Anemia by Convective Treatments. *Contributions to Nephrology*, H. Kawanishi, A.C. Yamashita, Eds., 168, 162-172.

[15] Winkler, R. E, & Ahrenholz, P. Freivogel K: Influence of Online Hemodiafiltration on Hemoglobin Level, ESA-Dosage and Serum Albumin- Retrospective, Multicenter Analysis. *Progress in Hemodialysis- From Emergent Biotechnology to Clinical Practice.* A. Carpi, C. Donadio, G. Tramonti, Eds., published by InTech, 978-9-53307-377-4free online: www.intechopen.com

[16] Ahrenholz, P, Winkler, R. E, Ramlow, W, & Tiess, M. Müller W: On-line hemodiafiltration with pre- and postdilution: a comparison of efficacy. *The International Journal of Artificial Organs/* (1997). (2), 81-90.

[17] Borawski, J, Naumnik, B, & Rydzewska-rosolowska, A. Mysliwiec M: Myeloperoxidas up-regulation during haemodialysis: is heparin the missing link? *Nephrol. Dial. Transplant* (April (2006).

[18] Hörl WH: Die Antikoagulation mit Zitrat reduziert die Mortalität und verbessert die Erholung der Nierenfunktion bei Patienten mit akutem Nierenversagen *Nephro-News*, Ausgabe 5/08

[19] Gritters, M. Grooteman MPC, Schoorl M, Bartels PCM, Scheffer PG, Teerlink T, Schalkwijk CG, Spreeuwenberg M, Nubé MJ: Citrate anticoagulation abolishes de-

granulation of polymorphonuclear cells and platelets and reduces oxidative stress during haemodialysis. *Nephrol. Dial. Transplant* ((2006).

[20] Daphna, E. M, Michaela, S, Eynat, P, & Irit, A. Rimon S: Association of myeloperoxidase with heparin: oxidative inactivation of proteins on the surface of endothelial cells by the bound enzyme. *Mol Cell Biochem.* (1998). Jun;183(1-2):55-61

[21] Maruyama, Y, & Lindholm, B. Stenvinkel P: Inflammation and oxidative stress in ESRD- the role of myeloperoxidase. *J. Nephrol 2004*Suppl. , 8, 72-76.

[22] Bauer, E, Derfler, K, & Joukhadar, C. Druml, W: Citrate Kinetics in Patients Receiving Long-Term Hemodialysis Therapy. *Am J Kidney Dis 2005* , 46(5), 903-907.

[23] Ahmad, S, Callan, R, & Cole, J. J. Blagg CR: Dialysate made from dry chemicals using citric acid increases dialysis dose. *Am J Kidney Dis 2000* , 35, 493-499.

# Permissions

The contributors of this book come from diverse backgrounds, making this book a truly international effort. This book will bring forth new frontiers with its revolutionizing research information and detailed analysis of the nascent developments around the world.

We would like to thank Professor Hiromichi Suzuki, for lending his expertise to make the book truly unique. He has played a crucial role in the development of this book. Without his invaluable contribution this book wouldn't have been possible. He has made vital efforts to compile up to date information on the varied aspects of this subject to make this book a valuable addition to the collection of many professionals and students.

This book was conceptualized with the vision of imparting up-to-date information and advanced data in this field. To ensure the same, a matchless editorial board was set up. Every individual on the board went through rigorous rounds of assessment to prove their worth. After which they invested a large part of their time researching and compiling the most relevant data for our readers. Conferences and sessions were held from time to time between the editorial board and the contributing authors to present the data in the most comprehensible form. The editorial team has worked tirelessly to provide valuable and valid information to help people across the globe.

Every chapter published in this book has been scrutinized by our experts. Their significance has been extensively debated. The topics covered herein carry significant findings which will fuel the growth of the discipline. They may even be implemented as practical applications or may be referred to as a beginning point for another development. Chapters in this book were first published by InTech; hereby published with permission under the Creative Commons Attribution License or equivalent.

The editorial board has been involved in producing this book since its inception. They have spent rigorous hours researching and exploring the diverse topics which have resulted in the successful publishing of this book. They have passed on their knowledge of decades through this book. To expedite this challenging task, the publisher supported the team at every step. A small team of assistant editors was also appointed to further simplify the editing procedure and attain best results for the readers.

Our editorial team has been hand-picked from every corner of the world. Their multi-ethnicity adds dynamic inputs to the discussions which result in innovative outcomes. These outcomes are then further discussed with the researchers and contributors who give their valuable feedback and opinion regarding the same. The feedback is then collaborated with the researches and they are edited in a comprehensive manner to aid the understanding of the subject.

Apart from the editorial board, the designing team has also invested a significant amount of their time in understanding the subject and creating the most relevant covers. They scrutinized every image to scout for the most suitable representation of the subject and create an appropriate cover for the book.

The publishing team has been involved in this book since its early stages. They were actively engaged in every process, be it collecting the data, connecting with the contributors or procuring relevant information. The team has been an ardent support to the editorial, designing and production team. Their endless efforts to recruit the best for this project, has resulted in the accomplishment of this book. They are a veteran in the field of academics and their pool of knowledge is as vast as their experience in printing. Their expertise and guidance has proved useful at every step. Their uncompromising quality standards have made this book an exceptional effort. Their encouragement from time to time has been an inspiration for everyone.

The publisher and the editorial board hope that this book will prove to be a valuable piece of knowledge for researchers, students, practitioners and scholars across the globe.

# List of Contributors

**Paulo Roberto Santos**
Federal University of Ceará, Brazil

**Konstantinos Pantelias**
Nephrology Department, Aretaieio University Hospital, Greece

**Eirini Grapsa**
Athens Medical School, Nephrology Department, Aretaieio University Hospital, Greece

**Sandra Ribeiro**
Faculdade de Farmácia, Universidade do Porto, Portugal
Instituto de Biologia Molecular e Celular, Universidade do Porto, Portugal

**Elísio Costa**
Faculdade de Farmácia, Universidade do Porto, Portugal
Instituto de Biologia Molecular e Celular, Universidade do Porto, Portugal

**Luís Belo**
Faculdade de Farmácia, Universidade do Porto, Portugal
Instituto de Biologia Molecular e Celular, Universidade do Porto, Portugal

**Alice Santos-Silva**
Faculdade de Farmácia, Universidade do Porto, Portugal
Instituto de Biologia Molecular e Celular, Universidade do Porto, Portugal

**Flávio Reis**
Instituto de Farmacologia e Terapêutica Experimental, IBILI, Universidade de Coimbra, Portugal

**Ayman Karkar**
Kanoo Kidney Centre, Dammam Medical Complex, Dammam, Kingdom of Saudi Arabia

**Bernard Canaud**
Medical Board EMEALA, Fresenius Medical Care Deutschland GmbH, Bad Homburg, Germany

**Ciro Tett**
Medical Board EMEALA, Fresenius Medical Care Deutschland GmbH, Bad Homburg, Germany

**Daniele Marcelli**
Medical Board EMEALA, Fresenius Medical Care Deutschland GmbH, Bad Homburg, Germany

**Katrin Koehler**
Medical Board EMEALA, Fresenius Medical Care Deutschland GmbH, Bad Homburg, Germany

**Guido Giordana**
Nephrocare Coordination EMEALA, Fresenius Medical Care Deutschland GmbH, Bad-Homburg, Germany

**Stefano Stuard**
Nephrocare Coordination EMEALA, Fresenius Medical Care Deutschland GmbH, Bad-Homburg, Germany

**Miryana Dobreva**
Nephrocare Coordination EMEALA, Fresenius Medical Care Deutschland GmbH, Bad-Homburg, Germany

**Andrea Stopper**
Nephrocare Coordination EMEALA, Fresenius Medical Care Deutschland GmbH, Bad-Homburg, Germany

**Carlo Barbieri**
Healthcare and Business Advanced Modeling Fresenius Medical Care DeutschlandGmbH, PalazzoPignano, Italy

**Flavio Mari**
Healthcare and Business Advanced Modeling Fresenius Medical Care DeutschlandGmbH, PalazzoPignano, Italy

**Emanuele Gatti**
CEO EMEALA, Global Chief Strategist, Fresenius Medical Care, Bad Homburg, Germany
Center for Biomedical Technology, Danube University, Krems, Austria

**Rodolfo Valtuille**
Centro Hemodialisis Burzaco, Buenos Aires, Argentina

**Manuel Sztejnberg**
Instrumentation and Dosimetry Division, National Atomic Energy Commission, Argentina

**Elmer A. Fernandez**
Catholic University of Cordoba, Cordoba, Argentina

**Fabio Grandi**
Bellco S.r.l., Mirandola, Italy

**Giuseppe Palladino**
Bellco S.r.l., Mirandola, Italy

**Luisa Sereni**
Bellco S.r.l., Mirandola, Italy

**Mauro Atti**
Bellco S.r.l., Mirandola, Italy

**Paolo Maria Ghezzi**
Bellco S.r.l., Mirandola, Italy

**Piergiorgio Bolasco**
Territorial Department of Nephrology and Dialysis, ASL Cagliari, Italy

**Marialuisa Caiazzo**
Laboratory Diagnostics and Forensic Medicine University of Modena and Reggio Emilia, Italy

**Kyungsoo Lee**
Nephrology Division, Department of Internal Medicine, University of Michigan, Ann Arbor, Michigan, USA
AnC Bio Inc, Seoul, Korea

**Pierpaolo Di Cocco, Antonio Famulari, Francesco Pisani, Linda De Luca, Vinicio Rizza and Katia Clemente**
The Royal London Hospital, University of L'Aquila, United Kingdom

**Roland E. Winkler**
Praxisverbund für Dialyse und Apherese, Rostock, Germany

**Wolfgang Paetow**
Praxisverbund für Dialyse und Apherese, Rostock, Germany

**Grit Waitz**
BioArtProducts GmbH, Rostock, Germany

**Peter Ahrenholz**
BioArtProducts GmbH, Rostock, Germany

**Hartmut Wolf**
Biomedical Consulting, Hohen Neuendorf, Germany

CPSIA information can be obtained at www.ICGtesting.com
Printed in the USA
LVOW05*1313040215

425684LV00003B/42/P